# ACCIDENTAL
# LOGICS

# ACCIDENTAL
# LOGICS

The Dynamics of Change
in the Health Care Arena
in the United States, Britain, and Canada

CAROLYN HUGHES TUOHY

New York    Oxford
Oxford University Press
1999

Oxford University Press

Oxford   New York

Athens   Auckland   Bangkok   Bogotá   Buenos Aires   Calcutta
Cape Town   Chennai   Dar es Salaam   Delhi   Florence   Hong Kong   Istanbul
Karachi   Kuala Lumpur   Madrid   Melbourne   Mexico City   Mumbai
Nairobi   Paris   São Paulo   Singapore   Taipei   Tokyo   Toronto   Warsaw

and associated companies in
Berlin   Ibadan

Copyright © 1999 by Oxford University Press, Inc.

Published by Oxford University Press, Inc.
198 Madison Avenue, New York, New York 10016

Oxford in a registered trademark of Oxford University Press

Library of Congress Cataloging-in-Publication Data
Tuohy, Carolyn, 1945–
Accidental logics: the dynamics of change in the health care
arena in the United States, Britain, and Canada /
Carolyn Hughes Tuohy.
p.   cm.
Includes bibliographical references and index.
ISBN 0-19-512821-4
1. Medical policy—United States—Decision making.
2. Medical Policy—Great Britain—Decision making.
3. Medical policy—Canada—Decision making.
4. Medical care—United States—Finance—Decision making.
5. Medical care—Great Britain—Finance—Decision making.
6. Medical care—Canada—Finance—Decision making.   I. Title.
RA394.T86   1999
362.1—dc21                          98-28698

2 3 4 5 6 7 8 9

Printed in the United States of America
on acid-free paper

To Walter

# Preface

Cross-national discourse in public policy is marked by an ongoing tension between the common and the particular. At one extreme, we identify common trends and challenges in a given policy arena, and view national systems as laboratories in which responses to these challenges can be tested and, if successful, emulated. At the other extreme, we see national systems as so idiosyncratic that only "home-grown" solutions are possible.

In the health care arena of the 1990s, this tension was clearly apparent. On the one hand, cross-national attention was drawn to the alleged potential of market mechanisms to squeeze greater efficiency from health care delivery systems, as both public and private payers became more cost- and price-conscious. Experiments in Britain, the Netherlands, New Zealand, Sweden, and elsewhere, themselves influenced by developments in the United States, were closely watched for their lessons for other nations. At the same time, national debates about health care reform, particularly in the United States but also in other nations, were marked as well by skepticism about the applicability of foreign models to domestic circumstances.

Like policy makers, students of comparative public policy also debate the relative importance of common or distinctive features of national policy arenas. Countless conferences and symposia have been devoted to the question of whether advanced capitalism is driving toward a common model in economic and/or social policy arenas, or whether the particular characteristics of national arenas continue to channel policy development along distinctive paths.

In fact, as wisdom would counsel, both common and particular features need to be taken into account in cross-national discourse and in the comparative study of public policy. Awareness of experience in a variety of nations can illuminate the dynamics that create common challenges, and can stimulate the imagination as to possible responses. But enthusiasm for cross-national learning needs to be tempered by the recognition thet the working out of the common logic of a given policy arena will be mediated by the particular logics of national systems. And those national systems, with their distinctive logics, are products of the eras of their birth, when broad political forces created windows of opportunity for policy change. These particular logics, then, are in an important sense "accidents" of history. Common challenges will be experienced somewhat differently in these different national systems; and responses to those challenges will play out differently when transposed from one national context to another.

Nowhere, indeed, was this relationship between common and particular logics better illustrated than in the health care arena of the 1990s. The wave of enthusiasm for market-type mechanisms that spread across OECD nations was certainly driven by some common features of the evolving microeconomics of health care delivery, which elevated the significance of bargaining among large, relatively sophisticated entities on both supply and demand sides of the arena. But the interpretation and implementation of market mechanisms, and the occupants of bargaining roles, varied dramatically across nations, in ways that can be understood only by analyzing the particular logic of the system in place in each nation.

Exploring the common and the particular logics of the health care arena, as this book does, sheds light on the ongoing debate about the role of the "state" and the "market" in health care and more broadly. Specifically, this book provides a way of thinking about the state and the market that distinguishes between the balance of *influence* among various types of actors (state, private finance, and health care professional) and the mix of *instruments* of social control (hierarchy, market, and collegiality). In this framework, the "state" and the "market" can be seen as belonging to two analytically distinct dimensions.

Traditionally, the relationship between these two dimensions has been assumed to be marked by a fairly stable set of affinities: state actors operate through hierarchical instruments, private financial actors through market mechanisms, and professional actors through collegial bodies. What is remarkable about the 1990s is the degree to which these affinities were shuffled. Most notably, state actors were increasingly attracted to the use of "market," exchange-based mechanisms, even while privately financed organizations were drawn increasingly into vertically and horizontally integrated forms. In this context, collegial mechanisms, and with them the influence of professionals, were progressively squeezed and contracted.

Yet in this process, it became apparent that the impact of market and hierarchical instruments depends very much upon who is wielding them. As this book demonstrates, it depends in particular upon the balance of public and private finance, and upon the organization of private finance. The state's embrace of market mechanisms in Britain, for example, did not change the requirement for political actors to maintain complex coalitions of support. And it was the rise of for-profit investor-owned corporations, driven by the logic of the American health care system, that more than any other factor propelled the turbulent transformation of the system in the 1990s. In these processes, the influence of medicine proved greater in alliance with the state than with private finance—a finding borne out as well in the more stable Canadian system.

In illuminating the intersection between instruments and influence, the study of the health care arena can cast light on other policy arenas as well. As I note in the conclusion to this book, some care needs to be taken in drawing heuristic analogies to other arenas. But as much as any policy arena I can think of, health care throws into high relief key features of policy-making: the relevance of competing bases of power—authority, wealth, and skill: the relationship of technological development to policy change; and the capacity of the policy process to deal with matters central to the human condition. I am grateful to the intellectual muse that led me almost thirty years ago to choose the health care arena as an object of inquiry, and that has kept it in my sights, centrally or peripherally, ever since.

This book would not have been possible without the generosity of a number of institutions and individuals. The Connaught Fund of the University of Toronto, as well as the Office of the Vice-President and Provost, provided essential research support and made it possible for me to take a year's research leave in 1995–96. My colleagues in the Provost's Office, most notably Provost Adel Sedra, accommodated this leave in the collegial spirit that distinguishes this remarkable group. The School of Social Sciences at the University of Bath, under the leadership of Graham Room, and the King's Fund Policy Institute, under the leadership of Ken Judge, were kind hosts and facilitators of my research in England. The Center for International Affairs at Harvard University, under Bob Putnam's leadership, provided a similarly welcoming and helpful venue for my research in the United States.

Several close colleagues and friends have been important reference points, sounding boards, and constructive critics through this project. Among these certainly Rudolf Klein and Ted Marmor must take pride of place: their contributions to my thinking go well beyond the liberal citations to their published work in my bibliography. Keith Banting provided a thoughtful, deep, and invaluable commentary on the penultimate draft of the manuscript. Two colleagues—Peter Hall at Harvard and Carol Propper at Bristol—may be surprised to learn that my individual conversations with each of them proved to be critical moments in the formulation of the framework and argument of this book. Such is the serendipitous nature of our academic enterprise—I thank them for their penetrating questions and hope they recognize the results of our discussions here. Finally, the many people in Britain, the United States, and Canada whom I interviewed in the course of my research are too numerous to mention here—but not too numerous to be remembered with gratitude. I trust that I have done justice to their thoughts.

There is, in the end, one person who lived with the preparation of this book almost as closely as did I. While our children, Laura and Kevin, observed the process this time from the bemused distance of their own academic perches, my husband, Walter, bore the brunt of my preoccupation, absences, and periodic and unpredictable spurts of enthusiasm to share the latest insight. We are students of social policy together; and he has helped, more than he knows, to enrich and distill my thinking. To him, with love, I dedicate this book.

# Contents

# ACCIDENTAL
# LOGICS

# Understanding the Dynamics of Change in the Health Care Arena

In the last two decades of the twentieth century, health care was not far from the top of the policy agenda in any advanced industrial nation. As governments sought to reduce or stabilize expenditures in the prevailing climate of fiscal stringency, state-sponsored programs of universal health insurance in most nations presented large but politically risky potential targets. In the minority of nations (notably the United States, but also the Netherlands) in which state-sponsored programs were not universal, major policy initiatives were undertaken to extend the scope of public programs and to better integrate public and private coverage. In nations emerging from the era of communist regimes, the restructuring of health care was caught up in the wrenching readjustments of the move to market economies. Everywhere, the centrality of health care to social well-being—and the appropriate roles of the "state" and the "market," the "public" and the "private" sector in the health care arena—were debated with new vigor.

These debates about health care formed part of the larger debate about the welfare state in the late twentieth century. The challenges to the welfare state in this period—economic, fiscal, and political—grew as the cushion of economic growth in the 1960s deflated under the pressure of international economic developments. Cross-nationally, the rate of expansion of the fiscal scope of the welfare state slowed on average in the 1980s, and public spending on health care was no exception to this phenomenon.[1] (There were, however, some significant national exceptions to this cross-national trend.) Potentially more significant than this fiscal restraint, moreover, was the development of a set of agendas for redesigning welfare-state programs and institutions. Neoconservative governments were loudest in announcing this agenda; but over the 1980s and 1990s reform was championed by governments of varying partisan complexions across advanced industrial nations. Although these reform agendas varied themselves, they had in common a concern with the structure of incentives embedded in welfare-state programs, and the declared objective of redesigning programs to provide incentives to efficiency and effectiveness.[2]

This type of reform agenda has profound implications for the health care arena. Pursuing this agenda meant moving beyond the blunt instruments of budget constraint and cost-shifting that governments relied upon in the past, and attempting to change the systems of decision-making in health care—the systems through which day-to-day decisions were made about the production and consumption of health care services. As the Organization for Economic Cooperation and Development (OECD) (1994) noted, this represented an expansion of policy perspective from a macro-level focus on global budget allocation to include micro-level considerations of the relationships between providers and purchasers of care. And in confronting these relationships, policymakers had to deal with the structures of decision-making in health care, and with issues unique to the health care arena.

Large areas of the welfare state—those relating to income maintenance—involve income transfers between the state and the individual recipient. Others, such as housing, social services, and education as well as health care, offer goods and services whose production requires the participation of intermediate producers with varying levels of technological skill and hence labor market power. Perhaps only postsecondary education, however, rivals the health care arena in the level of education and technological expertise required of providers, and the extent to which those providers can insist upon their autonomy to make decisions according to the norms of their disciplines, regardless of the source of their remuneration. Unlike many forms of postsecondary education, moreover, health care delivery rests upon the individual encounter between the highly skilled practitioner(s) and the recipient of care. It is a system in which trust networks—between patients and providers, and among providers themselves—have traditionally characterized the decision-making system.

Given the density and complexity of the networks that characterize the decision-making system in health care, it is not surprising that attempts to implement health care reform agendas met with widely varying degrees of success across nations. Nor is it surprising that the agendas themselves varied across nations, although there were some important common themes. Indeed, only in Britain was sweeping change in the public policies governing the decision-making system enacted and implemented. More modest versions of the British reforms took place in Sweden and New Zealand, but in both cases more ambitious reform proposals sputtered. Sweeping changes in the Netherlands to integrate public and private insurers within an overarching framework of regulated competition were proposed in 1988 and 1991 but were progressively scaled back in the 1990s. In other countries, such as Canada, Germany, and France, no sweeping redesign of the system was attempted, although governments made a number of strategic interventions with varying degrees of success.

Perhaps the most intriguing case is presented by the United States. There, attempts to expand coverage and to reshape health care decision-making systems failed spectacularly at the federal level in 1994 and subsequently in a number of states. Yet in the absence of major policy change, decision-making systems in health care underwent a dramatic and turbulent transformation with the rise of "managed care" entities and the growing role of the private sector.

Whether or not a nation attempted bold policy change in this period, let alone the likelihood of success, bore little relationship to overall levels and trends in spending on health care, or to the share borne by the public treasury. Change was attempted unsuccessfully in the United States, which, with the lowest share of public spending other than Turkey, nonetheless had the highest level of total health spending relative to gross domestic product (GDP) in the OECD in 1992, as well as the highest rate of growth in this measure from 1980 to 1992 (table 1.1). But change was also attempted with varying degrees of success in Britain (almost the mirror image of the United States, with a high public share but one of the lowest levels of total health spending among the family of OECD nations and an intermediate rate of growth in spending), as well as in the Netherlands and New Zealand (with relatively low public shares, intermediate levels of expenditure, and relatively low rates of growth). Meanwhile Canada, with levels of expenditure and a growth rate second only to the United States, as well as a public share approximating the OECD average, experienced no attempt at major policy change.

TABLE 1.1  Health Expenditures in Selected OECD Countries, 1980–1992

| | Total Health Spending as Percent of GDP, 1992 | Average Annual Increase in Ratio of Total Health Spending to GDP, 1980–92 | Public Health Spending as Percent of Total Health Spending, 1991 |
|---|---|---|---|
| Australia | 8.8 | 1.6 | 67.8 |
| Canada | 10.3 | 2.8 | 72.2 |
| France | 9.4 | 1.8 | 73.9 |
| Germany | 8.7 | 0.3 | 71.8 |
| Italy | 8.5 | 1.8 | 77.5 |
| Japan | 6.9 | 0.4 | 72.0 |
| Netherlands | 8.6 | 0.6 | 73.1 |
| New Zealand | 7.7 | 0.6 | 78.9 |
| Sweden | 7.9 | −1.4 | 78.0 |
| United Kingdom | 7.1 | 1.7 | 83.3 |
| United States | 13.6 | 3.2 | 43.9 |
| OECD Average | 8.1 | 1.2 | 75.4[a] |

*Sources:* Schieber et al. (1994: 101); OECD (1993, vol. 1: 252).

[a] Except Turkey and Luxembourg.

How are we to make sense of the commonality and the differences across nations in their experience with the health care arena in the 1990s? What drives change in health care systems, and why do certain types of change occur in some nations and not in others? This book is an attempt to answer those questions, by focusing in particular on the experiences of Britain, Canada, and the United States. The answer, I will argue, lies in an understanding of the "accidents" of history that shaped national systems at critical moments in time, and in the distinctive "logics" of the systems thus created. This chapter will lay out the elements of that argument, and will introduce the puzzles of policy development in Britain, the United States, and Canada to which the argument will be applied.

## The Conceptual Framework: The Accidental Logics of Change in Policy Arenas

This book presents a way of thinking about and understanding change in the health care policy arena, and in policy arenas more generally. The framework developed here, as in other recent interpretations of public policy (e.g., Pierson 1994, esp. 174–75), draws upon the insights of two strains of analysis in political science: "historical institutionalism" and "rational choice." It explores the distinctive logics of particular decision-making systems, within which actors respond, rationally, to the incentives facing them given the resources they can bring to bear. But it also recognizes that the dynamics of change in decision-making systems cannot be understood entirely in terms of the "rational choice" of the actors within them. Periodic episodes of policy change establish the parameters of the systems within which actors make their choices. And those episodes are best understood as products of particular historical contexts.

This line of argument has much in common with the growing literature on "path dependency" in political science. Various scholars, such as Krasner (1984), Baumgartner and Jones (1993), Putnam (1993), Wilsford (1994), Rothman (1997), and Pierson (1997), have argued "that specific patterns of timing and sequence matter; . . . that particular courses of action, once introduced, can be virtually impossible to reverse; and that consequently political development is punctuated by critical moments or junctures which shape the basic contours of social life" (Pierson 1997: 1). Or in Putnam's words, "History matters. . . . What comes first (even if it was in some sense 'accidental') conditions what comes later. Individuals may 'choose' their institutions, but they do not choose them under circumstances of their own making, and their choices in turn influence the rules within which their successors choose" (Putnam 1993: 8, cited in Rothman 1997: 13).

This book recognizes and seeks to explain this pattern of "path dependence" or "punctuated equilibrium" in the dynamics of policy change. It will demonstrate why particular windows of opportunity for change in health policy opened at certain times and not at others—a pattern of timing that derived from factors in the broader political system, not the health care arena itself. It will demonstrate through comparisons across nations and across time that the timing of these windows affected not only what did happen in these systems but also, arguably, what did not happen. It will show, accordingly, that key features of health care systems are "accidental" in the sense that they were shaped by ideas and agendas in place at the time a window of opportunity was opened by factors in the broader political system. And it will develop an argument that explains the path dependence of these systems *between* episodes of major change by exploring the logic of decision-making that each put in place, a logic that shapes the rational behavior of actors within them.

Periodic episodes of policy change establish what I shall call here the *structural* and *institutional* parameters of the decision-making system. The structural dimension relates to the balance of influence across key categories of actors: in the case of health care, the balance across the state, the medical profession, and private finance. The institutional dimension refers to the mix of various instruments of social control—hierarchy, market, and collegiality. Change in the policy parameters establishing the structural balance and the institutional mix of the health care system requires an extraordinary mobilization of political authority and will—on the scale, as we shall see, of the Labour majority government at the end of World War II in Britain, the Democratic landslide in the 1964 presidential and congressional elections in the United States, or the era of "cooperative federalism" in the 1960s in Canada. Accordingly episodes of policy change have required a confluence of factors in the broader political arena; the resultant systems have been shaped by the climate of ideas and the constellation of interests that exist at the time that such a confluence occurs. Once established, the institutional mix and structural balance of these systems intersect to generate a distinctive logic that governs the behavior of participants and the ongoing dynamic of change.

These logics derive from two essential characteristics of institutional mixes and structural balances—their implications for information flows and for lines of accountability respectively. Hierarchical and collegial systems economize in different ways on information—that is, they reduce information costs—but they run the risk of excluding certain information which can be overlooked by the normal channels of transmission. Market mechanisms provide incentives for acquiring necessary information, but because of the number, variety, and independence of the sites at which information is held, they make it costly for participants to do so. Similarly, state actors, professionals, and private financial interests derive their influence from different sources, and accordingly respond to different demands, through different channels of accountability. In very broad terms, state actors function within systems in which those in command are ultimately dependent upon political support; therefore they seek to accommodate a sufficient range of interests and opinions to maintain a coalition of support. Actors whose influence is based on access to private finance must respond to the demands of owners of private capital to realize rates of return comparable to those in other areas of investment. And professionals, who derive their influence from membership in the professional group, must maintain standing in the group by continuing to meet its standards and norms.

What this means is that understanding the logic of decision-making systems in health care requires an understanding of the *intersection* between institutional mix and structural balance. As a beginning, and although the particular combinations of institutional mix and structural balance that we observe across nations are numerous and varied, it is possible to identify certain "ideal types" in order to develop some hypotheses about the dynamics of change in different types of systems. These ideal types are based upon the affinity between certain categories of actors and certain institutional mechanisms: between state actors and hierarchies, professional actors and collegial systems, and private financial interests and markets. A hierarchical system lends itself to the exercise of authority, an exchange system to the investment and deployment of wealth, and a collegial system to the exercise of skill. Hence a heavy weight for hierarchical, market, and collegial instruments may enhance the influence of state actors, private financial interests, and professionals, respectively.

These "ideal types"—state hierarchy, private market, and professional collegial institutions—will be fleshed out in what follows. It is important to note here, however, that one of the most remarkable phenomena of the health care arena of the 1990s was the *shuffling* of the natural affinities just described. As part of the emergence of a "new paradigm" for the financing and delivery of health care, to be discussed later, the state in some cases sought to avail itself of exchange-oriented instruments; private financial interests increasingly experimented with vertical and horizontal forms of integration; and professional groups became more and more divided as to whether to become more managerial or more entrepreneurial, and whether to ally with the state or with private finance. Where such shuffles occurred, they generated their own distinctive logics. As we shall see, "market" instruments operate differently when the preponderance of influence is held by state actors (or medical professionals) than when influence is held by entrepreneurs responding to shareholders. Similarly, the dynamics of change in hierarchies whose senior officers are ultimately accountable to shareholders differ from those in hierarchies whose lines of accountability run to the political system.

The logics created by different structural balances and institutional mixes cannot be understood in isolation from the particular characteristics of the policy arenas in which they operate. Hence one of the sections of this introductory chapter is devoted to an exploration of the essential microeconomic logic of health care delivery. That logic derives, fundamentally, from the disparities in the distribution of information between potential providers and potential recipients of health care. That fundamental disparity creates an imbalance of influence between providers and recipients of care; that disparity underlies the establishment of agency relationships, whereby potential recipients of care delegate decision-making authority to selected providers. Moreover, other important dimensions of the microeconomics of health care delivery—the risk and uncertainty of the need for health care—introduce another category of actors into the decision-making system; namely, the "third-party payers," public or private, who undertake to administer risk-pooling arrangements. Because agency relationships assign broad discretion to providers of care, it is necessary to guard against the abuse of such discretion. Control mechanisms are typically put in place by those whose interests might be compromised—either potential recipients of care or third-party payers. These mechanisms, like other mechanisms of social control, fall into the three broad categories already noted: hierarchical, market-based, and collegial. The structural balance of interests and the institutional mix of instruments of control in any given national context, then, must be established within the constraints set by the fundamental need to establish and to control agency relationships that give broad discretion to providers of care.

The microeconomic logic of the health care arena is, however, itself in flux. Technological change has contributed both to increasing health care costs and to decreasing the costs of amassing and analyzing large amounts of information. Together these changes have led to the rise of increasingly cost-conscious and educated purchasers of health care, and to arenas characterized by bargaining relationships among relatively large and sophisticated players. The occupants of the bargaining roles, and the nature and pace of change, have nonetheless varied considerably across nations.

The remainder of this chapter fleshes out this framework. It first explores in more detail the two key dimensions of decision-making with which this book is concerned: structural balance and institutional mix. It then looks at the two primary ways in which the structural balance and institutional mix of a given system may change over time: through periodic policy episodes in which fundamental structural and institutional parameters are changed, and through the playing out of the inherent logic of the prevailing system through the rational behavior of the actors within it, between episodes of major policy change. Next, it explores the microeconomic logic of health care delivery—and in particular the central role of agency relationships—that provides the common context in which balances of influence and mixes of instruments must be established. Finally, it summarizes the health policy agenda as it emerged cross-nationally in the latter half of the twentieth century (and particularly in the 1990s), sets out three puzzles posed by the experience of Britain, the United States, and Canada in the 1990s, and positions those puzzles to be explained through an understanding of the "accidental logics" of the three systems in the rest of the book.

## Dimensions of Decision-Making Systems: Institutional Mix and Structural Balance

My concern in this book is with the dynamics of change in the decision-making systems of the health care arena—that is, the systems through which day-to-day decisions are made about the production and consumption of health care services. The first step in understanding those dynamics is to identify the two dimensions that define the essential character of such decision-making systems.

The first of these dimensions refers to the mix of hierarchical, market-oriented, and collegial elements that characterize the decision-making system. It refers to the ways in which human interactions are "institutionalized"—that is, systematized and legitimized for purposes of social control. Hence I term this dimension the "institutional mix." As Victor Fuchs (1993) has pointed out, "[E]very society must have control mechanisms for determining how much health care to produce, how to produce it, and how to distribute it among the population. In principle, only three types of mechanism are available: the market, central direction, and traditional norms" (165). Fuchs's trilogy of control mechanisms is similar to those identified by Kenneth Boulding (1968) who characterized them as the exchange system, the threat system, and the integrative system, and by Charles Lindblom (1977), whose framework comprised the mechanisms of exchange, authority, and persuasion. In the context of the health care arena, these distinctions are best captured by the concepts of market, hierarchy, and collegiality.

In a pure market system, the overall pattern of the production and distribution of health care (as any other good) would be the result of voluntary trades between multiple investors, providers, and consumers: it would be determined by the decisions of owners or controllers of capital to invest in the provision of health care facilities and personnel, and the decisions of consumers to purchase such care. In a pure system of hierarchy, that pattern would be centrally planned and implemented through the establishment of rules—under, in Lindblom's terms, the operation of a generally accepted "rule of obedience." And in a pure system of collegiality, the pattern of health care provision would be the aggregate of the results of numerous professional decisions made in individual clinical encounters, in accordance with norms developed by the body of practicing professionals and enforced through professional trust networks. In practice, of course, real-life systems are admixtures of these pure types.

The second definitive dimension of decision-making systems relates to the balance of influence across three broad categories of actors—the state, health care professionals (and particularly the medical profession), and private financial interests. That is, it relates to the politicoeconomic structure of interests in the arena; hence I refer to this dimension as the "structural balance" of the arena. The three categories of actors represent the fundamental bases of power in the health care arena—authority, skill, and wealth. It is the balance among these categories that determines how the influence of other interests will be mediated. Notably, depending on the balance of influence across these categories, the interests of recipients and potential recipients of health care will be exercised to varying degrees through representation in the public policy process (as "citizens" within the state), through individual interactions with health care professionals (as "patients"), and through the exercise of consumer sovereignty in private markets (as "consumers").

Changes may occur *within* institutional or structural categories: hierarchies may become more or less decentralized, for example, or markets more or less concentrated; certain types of state actors or health care providers or private financial interests may gain or lose in influence. But such shifts are less radical and less definitive of the character of the system than are changes in the mix of hierarchy, collegiality, and market instruments and the balance across state, provider, and private financial actors. It is these two dimensions that define the essential character of decision-making systems. Together they establish a logic of decision-making that shapes the expectations of participants and the ways in which they will respond, rationally, to challenge. It is these powerful logics that explain the durability or volatility of particular institutional configurations.

## Policy Episodes and System Logics

The institutional mix and structural balance of health care systems is a product of two factors: public policies that establish the institutional and structural parameters of the system, and the behavior of actors within these parameters over time. Each of these factors involves a particular dynamic of change.

### Policy episodes

Major policy initiatives altering the fundamental institutional mix and structural balance in health care decision-making systems are episodic and rare. Such initiatives have required an extraordinary mobilization of political authority and will, and accordingly they have depended upon factors largely external to the health care arena. The timing of these episodes has been critical in determining the design of health care decision-making systems: changes made in these episodes have established distinctive institutional mixes and structural balances in each nation that bear the mark of the constellations of power and the policy ideas current in national contexts at the time.

Such episodes occur only when a coincidence of external forces is strong enough to overcome the resistance of interests within the arena to such change. As already argued here, it is in the nature of health care delivery systems to generate a profoundly uneven distribution of a central resource—information. Those who control this resource have a substantial power base from which to resist state action to change the balance of influence. Hence state action is likely to occur only when factors external to the health care arena coalesce to bring it about. Essentially, two conditions must obtain in order for a "window of opportunity" for major policy change affecting the institutional mix and structural balance of health care decision-making systems to occur. Each of these is necessary, but neither one alone is sufficient.

First, the political system must provide a consolidated base of authority for policy action. That is, those who command the key levers of state authority must be willing and able to act in concert. Political systems vary in their potential to consolidate authority. In Westminster parliamentary systems, a consolidation of authority requires either a majority government or a multiparty consensus in a minority government. In congressional systems, it means either single-party control of both legislative and executive branches sufficient to ensure the achievement of the party's agenda, or a multiparty consensus. Where the necessary authority is divided among levels of government, moreover, there needs to be a consolidation of intergovernmental authority—a propitious climate of intergovernmental relations. The conditions under which the political authority that is necessary to effect institutional change in the health care arena can be mobilized are more likely to occur in some nations than in others. It has often been pointed out that the institutional structure of government in the United States makes such action particularly difficult (Steinmo and Watts 1995). But in this sense the United States is different in degree but not in kind from other systems—the mobilization of authority sufficient to bring about change in the structural and institutional parameters of the welfare state in the health care arena is a rare occurrence in most systems.[3]

Second, the opening of a window of opportunity for policy change requires that substantial change in health care policy hold a high priority within the broader agenda of those who command the levers of authority. That is, there must be a commitment to policy change on the part of key political actors—a willingness to elevate the issue above the myriad others that might be accomplished given the consolidation of authority.

Major policy change affecting the institutional mix and structural balance of health care decision-making systems, then, requires an extraordinary mobilization of political authority and will. And this argument has some important corollaries:

First, episodes of major change in health care policy, generated as they are by factors external to the arena, arise independent of the evolution of policy ideas about health care delivery. But the type of change attempted is likely to be shaped very much by the prevailing climate of policy ideas in the health care arena. To put it another way, the "window of opportunity" for change may be created and opened by factors in the broader political system. But that window will open onto a landscape of policy ideas within the health care arena that is in a constant state of evolution. The particular changes that are considered will depend in large part upon that landscape.[4] Rarely, however, will the landscape yield one unambiguous policy option. The choice among the alternatives that are offered will depend in large part on the nature of the external forces that caused the window to open. That is, it will depend on the broader agenda of which health policy change forms a part.

Finally, the success of these attempts at change will depend on the durability of the forces that created the window of opportunity, and the "goodness of fit" between the strategy of change proposed and the internal logic of the system to which it is addressed. The logic of particular systems is a legacy of past episodes of policy change, and the playing out of these logics thus acts as a "rolling restraint" on the impact of policy change.[5]

### System logics

Episodes of major policy change establish the institutional and structural parameters of systems of decision-making for health care. Between such episodes, the system is shaped by the behavior of key groups of actors within these parameters. In each case, this behavior follows a distinctive logic. These logics differ in their capacity to mitigate the impact of exogenous policy initiatives or to generate endogenous change in the institutional mix and structural balance of the decision-making system. As we shall see later, the logic of the decision-making system has both facilitated and mediated the impact of major policy intervention in Britain, has transformed decision-making structures in the absence of major policy intervention in the United States, and has kept the decision-making system remarkably stable in Canada.

The logics of different institutional mixes—the ways in which they shape the rational behavior of actors—derives from the different ways in which they handle the actors' needs for information. Market-based instruments are information-intensive: an actor (such as a purchaser) who would control the behavior of another (such as a supplier) purely on the basis of voluntary exchange must be able to specify exactly what is expected and exactly how it will be rewarded. It must be possible, in other words, to write a specific contract, to assess the performance of the provider against that contract and to exit the relationship if not satisfied. In a number of areas (including health care), however, information gaps make it very difficult to specify and to monitor contracts. Such difficulties can lead to a redoubling of effort to specify every contingency and to increase monitoring until the marginal cost of acquiring information exceeds its marginal benefit. They can also lead to a search for alternative forms of control.

A second option is to establish relationships that achieve the objectives of purchasers without the need to contract with independent entities. The logic behind this second option has been perceptively traced out by Oliver Williamson and a number of other scholars who have followed his lead (Williamson 1975; Bartlett 1991). They have described the difficulty of writing, executing, and enforcing the "complex contingent claims contracts" as required in areas in which "transactions are multidimensional and outcomes are contingent upon an uncertain environment" (Bartlett 1991: 3). In such circumstances, faced with the costly and perhaps impossible task of acquiring the information necessary to specify all possibilities in advance, it is rational for economic actors to establish forms of organization which allow them to "deal with uncertainty and complexity in an adaptive and sequential fashion" (Bartlett 1991: 4). It is not, of course, feasible for individual recipients of care to establish such organizational forms, but they can seek out agents associated with such organizations in order to increase the likelihood that the agency relationship will not be abused. These organizations, that is, assume a collective agency role—a responsibility for ensuring the trustworthy behavior of individual agents.

There are essentially two forms of such organization, one hierarchical and one collegial. The collegial form is the "peer group," an organization based on the ability of professionals to assess each other's competence and their commitment to a common set of professional norms. The peer group, Williamson argues, is a feasible form of organization when the numbers of professionals involved is relatively small. Beyond a certain point, however, the bonds of professionalism become attenuated, and more structured forms of organization, allowing for feasible spans of control, become necessary.

The second form of organization discussed by Williamson, Bartlett, and others—and the one to which they devote most attention—is the hierarchical firm. In this case, administrative rules and processes, enforced by sanctions related to job security and career advancement, provide the control mechanism and allow for sequential adaptation to uncertainty. And as sociologists such as Granovetter (1992) have argued, hierarchies also provide for a stability of relationship which allows for the development of trust networks over time—based not on common identification with professional norms as in the case of peer groups, but on a history of dealings and the anticipation of future dealings.

The vertical integration of functions in a hierarchy allows instructions to be given as eventualities occur, rather than being specified in advance. It also allows, at least in theory, for the development of an information system consistent with the "bounded rationality" of participants: "front-line" service providers have extensive information about individual cases, which can then be progressively aggregated, abstracted from, and distilled as information moves up the levels of the hierarchy. (The best exposition of this logic is still Simon's classic work [Simon 1956: 79–109].) But hierarchies, like other approaches to controlling agency relationships, also have their limitations and costs. Vertical information flows can lead to distortions and imperfections in transmission. The development of organizational routines may establish a fixed repertoire of responses and discourage innovation and flexibility.

Each of these mechanisms, then, has its pros and cons. But each does provide actors with a rational way of seeking to control the behavior of others in a world of costly information. The ways in which hierarchical, market-oriented, and collegial systems function, however, will also depend on the balance of influence of the actors within them. As already noted, state actors, private financial interests, and professionals respond to different demands through different lines of accountability. This discussion, then, generates the following speculations about the dynamics of change in the three ideal types:

*State hierarchies*    Hierarchical systems dominated by state actors, given their grounding in a "rule of obedience" and their established channels of communication, are in theory capable of periodic abrupt and dramatic change ordered and communicated from the top—including change in the very weight of state actors and hierarchical mechanisms themselves. To order such change, state actors must have a political coalition of support that is stable over the period of time necessary for change to be implemented. Implementation may, however, be delayed even in an "obedient" hierarchy when information necessary to implement centrally ordered change in local circumstances is lacking. And with delay, as Pressman and Wildavsky (1973) classically observed, may come the erosion of political support. To summarize, state hierarchies can generate abrupt strategic changes, but they are vulnerable to problems of delay.

*Private markets*    Markets in which entrepreneurs are seeking to respond to the demands of owners of private capital for competitive rates of return are likely to generate ongoing, often rapid and turbulent organizational change in the health care arena, given the high mobility of capital, the uncertainty among relatively uninformed consumers about the quality of the product, and the swift pace of technological innovation. Again, such change may involve the institutional mix and structural balance of the system—for example, as hierarchical mechanisms arise to reduce transaction costs, or as the relative influence of state actors ebbs and flows through a series of regulatory initiatives to deal with perceived market failures and market responses to those initiatives. One constraint on such turbulent change in markets such as health care is the significance of "brand names" in a context in which consumers lack the information necessary to judge the quality of the product. Consumer loyalty to "brand name" producers may provide a source of stability. Alternatively, the problem of uninformed individual consumers may generate change on the demand side of the market such as the rise of sophisticated purchasing organizations. In theory, countervailing or complementary changes in organization on the supply and the demand sides of the market could yield a degree of stability over time. To summarize, private markets in the health care arena are likely to generate turbulent structural and institutional change unless stabilized through a degree of cartelization on the demand or the supply side.

*Professional collegial institutions*    Collegial bodies and institutions dominated by professionals are likely to yield a relatively slow pace of incremental change. The slow pace is in part a function of the need to achieve a substantial degree of consensus among peers before changes are made. It also reflects an important implication of peer-group identification: a change threatening any given segment of the group is likely to be perceived, and accordingly resisted, as a threat to all. Incremental change may involve experimentation with hierarchical mechanisms as the group becomes too large to rely exclusively on the subscription of members to common norms. Or it may involve the adoption of market strategies as individual professionals seek to advance their positions as independent practitioners. But norms of peer equality and cooperation constrain professionally dominated collegial systems from moving far in either of these directions. To summarize, the internal logic of such systems is one of incremental consensually driven change.

In the real world, decision-making systems are admixtures of these ideal types, and explaining the dynamics of change is accordingly more complicated. Moreover, as noted, a key feature of the developments of the 1990s was the shuffling of the "natural affinities" underlying these ideal types. The general argument of this book—that decision-making systems in health care, established during particular episodes of policy change, develop distinctive logics that condition future changes—can hence be illustrated only by close examination of specific examples. Before doing so, however, we need to establish one more component of the argument. However distinctive are the logics of particular health care decision-making systems, they must all respond to certain underlying elements of the microeconomics of health care delivery. The next section presents a brief overview of those elements.

## The Economics of Health Care Delivery: Agency, Risk, and Localism

Certain fundamental characteristics of the economics of health care delivery are common across nations. These characteristics do not determine the nature of public policies regarding the organization and financing of health care, nor of the behavior of actors within the parameters established by public policy, as is evidenced by wide cross-national variations in these respects. But they do establish the conditions in which the policy "problem" and the range of behavioral responses are defined.

At the heart of the economics of health care delivery is the "agency" relationship between the health care provider (quintessentially the physician) and the patient. Three characteristics of health care—information asymmetry, the difficulty of evaluating the product, and high costs of error—mean that it is rational for consumers of health care to establish agency relationships with providers, that is, to delegate decision-making authority to providers to choose the care required by the consumer. Diagnosing the nature of an ailment, determining the appropriate therapeutic response, and providing the necessary service typically require access to a specialized and systematic information base. For an individual consumer, the marginal costs of acquiring the necessary information in his or her particular case would be extremely costly or infeasible. Furthermore, it is difficult for the consumer to evaluate the quality of the service offered by competing practitioners, at least until possibly irreversible results have occurred. Because the outcome of treatment in any given case depends on a number of factors beyond the care provided (including, as Fuchs [1993: 34] has pointed out, the patient's own "knowledge, skill and motivation and the level of trust between patient and physician") it would again be very costly or infeasible for an individual patient to "shop" for care by investigating the experience of other patients in similar situations. Finally, the costs of error in attempting to deal with the problem in the absence of the necessary information may be very high or, indeed, irreversible and incompensable.

In such circumstances, it is rational for the individual consumer of health care to delegate decision-making authority to an agent with the information necessary to determine the requisite care and to provide that care or to select among alternative providers, and to trust that agent to act in the consumer's interest. This fundamental logic has traditionally placed physicians at the center of the decision-making system for health care. It has meant that supply and demand are not independently determined in the health care market. And it has also generated attempts to find mechanisms to ensure that physicians as agents do not abuse their positions of trust.

There are essentially three types of such mechanisms, corresponding to the institutional mechanisms of control already set out—market, hierarchy, and collegiality. In the first place, the potential recipient can attempt to specify his or her interests and objectives as tightly as possible in the contract with the provider. Such would be a classic "market" response. There are major constraints on drawing up specific contracts for health care, however. Indeed, these constraints—imperfect information on the part of consumers as to what care will be required in a given incident, and uncertainty about the very incidence of demand—are the factors that give rise to agency relationships with providers in the first place.

Second, the state could seek to regulate providers, establishing rules to govern behavior—an essentially hierarchical response. Cross-nationally, physicians are indeed subject to the control of state-sanctioned regulatory bodies. But state actors themselves face information gaps in regulating the behavior of professional groups such as physicians.

Accordingly a third way—which in fact characterizes most state-sanctioned systems for the regulation of medical professionals—is self-regulation: placing the control of medical behavior essentially in the hands of the professional group itself. Self-regulation, in fact, amounts to the establishment of a second-level agency relationship between the state and the profession, which follows a logic analogous to that which underlies the individual physician–patient relationship and is grounded in the profession's access to the body of knowledge necessary to judge the quality and appropriateness of care required in individual cases (Tuohy and Wolfson 1977). That is, the state delegates decision-making authority to the professional body to regulate its own members. And like the relationship between individual physicians and their patients, the relationship between the profession and the state under the self-regulatory model, although hedged about with accountability mechanisms, is essentially one based on collegiality and trust.

As we shall see, this model has come under great pressure in the late twentieth century. Before turning to recent developments, however, it is necessary to discuss two other fundamental features of the health care market, and their policy implications—the stochastic nature of demand and the local base of the market.

For the individual, the occurrence of the need for health care and the type of health care required is an uncertain risk. As in other markets characterized by risk and uncertainty, especially where the costs incurred may well be very large, the response has been the rise of insurance mechanisms. As Fuchs has pointed out, there are two basic models for insuring against the costs of health care: casualty insurance and social insurance. They differ essentially in the degree of cross-subsidization across different risk groups that they entail. Under the casualty insurance model, individuals are grouped into risk pools according to their level of risk, and premiums are established accordingly. Social insurance is fundamentally a system of broad cross-subsidization: in the limit, all members of society form a common risk pool.

Casualty insurance markets face two problems that can greatly skew the composition of risk pools. On the one hand, high-risk individuals will be more likely to take out insurance than will low-risk individuals. Since premiums are set to reflect expected loss, this phenomenon of "adverse selection" may lead to a spiral of escalating premiums whereby more and more low-risk individuals drop out of the market and risk pools become less and less diluted until, in the extreme case, the principle of pooling is lost. The mirror image of the problem of adverse selection is the problem of "cream-skimming," in which insurers establish eligibility requirements that allow them to select low-risk customers and hence reduce their expected losses, thus drawing those individuals out of broader risk pools and leaving those pools more concentrated with high risks.

States have typically reacted to these problems by establishing various regulatory mechanisms that attempt to control either the level of premiums or the composition of risk pools or both. As we shall see in the case of the United States, however, attempts to regulate the insurance market can provoke market responses that provoke further regulatory action in an escalating spiral of complexity.

The alternative to regulating the health "casualty" insurance market is effectively to supplant it through a system of social insurance. (I use the term here broadly to include systems in which the state directly employs the providers of care as well as those in which it underwrites the provision of care by privately organized providers.) This approach overcomes problems of adverse selection and cream-skimming, but it is likely to be motivated by equity considerations as well as those of market failure. Essentially, it rests on the premise that health care should be distributed according to need rather than according to ability to pay. In theory, this could also be accomplished through state subsidization of premiums in private insurance markets. The latter approach, however, leaves in place the problems of adverse selection and cream-skimming, with the associated regulatory complexity.

Both casualty and social insurance, moreover, suffer from the potential problem of "moral hazard": the likelihood that individuals will overconsume health care since the costs of care for any individual are spread across the pool of insured individuals. In the context of uncertainty about the outcome of a given intervention in a particular case and in the absence of a budget constraint, there is an incentive for providers to provide and consumers to consume health care to the point that the marginal benefit is equal not to the marginal cost of provision, but to zero. As long as the resulting increase in costs can be passed on to consumers in the form of higher premiums or taxes, this problem remains. One response to the problem, which has characterized most systems of social insurance or public finance, has been to establish global budget constraints while relying upon the agency relationship between the state and the medical profession to ensure that budgets are allocated cost-effectively. But third-party payers in both the public and private sectors have increasingly sought ways of establishing specific incentives to require those who make consumption decisions to be more conscious of cost-benefit trade-offs.

Attempts to establish a locus for cost-benefit decisions ran up against a central dynamic of health care economics—the dynamic created by the incentives for all participants to hedge against the open-ended costs associated with unpredictable needs for health care by shifting the risk of cost-bearing to others. Each of the nations with which we are concerned exhibited its own variant of risk-shifting behavior in the 1990s. And this risk-shifting behavior generated a major irony of the health care arena in the emerging environment of cost-conscious purchasers: those who ended up with the burden of cost-bearing risk also assumed the central role in decision-making, the role of weighing costs against benefits. In the United States this role came to be played by managed care entities; in Britain and Canada it was played in different ways by health care providers themselves (particularly by physicians).

A final characteristic of the health care market that is important to the understanding of the policy context is its essentially local base. Highly specialized tertiary or quaternary services may draw patients from a wide geographic area, but for the most part "catchment areas" for hospital and medical services are local in nature. This feature has a number of implications. It means that there are not the economies of scale that would favor the rise of large corporations; hence the industrial organization of health care delivery has tended to be decentralized. It also makes for locally based monopolies or oligopolies: even given the ability of providers to generate demand for their services, small- to medium-sized local communities can support only a limited number of hospitals or medical specialists. Even this characteristic is, however, vulnerable to the feedback effects of public policies. In the United States, for example, as we shall see, the heavy reliance on regulatory instruments over time has generated a complex environment of rules which has favored the rise of large multi-institutional and multistate corporations, in defiance of the diseconomies of scale in health care provision per se. And this effect has in turn fed back into the policy process, as these large entities have become important political actors.

Each of these characteristics of the health care market—the asymmetry of information between providers and patients, the stochastic nature of demand, and the local base of the catchment area for service—have historically shaped decision-making systems in the health care arena. The first and third characteristics have traditionally yielded decision-making systems in which locally based groups of physicians have, both individually and collectively, played the dominant role in determining the pattern of production and consumption of health services. The second characteristic has led to the widespread existence of health care insurance, and the presence of "third-party payers" as key economic and political actors. But each of these characteristics has also called forth policy responses from the state. And those responses, varying in design for reasons to be explored later in this book, have reshaped the political economy of health care in different ways in different nations. Different institutional mixes of hierarchical, collegial, and market instruments, and different structural balances across the state, the medical profession, and private finance have emerged in different nations and have evolved in different ways over time. These mixes and balances positioned nations to respond differently to the evolving health policy agenda.

## The Health Policy Agenda of the 1990s

In the post–World War II period, the agenda of health policy can be described in very broad terms as having evolved—at different paces and to different degrees in different nations—from ensuring equity in access to health care, to controlling the overall costs of care (or at least those costs borne by public sources), to achieving microeconomic efficiency. These concerns were cumulative: those arising later did not displace those arising earlier, although they have confronted policy-makers with new trade-offs (OECD 1992: 14). Hence the agenda of health care reform in the 1990s was marked early on by attempts by governments to maintain or even to increase the proportion of their populations with coverage against health care costs while limiting their own fiscal exposure; this was done by establishing budget caps and/or by shifting some costs to other levels of government or to private sources of funding. These aspects of the agenda were not new, but they increased in salience on the political agenda. In addition, there were attempts in a number of nations to change the economic incentives facing various actors in the system, notably by introducing various types of market or marketlike mechanisms. Examples of these various aspects of the agenda can be briefly sketched as follows.

*Access*

By and large, state-sponsored health care programs were established or dramatically expanded during more buoyant fiscal times. Under the fiscal pressures of the 1980s and 1990s, one policy response might have been a contraction of eligibility for publicly financed health care, as occurred in a number of nations in other welfare-state programs such as unemployment insurance and public assistance. This course, however, was not chosen; no OECD nation reduced eligibility under its state-sponsored health care programs, although there were modest reductions in the package of *benefits* provided under these programs, and some increases in the proportion of costs borne by recipients of care themselves. The most notable initiatives with respect to access, on the contrary, had to do with *expanding* eligibility for health insurance by expanding the role of the state and better integrating public and private insurance. In the United States, where about 15% of the population lacked health insurance at any given time and a variety of limitations on coverage existed for a substantial proportion of the remainder, the failed Clinton proposal of 1993 would have expanded health insurance coverage through a number of reforms: requiring employers to purchase health insurance for their employees and to contribute a certain proportion of the cost; adopting a number of reforms to the insurance market; establishing regional purchasing alliances to purchase insurance on behalf of individuals and small groups; and integrating the existing Medicaid program for the poor into the new arrangements. In the Netherlands, where health insurance coverage was near universal but divided between social insurance funds and private insurers, reforms proposed in the late 1980s and early 1990s sought to establish an integrated system of compulsory basic insurance and voluntary supplemental insurance, both to be offered through competing social insurance funds and private insurers. Neither the American nor the Dutch plan succeeded, however—a phenomenon that underscored the difficulty of expanding eligibility for public programs in the climate of the 1990s. A number of U.S. states expanded access to health insurance for their low-income populations (Holahan et al. 1995b), and both federal and state legislation attempted to expand access through reform of private insurance markets, as will be discussed later in this book. In general, however, the proportion of the population without health insurance continued to grow in the absence of a universal plan (Thorpe 1997: 354–58).

### Cost control

The period since the mid-1970s saw a progressive tightening of budget caps at the sectoral, institutional, and individual levels, and in some cases an increased reliance on cost-shifting. The scope and stringency of budget limits has varied across nations, but most OECD nations had established global budgeting in at least some subsectors of health care by 1990 (Taylor-Goodby 1996: 208; OECD 1992: 140–41). In Britain, for example, the health care budget (for other than general practitioners) was subjected to "cash limits" beginning in 1976; in Canada, provincial governments introduced global budgets for hospitals in the 1970s, global limits on physician billings in the 1980s, and graduated caps on individual physician billings in the 1980s and 1990s. In Germany, global ceilings for payments to physicians were negotiated on a national basis and at the level of sickness funds since the 1970s; global operating budgets for individual hospitals were negotiated between sickness funds and hospitals since 1986; and in 1993 caps were temporarily placed on the prescribing budgets of individual physicians (Henke et al. 1994). In France, global budgeting for public hospitals was established in 1984; and a plan to establish graduated caps on payments to individual physicians was announced in 1996. This list could be extended; but it serves to indicate both the pervasiveness and the variety of budget capping strategy. Even in the United States, an analogue can be seen in the private sector, where the increasing popularity of various forms of prepaid care established de facto annual budget limits for some providers.

### Cost-shifting

A strategy of considerable duration in some nations is the attempt to shift costs to other levels of government or to the private sector. In Canada, the federal government moved from its open-ended cost-sharing arrangement with provincial governments to a formula-limited block grant system in 1977, and subsequent changes led to a progressive diminution of the federal share. Most Canadian provinces established regional health authorities, but these were creatures of the provincial government without taxing authority (although consideration has been given to granting them such authority in at least one province, Saskatchewan). In Sweden, considerable tension marked the relationship between the central government, county councils, and municipalities over the financing of health care throughout the 1980s and 1990s. Increasing authority and fiscal responsibility for health care services had been transferred to county councils over the course of the twentieth century, culminating in an integrated health care financing and delivery model at the county level in 1983. The Swedish central government continued to exert influence over health care spending, however, through blunt mechanisms such as the freezing of local taxation. Conflict among the three levels of government led to an elaborate review exercise in the early 1990s, which generated a range of possible models but in the end left the county council model essentially intact (Garpenby 1995).

The shifting of costs to the private sector was, despite alarmist media commentary in a number of nations, relatively modest. On average, the public share of total health expenditures in OECD nations was 73.2% in 1970. By 1980, this figure had climbed to 77.9%, and by 1991 it had declined slightly to 75.4%.[6] Cost-shifting took a number of forms. In some nations, more-or-less uniform "user fees" for physician visits and/or hospital stays were instituted, increased, or proposed. In Sweden, user fees were increased in the late 1980s; in New Zealand, user fees were instituted for hospital services in 1991, although user fees for inpatient services were abandoned shortly thereafter (in 1993) in response to public opposition (Flood 1996). A regime of user fees was also proposed in the Netherlands in 1994 (van der Wilt 1995: 621). Various forms of user charges for pharmaceuticals have been instituted or increased in a number of nations, including New Zealand and Germany, plus several Canadian provinces with drug plans for elderly or low-income groups.

Other types of private charges, in the form of unregulated billing above the rates covered by public insurance, actually decreased in a number of nations in the 1980s and early 1990s. In Canada, such charges for medical and hospital services were disallowed under federal legislation establishing the criteria for federal contributions to provincial health insurance plans in 1984. In Australia, the incidence of such charges for medical services outside hospitals decreased steadily after the reintroduction of universal health insurance by the Labour government in 1984, although the issue, as well as that of the role of private insurance, has continued as a prominent issue of political debate (Gray 1996). In New Zealand, by contrast, the proportion of charges not covered by public insurance in the small general practice sector rose steadily in the 1980s and 1990s (Flood 1996). Indeed, after 1991 a "targeted" user fee regime for general practitioner services (as well as for hospital services and pharmaceuticals) was introduced; among other things, this change reduced the rate of government subsidization of fees paid by members of upper income groups (Brown 1996: 295–98).

Yet another "cost-shifting" strategy involved reductions in the package of benefits covered by state-supported programs. The definition of a "core" benefit package was a focus of public policy in a number of jurisdictions, including the United Kingdom, the Netherlands, New Zealand, Canada, and the United States. The results were, however, incremental and modest (Klein et al. 1996: 109–19). Services "delisted" (that is, removed from the list of publicly insured services) in a number of Canadian provinces related primarily to cosmetic procedures and some services related to reproduction, such as reversal of vasectomies and in-vitro fertilization. As Klein and his colleagues noted, these exclusions were "remarkably similar" to the few procedures that various health authorities in Britain chose to remove from the package of services they purchase on behalf of their respective populations (Klein et al.: 118). In Sweden, the Netherlands, and New Zealand, government commissions appointed to consider the appropriate scope of a basic package of publicly insured services produced sets of criteria, without defining the actual services to be included or excluded.

The policy initiative regarding the definition of a basic list of insured services that attracted the greatest international attention was the project in the U.S. state of Oregon to identify a list of procedures, in order of priority, to be covered under a program to provide health insurance to all individuals and families with incomes below the federally defined poverty level (Garland 1991; Klein et al. 1996: 111; Jacobs et al. 1998). The availability of public funds would determine how far down the list coverage would extend. It is important to note that this project was not carried out in the context of a universal health insurance program. Rather, it was adopted as a way of expanding health coverage to the uninsured population within budget limits—that is, the population covered was expanded while the benefit package was restricted (meaning that some beneficiaries of existing programs would be left at least potentially worse off). After considerable negotiation with the federal government,[7] the program went into effect in 1994 (Holahan et al. 1995b). Despite having become the cynosure of international attention, however, the Oregon experiment was not repeated in any other jurisdiction.

Finally, depending upon the design of public programs, a process of "passive privatization" may occur as a by-product of technological change. This was a matter of some commentary in Canada, for example, where a number of goods and services, such as drugs, were covered (as "hospital services") if they were provided on an inpatient basis but not if they were provided outside the hospital. As technology made possible shorter hospital stays, day surgery, or medical as opposed to surgical interventions, a number of costs once borne by the public plan were shifted to the private sector. Over the 1980s, the public share of total health spending in Canada contracted at a rate only slightly above the average rate for the OECD; but, as we shall see, the phenomenon gave rise to concerns about future trends.

### Changing decision-making systems

None of these aspects of the health policy agenda was new in the 1990s—each represented an extension of strategies employed in the past. (Attempts at explicit definition of the scope of the public benefit package, however—represented in their most extreme form by the Oregon experiment—arguably pushed previous definitions of public coverage into new territory.) What was new in the 1990s, as noted earlier, was an increased attention to the incentive structures embedded in existing decision-making systems, and a variety of attempts to change those systems in order to promote greater efficiency and effectiveness.

Although attempts to modify the relationship between payers, providers, and recipients of care varied considerably across nations both in their design and in their degree of success, there were common themes in a number of these initiatives. First, various mechanisms were proposed to counterbalance the expertise-based power of providers by creating more sophisticated planning or purchasing entities intermediate between the state and providers. These entities were to operate on behalf of population groups, often geographically defined.

The creation of regional health service planning and management boards in nine of the ten Canadian provinces represented one variant of this approach, although it essentially involved a reorganization of state authority more than it did a change in the nature of the relationship between payer and provider groups. Policies directed at shifting power from providers to sickness funds in Germany represented another variant—a subtle shift of power within an existing relationship, but not a redefinition of the relationship (Döhler 1994).

More dramatic, however, were the attempts to redefine the relationship among payers, providers, and recipients by introducing "quasimarket" or "internal market" mechanisms into public-sector programs. The key theme of these reforms was to move from a managerial relationship between the payer and the provider to one of *contract*. The reorganizations of geographically based authorities in the United Kingdom, Sweden, and New Zealand by splitting their "purchasing" and "providing" functions are examples of this trend. Under reforms adopted in the United Kingdom in 1991 (which will be discussed at much greater length later in this book), geographically based Health Authorities were divested of most of their managerial functions, and they became "purchasers" of services from hospital and community care units they had previously managed; general practitioners were given the option of becoming "fundholders" to purchase a range of hospital and community services for their patients within a defined budget. Hospitals and other provider units were given the option of becoming self-governing trusts. The 1991 New Zealand reforms largely mirrored those in Britain, although they were mostly confined to the hospital sector. Geographically based health boards in New Zealand were consolidated into four Regional Health Authorities (RHAs), which became purchasers of primary and secondary care on behalf of their populations; while some 100 public hospitals were restructured into twenty-three Crown Health Enterprises to compete for RHA contracts (Flood 1996). (In 1997, a change in government resulted in plans for further consolidation, with a single central agency replacing the RHAs and new regional hospital and community services agencies to replace the Crown Health Enterprises [Ham 1997].) In Sweden in the early 1990s, while intensive consideration was being given at the national level to a variety of models, a version of "internal market" reforms, based on increased consumer choice and increased managerial autonomy for hospitals, began to be implemented by some county councils. By 1993, however, such reforms had been implemented in the hospital sector in only six of twenty-four counties, representing less than 40% of the population (Rehnberg 1995: 55), and enthusiasm for these reforms subsequently cooled (Garpenby 1995). In Italy, a more modest version of this model gave large public hospitals greater managerial autonomy from local health units (which were in turn given greater autonomy from local political bodies) (Ferrara 1995).

A second common theme, linked to these attempts to develop sophisticated purchasing entities, was the attempt to enhance competition among providers—both public and private. In the reforms in the United Kingdom, Sweden, and New Zealand, the intention was that provider units organized as "trusts" or crown enterprises would compete not only with each other but with private providers for the contracts of purchasing agencies. In Sweden, a major aspect of county-level reform was to allow individual patients to choose hospitals for service, regardless of where purchasing authorities placed their contracts.[8] The choices of patients were then to constitute "guidance" to purchasers in negotiating contracts. In addition, national legislation relating to the small primary-care sector allowed patients free choice (subject to certain user charges) among providers in public clinics and in private practice (Rehnberg 1995: 54–56).

In other nations, the focus was on increasing competition among insurers. Proposals in the Netherlands in the late 1980s and early 1990s were aimed at introducing competition among social insurance funds and private insurers within an overarching integrated fiscal and regulatory framework, although the proposals were substantially scaled back and focused essentially on the social insurance funds themselves in the face of political opposition and the difficulties of designing a "risk-adjustment" formula that would allow competition while meeting equity concerns (van de Ven et al. 1994; Schut 1995). In Germany, legislation that came into effect in 1993 provided for a phased transition toward competition among social insurance funds, with a view to allowing beneficiaries free choice among at least a substantial proportion of funds beginning in 1996. Crucial to the success of these proposals, however, was the development of a risk-adjustment formula, such as bedeviled the Dutch reforms (Hinrichs 1995). Initially, the risk-adjustment formula was based simply on the profile of subscribers based on income, age, sex, and number of dependents; experience under this system is too recent to be assessed (Pfaff 1996). In New Zealand, a provision of the 1991 reforms that would have allowed individuals to direct their (risk-adjusted) share of public funding to private insurers as opposed to their RHA was not implemented; in Italy the issue of allowing individuals to opt out, in whole or in part, of the public system in favor of private insurance was a matter of modest experimentation and hot political debate in the 1990s (Ferrara 1995).

Perhaps nowhere was the attempt to use market forces within an integrated public–private system more apparent than in the various proposals for "managed competition" that characterized the health care reform debate in the United States in the 1990s (this case will be addressed at much greater length later in this book). The proposals put forward by President Bill Clinton in 1993, as well as those advanced by a number of his opponents, were premised on the development of sophisticated "sponsors" or purchasing entities (large employers, regional health alliances, etc.) who would choose, on behalf of defined populations, among plans offered in a regulated market by competing insurers and providers. In the wake of the failure of these proposals, the employer-based market for health insurance continued to evolve in this direction.

### A new paradigm?

The common logic driving these various attempts to reorganize the relationships among payers, providers, and recipients of care has been perceptively traced out by Dov Chernichovsky (1995). He defines three "system functions"—financing, the "organization and management of care consumption" (a sophisticated purchasing function), and provision—and describes the emergence of a new "paradigm" in which two, but not all three, of these functions may be combined. This paradigm is a response to the mirror weaknesses inherent in the "old" opposing paradigms of state-driven systems on the one hand and market-driven systems on the other. Under a hierarchical state system, quintessentially represented by the British National Health Sevice (NHS) prior to 1990, all three functions were combined, and the incentives to innovation and efficiency associated with the market were allegedly lacking. Under traditional market-driven systems of medical insurance in which third-party payers played a more or less passive financing role, the three functions were completely separated, and those making the actual purchasing decisions were individuals lacking the resources to make sophisticated decisions. Simply substituting government as the third-party payer in this model did not resolve this problem.

Under the emerging paradigm, the financing and purchasing functions could be combined, as in the case of the acute care hospital sector in Canada and Germany and (under the 1990s reforms) in Britain, Sweden, and New Zealand in which state agencies negotiated "global budgets" or "contracts" with independently constituted hospitals. Another example of the combination of financing and purchasing functions in the private sector is provided by U.S. firms which self-insured to provide health care to their employees, and which entered into "preferred provider" agreements with certain providers.[9]

Alternatively, the purchasing and providing functions could be combined. The primary examples of such a combination were health maintenance organizations (HMOs) in the United States, which undertook to "manage" all the care required by an individual for a prepaid annual fee. In the public sector, such a combination was represented, at least in principle, by British general practitioner "fundholders" who provided primary care and purchased a range of hospital care on behalf of their patients. The American economist Alain Enthoven, whose thought had great impact in both Britain and the United States, has speculated on the potential analogy between American HMOs and British fundholders. Though both types of organizations combined purchasing and providing functions, British fundholders dealt with a narrower range of services than did HMOs, and generally did not compete with each other for patients, in contrast to the highly competitive HMOs in the American context (Newman 1995).

Not all contemporary developments in health care policy neatly fit Chernichovsky's emerging paradigm. But the paradigm does illuminate the thinking underlying the cross-national attractiveness of "market"-oriented policy options in the 1990s. It also draws attention to a significant and pervasive phenomenon of the 1990s: the growing importance of bargaining relationships among relatively large, sophisticated, and autonomous entities as a mode of decision-making in the health care arena. The occupants of these bargaining roles, and the rate at which these developments proceeded, varied across jurisdictions. But in general this phenomenon represented a significant transformation, if not a supplantation, of the model of decision-making that had prevailed in the past.

The emergence of these bargaining relationships represented change, to different degrees in different nations, in the structural balance and institutional mix of the health care arena. This book explores those changes (or lack thereof) in three nations in particular. Britain, the United States, and Canada provide not only three different structural and institutional models—approximating very roughly the ideal types of state hierarchy, private market, and professional collegiality—but they also evince very different histories of change in the 1990s.

## Britain, the United States, and Canada

As examples of health care decision-making systems which at the outset of the 1990s accorded a heavy weight to state actors and hierarchy, private finance and markets, and the medical profession and collegial instruments, respectively, Britain, the United States, and Canada have much to recommend them. Exploring these cases can illuminate the logic of our three ideal types and vice versa. Each of these systems, however, incorporates other elements to a substantial degree. Because none of these cases exactly fits an ideal type (nor would any other existing system), the analysis becomes richer and more complicated, if less definitive.

From its inception in the 1940s, the British NHS provided the classical model of a hierarchical, geographically organized system under the aegis of the state. In 1990, the proportion of total health care costs that was borne by the public treasury in Britain, at 83.5%, was among the highest in the OECD, exceeded only by four small states: Belgium, Iceland, Luxembourg, and Norway (OECD 1993: 252). Under the NHS, established in 1948, health care was financed and delivered through a centralized organization that controlled the great preponderance of the factors of production. Through two major reorganizations in 1974 and 1982, the essential features of this organization remained intact. Hospitals were state owned and run, and hospital-based consultant (specialist) doctors were state employees, albeit with the freedom to maintain private practices as well. General practitioners (GPs) were organized in independent practices but derived almost all their income from the state in the form of weighted capitation payments based on the number of individuals enrolled with their practices, weighted for a variety of patient and workload characteristics. Until the reforms of the 1990s there was very little potential for competition among providers. Patients enrolled with a local GP, from whom they received all primary care and who functioned as the gatekeeper to the consultant and hospital sector. Switching from one general practice to another on an episode-by-episode basis was not possible, and although in theory it was possible to switch from membership in one practice to another, such switches were rare.[10]

The British system nonetheless incorporated market elements in its small private sector. The private system (oriented primarily to certain "niche" areas of practice such as hip and knee replacements) operated in parallel to the public system—by paying private fees, individuals could avail themselves of privately provided alternatives to publicly funded services. More important, however, the NHS exhibited a strong dimension of collegiality, and provided a central role for medical professionals. As will be discussed at length later, the defining feature of the NHS was a form of "hierarchical corporatism"—a geographically defined hierarchy bringing together functional pillars of authority within structures of "consensus management" that gave physicians an effective veto at each level of the organization. Furthermore, while the budgetary parameters of the NHS were established in a hierarchical top-down manner, the clinical autonomy of physicians to determine patterns of care according to professionally determined norms was preserved, in what Rudolf Klein refers to as the "implicit bargain" between the medical profession and the state upon which the NHS was founded (Klein 1995: 75).

Britain, then, presents an illuminating case within a set of nations whose health care systems give heavy weight to state actors and hierarchical mechanisms, but which also incorporate other elements to varying degrees. The model of an integrated geographically based hierarchy for health care financing and delivery also developed in different variants in Ireland, the Scandinavian countries, and New Zealand, and through the transformation of the corporatist social insurance systems of Italy, Portugal, and Spain in the 1970s and 1980s (Elola 1996; Flood 1996; Ferrara 1995; Rodríguez 1995). Each of these national systems also accorded varying degrees of weight to other sets of actors and instruments as well: all, for example, continued to allow for various admixtures of public and private finance through copayments or parallel private sectors. The role of the medical profession and collegial institutions varies considerably across these nations. In Scandinavia, collegial elements were retained within the state system, and the effect of the growing role of the state was not so much to constrain the exercise of professional influence as it was to shift the balance of power within the medical profession itself (Erichsen 1995). In Spain, on the other hand, reforms in the 1980s that drew the system closer to the state hierarchical model reduced substantially the role of professional bodies and the influence of the medical profession (Rodríguez 1995: 156–58).

As for the second ideal type, the United States at the beginning of the 1990s provided the most extreme example in the OECD (other than Turkey) of a system heavily weighted to private finance and market mechanisms: in 1990, 58% of all health expenditures in the United States flowed through private markets, as against an OECD average of 24.5% (OECD 1993: 252). Unlike the British pattern of parallel public and private systems, moreover, in the United States the distinction between public and private financing was based essentially on population categories. The American system, in fact, comprised two contesting models for the financing of medical and hospital care. One, underlying the federal Medicare program for the elderly and disabled and the federal–state Medicaid program for the indigent, covering less than one-quarter of the population, was based on direct government subsidization of health care costs. The other model, establishing the financial conditions under which medical and hospital care was available to the remainder of the population, was based on government regulation (at both the federal and state levels) of the private insurance market (as well as indirect subsidization through the tax deductibility of employers' expenses for employee health benefits). The organization of health care delivery, moreover, was decentralized among myriad privately constituted and autonomous entities.

In each of these segments of the bifurcated U.S. system, the state clearly played an important though different role, both fiscal and regulatory. Furthermore, the prevailing market model in theory (and for most of its history in practice) allowed physicians both entrepreneurial discretion and clinical autonomy. For much of the twentieth century the overall pattern of the production of health care services was little more than the aggregate of decisions made by autonomous physicians in their local hospitals and practices, although both small-scale private practice and systems of collegial decision-making were threatened by the rise of large private hierarchical organizations in the 1970s and 1980s (Starr 1982; Salmon 1994). In addition, the heavy reliance on market mechanisms meant that attempts to control medical behavior increasingly took the form of explicit contractual arrangements.

If the United States was almost *sui generis* in the role it allowed for private finance and for market competition, it nonetheless constitutes an important case—and not only as a close approximation of an ideal type. Its sheer size commands attention: in 1994, total health expenditures in the United States roughly equaled the combined total for all twenty-six other nations in the OECD. Moreover, as we shall see, the United States provided the crucible for many of the ideas about the role of market forces in health care that have greatly influenced the policy agenda of the 1990s.

Finally, we need an example of a system that gave predominant weight to medical professionals and to collegial mechanisms. Here a quintessential example is not as apparent as in the cases of our other two types. Indeed, two important themes have emerged in this regard in the political science of health care: the persistence of medical power under a variety of modes of finance and delivery through the 1980s, and the threatened or actual decline in that power in the 1990s (Björkman 1985; Moran 1994). The decline of medical power in the United States, together with the rise of large corporate concentrations of private finance on both the supply and the demand sides of the market, was, as previously noted, given increasing attention by American scholars in the 1980s and 1990s. Indeed, contrasts between the U.S. system and other systems in which the state played a much larger role led several scholars to hypothesize that the clinical autonomy and the overall policy influence of the medical profession was better protected through accommodation with the state than in the fray of the market (Döhler 1989; Tuohy 1994b; Morone and Goggin 1995). In the 1990s, however, the incremental assertion of state power vis-à-vis the profession in state-sponsored systems was increasingly noted (Moran 1994; Wilsford 1995; Johnson 1995). Commenting on these observations, Donald Light has made the important point that these trends need to be understood in the context of the "historical dynamics" between the medical profession and other actors within the health care arena. He proposes that these relationships be conceptualized as occurring within a field of forces that is in a state of ongoing change. Such a framework

> focuses attention on the *interactions* of powerful actors in a field where they are inherently interdependent yet distinct. If one party is dominant, as the American medical profession has long been, its dominance is contextual and eventually elicits countermoves by other powerful actors, not to destroy it but to redress an imbalance of power. . . . In those states where the government has played a central role in nurturing professions within the state structure but has allowed the professions to establish their own institutions and power base, the professions and the state go through phases of harmony and discord in which countervailing actions take place. In states where the medical profession has been largely suppressed, we now see their rapid reconstitution once governmental oppression is lifted. (Light 1995: 26–27)

Light also highlights the importance of understanding alliances among parties in a field of countervailing powers, noting that these alliances, such as that between the medical profession and private corporations in the United States, are often characterized by "structural ambiguities" and ambivalence, given the conflicting as well as common interests of the parties (Light 1995: 27).

All this said, there are certain national systems that accord the medical profession and its collegial processes particularly strong positions. The social insurance systems of continental Europe present a likely set of possibilities, given the extent to which they incorporate formal roles for medical associations into the systems of finance and management as buffers between the state or sickness funds on the one hand and individual practicing physicians on the other (OECD 1992: chaps. 3, 5, 7; Wilsford 1995: 579–85; Schepers 1995). Germany in particular has received considerable attention in this regard, as the European system in which the medical profession is most cohesively organized and its channels of influence most institutionalized (Stone 1977; Döhler 1991; Wilsford 1995: 580–81).

For our purposes, however, Canada offers a more appropriate case. (Among other things, there are advantages, to be discussed shortly, to confining the comparison to Anglo-American countries.) Canadian medicare, as we shall see, rested from its inception in the 1960s on a fundamental accommodation between the medical profession and the state, under which physicians retained their status as independent professionals, trading off a degree of entrepreneurial discretion (particularly over price but not, as in Britain, over location and practice inputs) in order to retain substantial collective and individual autonomy in clinical matters (Tuohy 1976). Within broad budgetary parameters established by provincial governments, physicians have been central to decision-making systems at various levels from central joint profession–government "management" committees at the provincial level, to the level of autonomously constituted hospital medical staffs, to the level of independent individual medical practices.

Professionally dominated collegial mechanisms, that is, not only survived the introduction of state-sponsored health insurance, but they were also reinforced and supplemented by other mechanisms. Canadian medicare essentially froze in place the health care delivery system that existed in the 1960s, in which, as at that time in the United States, the distribution of health care was determined by the decisions of independent medical practitioners subject to the norms of the professional group. The federal legislation establishing the medicare program set very broad parameters, requiring that provincial programs, in order to qualify for federal financial contributions, conform to five principles—universality, comprehensiveness, accessibility, portability, and public administration. The resulting provincial programs centralized the financing of medical and hospital services in the provincial governments (with federal contributions), while leaving the decentralized delivery system in place. The distribution of physicians was governed by the decisions of individual practitioners as to where to locate their practices, subject only to the authority of independently constituted hospital medical staffs to grant hospital privileges. Medical fees were negotiated between provincial governments and provincial medical associations, but in most provinces the negotiations pertained only to across-the-board measures, leaving the fee schedule itself (the value of fees for particular services, and hence the economic incentives to provide particular services) to be determined by the medical associations themselves. When provincial governments moved to institute various limited mechanisms of utilization review of the volume and mix of services provided by individual practitioners, they located these mechanisms (with one exception) in the professional governing body or voluntary association (Tuohy 1992: 123–27). Only in the case of capital expenditures by hospitals (including the acquisition of new technology) did provincial governments play a strong role in case-by-case decision-making; otherwise the state role was essentially confined to establishing overall budgetary limits through the negotiation of rates of increase in the medical fee schedule and historically based hospital global budgets.

If physicians exercised substantial influence through collegial mechanisms, they also retained considerable entrepreneurial discretion through the market mechanisms that remained key elements of the Canadian medicare system. Indeed, from its inception Canadian medicare was characterized by a type of "internal market" and "purchaser–provider split." Hospital and medical providers were organized autonomously from the provincial government "purchaser," and consumers had free choice of provider, at least at the level of primary care. (Specialists were typically seen on referral from a GP.) The power of provincial governments was essentially that of the monopsonist. Almost the last vestige of the individual physician's discretion over the price of service disappeared in 1984, with the passage of federal legislation providing for fiscal penalties to any province allowing "extra billing" (billing beyond the amount covered by the government plan) for medical and hospital services. But physicians continued to have broad discretion over the location of their practices, the inputs to their practices, and the volume and mix of services they delivered.

In addition to this "internal market," more than one-quarter of Canadian health care was provided through private markets. The balance between public and private finance in Canada in 1990 (approximately 72% public and 28% private) was close to the OECD mean (OECD 1993: 252)—a larger private share than in the British case, but a substantially smaller private share than in the United States. But the area open to private finance was defined quite differently in Canada than in either the United States or the United Kingdom. As opposed to the parallel private market of the United Kingdom or the population-based public–private distinction in the United States, public and private expenditures in Canada were confined to different segments of the health care delivery system. Certain segments—notably medical and hospital services—were almost entirely publicly funded; others, such as dental care, drugs, and eyeglasses and other prostheses, were in the private sector.[11] In most provinces, private insurers were foreclosed from insuring medical and hospital services covered by the government plan, and they were effectively confined to the remaining segments of the health care system.

Britain, the United States, and Canada, then, represent the broad range of systems suggested by the ideal-typical categories of state hierarchical, private market, and professional collegial systems. But they also share important characteristics that can frame a comparative analysis. In the first place, they share a broadly similar tradition of state–society relations which, among other things, implies an autonomous base for professions vis-à-vis the state, in contrast to the more "statist" or "state-corporatist" model of continental Europe (Rueschemeyer 1986; Stone 1977: 38–39). They also share a roughly similar structure for the organization of capital, with a distinction between "real" and "financial" capital and a heavy reliance on equity markets, again in contrast to a more integrated continental European model (Zysman 1983; Hall 1986: 229–83). Hence for the three major categories of actors in the health care arena—the state, the professions, and private finance—Britain, Canada, and the United States share a roughly similar cultural and structural context when viewed in broad cross-national perspective. This selection of cases, then, while it misses some interesting questions,[12] allows us to focus on shifts in the balance of influence across the state, the medical profession, and private finance within relatively similar systems.

The distinctive characteristics of the health care arenas of Britain, the United States, and Canada reflect the timing of the major policy episodes that established their fundamental institutional and structural parameters. The British NHS was a product of its genesis in the 1940s, after the centralization and expansion of government authority in the wartime period. Canadian medicare bears the marks of its birth in the 1960s, an era of high public expectations and government expansiveness, in which the indemnity model of private insurance had become established and the public underwriting of the costs of a professionally dominated system appeared feasible. The U.S. Medicare and Medicaid systems were born in the same period, and were fashioned on a similar model. But as we shall see they were introduced in a national context in which the legacy of past policy failures conditioned policy-makers to adopt an incremental approach that ironically sowed the seeds of future policy failures.

If Britain, the United States, and Canada present a range of possible admixtures of hierarchy, collegiality, and market and possible balances across state, professional, and private financial actors in the health care arena, they also present different histories of change in the late twentieth century. Each has responded in different ways to the evolving logic of health care economics, with its implications for the development of bargaining relationships between relatively large, sophisticated, and autonomous entities. Britain presents the most sweeping policy change in the OECD, brought about in the 1990s: the National Health Service and Community Care Act of 1990 sought a radical transformation of the NHS hierarchy through the creation of an "internal market" made up of organizationally distinct "purchasers" and "providers" within the tax-financed system. The United States, in contrast, presents perhaps the most spectacular example of the failure of an attempt at sweeping policy change—the defeat of President Clinton's proposal for health care reform through "managed competition" in 1993. Yet it nonetheless stands as the most dramatic example of structural and institutional change. In the absence of major policy change, it is arguably the case that the institutional mix of hierarchical, collegial, and market instruments, as well as the balance of influence across the state, the medical profession, and private finance, have both shifted more dramatically in the United States in the late twentieth century than in any other OECD nation. The rise of large corporate entities on both the supply and the demand sides of the market has transformed the decision-making systems of the health care arena. And Canada presents a case in which policy development has generally yielded only incremental alterations in the basic institutional mix or structural balance of the health care arena. The state has undergone internal reorganization through the creation of regionalized structures in most provinces and has sought to assert its role more strongly through the extension of traditional blunt instruments (such as budget caps) and targeted intervention into the hospital sector to achieve some horizontal integration. But the basic structure of Canada's "internal market," the balance between public and private finance, and, most significantly, the influence of the medical profession and the importance of collegial mechanisms of decision-making remain essentially unchanged. Whether this relative stability can persist in the face of the unprecedented fiscal constraint of the 1990s, however, is a key question to be addressed.

Each of these observations, on its face, opens up a puzzle. First, why was it in Britain that the most radical policy change regarding the institutional mix and structural balance occurred in the 1990s? In cross-national perspective, the NHS in the 1980s appeared remarkably successful in providing universal access to comprehensive health care while restraining its rising costs—a policy goal to which most reform efforts were addressed. Yet it was in Britain, and not in nations in which health care was consuming a larger and rising share of GDP, in which ambitious policy initiatives yielded the most substantial results.

The second puzzle is presented by the United States. In the most expensive health care system in the OECD, yielding the least comprehensive coverage of its population, major public policy change failed in the 1990s. But dramatic structural and institutional change occurred nonetheless. What was it about the U.S. system that made for this degree of change without major change in public policy?

Finally, there is a Canadian puzzle. Canada had, after all, one of the most expensive publicly funded health care systems in the world. Yet it experienced one of the lowest levels of institutional and structural change in the 1980s and 1990s. What made for this relative stability in the face of strong fiscal pressures?

The framework sketched in this chapter begins to provide the tools for unraveling these puzzles. That framework draws attention to national differences—in the timing of key episodes of policy reform and in the resultant logic of each health care system. The following chapters develop this argument in detail. Part I demonstrates how factors in the broader political system of each nation opened (or failed to open) windows of opportunity for change over time, and how the timing of policy reform established the distinctive structural and institutional parameters of the three systems. Chapter 2 deals with establishment of the modern welfare state in the health care arena in Britain in the 1940s, and in Canada and the United States in the 1960s. Chapter 3 contrasts the experience of these three nations with policy change in the 1990s—the institution of internal market in Britain, the failure of the Clinton health care reform initiative in the United States, and the relative policy stability of Canada. Chapter 4 tests the "windows of opportunity" argument presented in the preceding two chapters against other ways of understanding these policy developments.

Part II traces out the logics of the resultant systems and the implications for their evolution in the 1990s. Chapter 5 analyzes the logic of the mixed market system of the United States to explain the turbulence of the health care arena of the 1990s and the shifting political terrain that greatly complicated any attempts at health care policy reform. Chapter 6 analyzes the response of the system of hierarchical corporatism in Britain's NHS to the internal market reforms imposed by the Thatcher government and explains how the impact of the reforms was moderated in practice by the operation of an established logic. Chapter 7 analyzes the relative stability of Canada's single-payer system, in which the logic of an accommodation between the medical profession and the state dissipated pressures for change through relatively generous and essentially open-ended funding, until the imposition of budgetary caps threatened the basis of that accommodation. The final chapter summarizes the argument of the book and extends it to offer some concluding observations about the role of information technology and the contrasting effects of public and private finance, and to draw some implications for policy-makers, in the health care arena of the late 1990s.

# Episodes of
# Policy Change

1

# The Establishment
## of the Welfare State in
## the Health Care Arena | 2

In the comparative history of health policy in the three nations with which this book is concerned, the 1940s, 1960s, and 1990s were critical epochs. In each of these periods, extraordinary episodes of policy change occurred in the health care arena of at least one of these nations—episodes in which the structural balance among interests and the institutional mix of instruments were altered in significant ways. In the 1940s in Britain and the 1960s in Canada and the United States, the essential features of the welfare state in the health care arena were put in place. In the 1990s attempts were made (successfully in Britain and unsuccessfully in the United States) to make major changes in the public policies governing these arrangements. A comparison of the experience of these nations in each of these periods can shed light on the conditions under which windows of opportunity for policy change in health care open. It can also demonstrate the importance of the timing of the opening of these windows in determining the types of changes that occur as a result.

This chapter deals with the events of the "founding" periods of the 1940s through the 1960s. Chapter 3 turns to the "reformist" period of the 1990s. And chapter 4 views these events through a variety of explanatory lenses to test the persuasiveness of the argument focused on windows of opportunity.

## The Immediate Postwar Period:
## Britain versus Canada and the United States

### Britain

In July 1945 the Labour Party won a decisive victory in the British general election, capturing 61.6% of the seats in the House of Commons. It was, as Lawrence Jacobs has put it, that "rarest of political events, a landslide upset" (Jacobs 1993: 168). It had not been widely anticipated, given the fact that the opposing Conservatives were led by the "War Hero," Winston Churchill. But the Labour victory revealed the extent of public unease with the perceived inertia of the Conservatives in matters of domestic policy (Jacobs 1993: 169–70; Timmins 1995: 61–62). And it opened a window of opportunity for major policy change. The Labour government had the consolidated authority afforded a majority government in a unitary Westminster system. Equally important, it had the political will to enact a broad program of bold changes in social policy after a period of wartime Coalition government marked by ongoing attempts to craft compromise positions between Labour and Conservative partners and among affected interests.

This window of opportunity opened at a time of remarkable consensus on social policy objectives. There was a growing sense of the need for change in the existing patchwork system. Local authorities had jurisdiction over public health services, as well as that segment of the hospital sector descended from the nineteenth-century workhouses. Voluntary hospitals, dominated by specialist physicians ("consultants"), constituted the elite and selective segment of the hospital sector. General practitioners functioned in independent practice, remunerated largely through capitation payments under the system of National Health Insurance, which was established in 1911 to provide medical care for workers and was overseen by local medical committees. Wartime experience had nonetheless demonstrated the potential for integrating these various pieces into a more coherent system.

There was general agreement, shared by state actors and health care providers, on the need for a state-sponsored plan that would provide a comprehensive range of health services free at the point of service (Klein 1995: 1–2, 24). There was even agreement that the hospital sector, ill-coordinated and in many cases financially nonviable, needed to be "rationalized" on a regional basis (Klein 1995: 3–4, Allsop 1995: 25, Ham 1992: 13–14; Fox 1986). More generally, the wartime ideological climate was a propitious one for social policy change, as epitomized in the favorable public reception that greeted the landmark Beveridge Report in 1942. Public opinion polls revealed strong support for Beveridge's broad objectives, including the establishment of a national health service, although opinion was more divided on the specifics of any given proposal (Jacobs 1993: 113).

Despite broad agreement on objectives, the wartime Coalition government was unable to translate that agreement into specific policies. Divisions between the Conservative and Labour partners frustrated action, and the government instead "agreed to plan but not legislate" (Jacobs 1993: 117) and to defer action until a postwar government was in place. A White Paper issued by the Coalition government in 1944 attempted to set out compromise positions which, according to Klein, "left most of the actors involved feeling dissatisfied (Klein 1995: 13). The White Paper offered the medical profession an institutionalized advisory role, but not on the terms the profession had sought. Professionally based local committees for the control of general practice were to be abolished, but in an uneasy compromise the White Paper proposed replacing that function with a Central Medical Board and not forcing general practice under the control of local authorities. Local authorities were to provide "health centers" in which general practitioners would be encouraged to practice (a model earlier recommended by the British Medical Association), but which would not employ GPs. The White Paper temporized on the hotly contested issue of whether GPs were to be remunerated by salary or capitation. Local authorities were to retain their hospital management functions but were to exercise these responsibilities through regional "joint authorities."

Differences between Conservative and Labour partners were reflected in the alacrity with which the White Paper proposals were revised by the Conservative government when Labour withdrew from the Coalition government in 1945 (Klein 1995: 14–15). Had the Conservatives won the 1945 election as expected, it is they who would have had the consolidated authority necessary to enact their version of the basic consensus regarding the need for a free and comprehensive service. The Labour landslide gave this opportunity to a Labour government instead.

The sweeping nature of the Labour majority, moreover, emboldened the government to pursue an activist agenda of social policy change. Notwithstanding the fact that the 62% majority of seats had been achieved with less than a majority (47.8%) of the popular vote, the Labour government interpreted the result as providing it with a broad mandate for change. Consolidation of authority, then, was matched by firmness of political will: a bold National Health Service (NHS) bill was integral to the political program of the Labour government (Jacobs 1993: 171–72, 177). The development of policy hence shifted from the domain of civil servants and interest groups into the domain of Cabinet government, and particularly into the purview of the Labour minister of health, Aneurin Bevan (Klein 1995: 15–27, 24). The government was hardly ignorant of the need to reach accommodations with key interests, particularly local authorities and the medical profession. Indeed, as chronicled by many observers of the period, in many respects the Labour proposals represented permutations and combinations of what had gone before. But in one key area the Labour government broke dramatic new ground—it nationalized the hospital sector and established a regional hierarchy for the management of hospitals as one of three pillars of the health care delivery system.

Establishing the hospital pillar of the NHS flew against the interests of the local authorities and occasioned much debate within the Labour Cabinet before this strategy prevailed. But it suited the powerful hospital-based medical consultants. It allowed for a rationalization of inadequate hospital facilities and ensured that the hospital sector would be controlled not by local authorities but through a nationalized structure of Regional Hospital Boards and local Hospital Management Committees on which consultants themselves would be key participants. As part of its accommodation with the consultants, moreover, Labour agreed to a system of "distinction awards" for consultants—remuneration over and above basic salaries, to be distributed on the basis of peer judgment. In addition, and most controversial within the government, consultants were allowed to maintain private practices, a decision which also entailed allowing some beds in NHS hospitals—so-called "pay-beds"—to be available for private patients.

This accommodation with the consultants effectively split the medical profession. General practitioners, represented primarily by the British Medical Association (BMA) (as opposed to the consultants who were represented mainly by the Royal Colleges) continued to resist the Labour program for the NHS well after the passage of the National Health Service Act in 1946, until just before the legislation went into effect in 1948. As Klein (1995) points out, the extent of opposition by general practitioners was somewhat paradoxical, given the degree to which, as regards general practice, the Labour proposals mirrored the negotiated compromises that had emerged under the Coalition government (20). In fact, the fierce opposition of general practitioners and the BMA demonstrated just how fragile the compromises of the Coalition government had been. The Conservatives had backed away from key elements of those compromises as soon as Labour left the coalition: the Conservative proposals had dropped the Central Medical Board envisaged in the Coalition's White Paper, which would determine the geographic distribution of general practitioners; they had reinstated local professionally dominated committees for the supervision of general practice; they had reduced local authority-administered health centers to the status of pilot projects; and they had provided that general practitioners, in health centers and in independent practice, were to be remunerated on the basis of capitation, not salary. The Labour proposals reinstated most of the White Paper "compromises" and went one step further by banning the sale and purchase of practices. Only when Bevan made it clear that capitation was to be the primary mode of remuneration for GPs were general practitioners sufficiently mollified to allow the NHS to come into being without a GP boycott.

The structure put in place by the postwar Labour government, then, was a tripartite one. Hospitals were organized in a regional hierarchy reporting to the minister of health: Regional Hospital Boards, appointed by the minister, in turn appointed local Hospital Management Committees, and budgets flowed from top to bottom down this hierarchy. General practitioners (along with other "primary care" providers such as dentists and pharmacists) retained their independent status as "contractors," whose contracts were administered by local "Executive Committees" comprising members appointed by local professional bodies, local authorities, and the minister of health. Finally, the public health function (including functions such as maternal and child welfare clinics, health education, vaccination and immunization, and ambulances) remained under the control of local authorities (Ham 1992: 15–16). These changes built upon elements of earlier arrangements, particularly the role of local authorities in public health and the status of general practitioners, but opted for the consultant-dominated voluntary hospitals as the center of gravity for the newly nationalized hospital sector.

The National Health Service Act established the structural and institutional parameters of the British health care delivery system that were to endure for the next four and a half decades. It was a system that gave heavy weight to state authority and hierarchical mechanisms in budgetary matters, but left much discretion in clinical matters to individual medical professionals operating through collegial decision-making networks. In these respects, it was a state-sponsored system of "hierarchical corporatism." Private finance and market mechanisms played a marginal role.

The process of establishing the NHS demonstrates the importance of the timing of windows of opportunity for policy change. A broad consensus, among policy-makers and in public opinion, regarding the need for substantial change in the health care arena was not sufficient to bring about policy change until the political authority and will to make specific policy change could be mobilized. During the Coalition government, the broad consensus provided only the ground for unsatisfactory compromises on detailed features. Only with the postwar Labour victory was a political leadership in place that had both concentrated authority and the determination to make specific policy changes as consistent with its interpretation of its popular mandate. Labour's broad agenda of bold change in social policy shaped the choices it made in health care, which, while consistent with the evolving climate of policy ideas in the health care arena, also broke new ground with the nationalization of the hospitals.

### Canada

Wartime and immediate postwar developments in Britain were closely watched in Canada, where a consensus on the need for a universal system of coverage for health care was also growing. In Canada, however, governmental action entailed an additional layer of constraint. Constitutionally, power to make health policy lay formally with the provincial governments. The federal government could influence health policy only through the exercise of its "spending power": that is, only by making transfer payments to provincial governments (or, for that matter, to institutions or individuals) and by attaching conditions to those transfers.[1] In practice, those conditions would be matters of federal–provincial negotiation. A national health insurance policy, then, would inevitably require a coalition of support not only within but between levels of government.

As in the British case, the issue of national health insurance was the subject of a number of policy inquiries throughout the 1930s. Several provinces established commissions of inquiry, and the government of British Columbia went so far as to introduce legislation in 1936 that would have established a program of governmental health insurance for all those with incomes below a specified level. The British Columbia legislation was ultimately stillborn—indefinitely postponed in the face of opposition from organized medicine regarding the level and mode of remuneration of physicians under the plan (Naylor 1986: 58–94). During the 1930s, however, a climate of ideas broadly sympathetic to governmental health insurance had developed. Most notably, in 1934 the Committee on Economics of the Canadian Medical Association (CMA) issued a policy statement supportive of government health insurance as necessary and perhaps "inevitable," and setting out nineteen principles which, in the view of the CMA, should guide the development of a government program (Taylor 1979: 23–25).

The role of the CMA deserves some introductory comment here. In Canada, as in other federal systems, federalism is a feature not only of governmental structures but of interest organizations. The CMA strengthened its position as the federated voice of provincial medical associations throughout the 1930s. By the early 1940s, despite periodic tensions with provincial medical associations, it had established itself as the representative body for Canadian medicine at the federal level and played a key role in the development of policy proposals in the wartime and immediate postwar environment. And unlike the British case, the CMA could claim to speak for specialists as well as general practitioners. The organizational division between GPs and specialists that characterized British medical politics never materialized in Canada. The Royal College of Physicians and Surgeons, established in 1929, was concerned almost exclusively with standardizing specialty requirements and very little with political representation (Naylor 1986: 27–31, 95–97).

In the early 1940s, under the wartime federal Liberal government, a series of official committees was struck to consider policy options in health care. In 1942, an Interdepartmental Advisory Committee on Health Insurance (the Heagerty committee), chaired by a senior official in the Department of Pensions and Health, was established. The committee conducted its work in a climate much influenced by the release of the Beveridge report in Britain soon after the committee was formed. Indeed, one of the members of the Heagerty committee, Leonard Marsh, had worked with Beveridge as a graduate student and was commissioned to undertake a parallel review of social security (Taylor 1979: 17). The Heagerty committee worked closely with professional associations in the health care arena, especially with the Canadian Medical Association.

The report of the Heagerty committee, issued in December 1942, recommended a program of compulsory governmental health insurance to be administered by the provincial governments. The federal government would participate in the financing of the program through conditional "grants-in-aid." The committee's report included two draft bills, one for the federal government and one a "model" bill for provincial legislatures. The design of the draft legislation revealed how similar discussions in Canada and Britain were at the time: it contemplated a national commission (on which physicians would have a majority) to oversee the plan, a physician as the chief administrative officer of each provincial plan, and administrative health regions within each province. Issues—

such as the imposition of an income limit above which individuals would not be eligible for coverage under the public plan, and the balance of modes of medical remuneration as between salary, capitation, and fee-for-service—which were matters of dispute within the profession and between the profession and government in Britain, were equally so in Canada. In a classic federal strategy, the draft legislation left these matters to be resolved through negotiations at the provincial level.

The Heagerty committee report occasioned considerable debate within the federal Cabinet and was referred to a committee chaired by the deputy minister of finance, which expressed great concern about its financial implications. It was then referred to a Special Committee on Social Security of the House of Commons. The Special Committee's hearings and discussions revealed, as in Britain, broad support for the principle of compulsory health insurance (not only from health care providers and labor groups but even from the private insurance industry) but ongoing dispute about issues of income limits for eligibility and modes of medical remuneration. It is worth noting, however, that there was considerable support within the medical profession for capitation payments for GPs and for the removal of an income ceiling for eligibility— hence the CMA by 1944 was advocating that such matters be determined at the provincial level (Naylor 1986: 103, 128).

British influences on the activities surrounding the Special Committee were substantial. Beveridge himself addressed the committee, an address that was less notable for its technical advice than for the inspiration that it provided (Taylor 1979: 34). The CMA paid close attention to British developments. Its position on medical administration of the plan derived in part from observation of the British debate; and it included an endorsement of the concept of "health centers" on the model proposed in Britain. The CMA, moreover, was much influenced by advice from Canadian doctors on active military service abroad; through the Royal Canadian Army Medical Corps, these doctors took a position strongly supportive of compulsory health insurance for the entire population, and cognizant of the need for negotiation of issues of medical remuneration. This advice contributed to a softening of the CMA's stand on the issues of income limits and modes of medical remuneration in 1943 and 1944 (Naylor 1986: 127–29).

The report of the Special Committee, which generally endorsed the proposals of the Heagerty committee before it, returned to the maw of the federal Cabinet, where it again occasioned questions as to its financial feasibility. The Cabinet decision was to present a proposal for compulsory health insurance as part of a broad package of program and fiscal proposals for postwar reconstruction to a Dominion–Provincial Conference on Reconstruction, bringing together the heads of the federal and provincial governments in 1945.

Before the conference was convened, a federal election was held in 1944, with results quite different from the postwar Labour landslide in Britain. The federal Liberals, indeed, had feared such a leftward shift in Canada: the social–democratic Cooperative Commonwealth Federation (CCF) party had had recent successes in provincial elections and was threatening a strong showing federally (Maioni 1995: 13–14). In the result, the CCF gains (from 8 to 28 seats) were not as strong as expected. The Liberals were returned to power, but with a bare majority (125 of the 245 seats in the House of Commons, down from their previous total of 178). The Liberals could hence not claim the broad popular mandate for bold policy change assumed by the Labour party in Britain; although each of the parties competing in the 1944 federal election made expanding health care coverage a plank in its platform, there was considerable divergence on the issues relating to the design of the program (Taylor 1979: 44–48).

Even if the Liberals had claimed such a mandate, moreover, they would still have had to face the hurdles presented by Canadian federalism. The provincial ministers of health had endorsed governmental health insurance in principle at a meeting in May 1944, while insisting upon considerable provincial discretion in the design, phasing, and financing of the program. But at the Dominion–Provincial Conference on Reconstruction that convened for five days in August of 1945, the arena was expanded to include provincial delegations headed by the premiers, and the proposals for health insurance were part of a complex package of proposed social programs and federal–provincial financial arrangements. The provinces entered the negotiations in a mood highly skeptical of federal intentions, in the wake of what was perceived at least by some as federal aggrandizement during the war years. Over the next eight months, a flurry of proposals and counterproposals was exchanged by the federal government and the various provincial governments through a network of committees under the aegis of a Continuing Committee of First Ministers. In April 1946, the full conference was reconvened for five days but ended without reaching agreement. In the inauspicious climate of federal–provincial relations that prevailed in the immediate postwar period, it had proved impossible to mobilize the authority to adopt a federal–provincial health insurance plan, despite what would prove to have been a high-water mark of consensus among key actors in the health care arena itself.

To summarize, then, in the Canadian health care arena in the mid-1940s, the ground was prepared for compromise in the development of a national compulsory health insurance program in a way that paralleled developments in Britain. If a window of opportunity for policy change had opened in Canada in the 1940s, the resulting scheme would undoubtedly have borne a closer resemblance to the NHS (though undoubtedly without the Labour-inspired nationalization of hospitals) than did the Canadian plan that developed twenty years later. But no such window opened in wartime or the immediate postwar period, given the state of federal–provincial relations. The failure of its proposals for governmental health insurance did not, however, entirely forestall action by the federal government. In 1948, the federal government unilaterally (but after consultation with the medical profession) adopted a program of grants to the provinces in support of hospital construction, certain public health measures, and surveys of the health status and health care needs of the population. As was the case in the United States at the same time, the grant program was seen by its progenitors in the federal government as an incremental step toward national health insurance after what they hoped would prove to be a temporary setback in 1945–1946 (Naylor 1986: 164).

### The United States

As in Canada, proposals for national health insurance failed in the United States in the immediate postwar period and yielded to incremental steps in the form of hospital construction grants from the federal government. But beyond these broad-brush similarities, experience in the two nations had little in common. No broad consensus within the health care arena in support of governmental health insurance developed in the United States, nor was the British experience leading up to the establishment of the NHS nearly so influential in the U.S. policy debate as it was in Canada. Nor, importantly, did state-level experimentation spring up in the wake of federal failure in the United States as was the case with Canadian provincial governments. The reasons for these dissimilarities bear some exploration.

The Beveridge proposals did not go without notice in the United States. In fact, a bill tagged "the American answer to Beveridge" was introduced in the U.S. Congress in 1943. Sponsored by Democratic senators Wagner and Murray in the Senate and Democratic Representative Dingell in the House, the bill would have reorganized social insurance and added a national medical and hospital insurance plan. The Democratic administration of President Franklin Roosevelt did not endorse the bill, however, and it died without reaching the hearing stage (Maioni 1995: 17). When President Harry Truman assumed office upon the death of Roosevelt in 1945, he brought a greater sympathy to the issue of national health insurance, in part through a desire to put his own stamp on the social policy legacy of Roosevelt (Maioni 1995: 18). Another Wagner–Murray–Dingell bill, this one with Truman's endorsement, was introduced, focusing on health insurance alone. Unlike proposals discussed in Britain and Canada, the Truman proposals embodied no change in the organization of health care delivery nor in the mode of remuneration of physicians; the Truman plan essentially involved an underwriting of the existing delivery system.

Nonetheless, the Truman plan occasioned the fierce and vehement opposition of American organized medicine. In part, this may be attributed to the process through which the proposals were developed. In contrast to the Canadian and British cases, where organized medicine was closely consulted by officials developing health insurance proposals, in the United States officials consulted predominantly with organized labor (Maioni 1995: 18–20). More fundamentally, however, the ideological complexion of the American profession, at least as represented by the American Medical Association (AMA), was markedly different from its Canadian and British counterparts. The British and Canadian professions were characterized by a strong streak of what has been characterized in the Canadian case as "red toryism." As I have described it elsewhere (following Horowitz 1966), red toryism is "an ideology that emphasizes the social responsibilities and obligations of those who hold privileged positions in society, as part of the justification of those privileges; and it encourages a collaboration between the leadership of corporate groups and the state in the pursuit of redistributive policies" (Tuohy 1992: 13). In the case of the Canadian medical profession, this ideology was held by a strategically located group of opinion- and decision-makers within the profession who were willing to accept constraints on the economic power and entrepreneurial discretion of individual physicians in order to retain collegial control of medical practice (Tuohy 1992: 118–19). In the mid-1940s, this view was in the ascendancy within the Canadian Medical Association and in provincial bodies such as the College of Physicians and Surgeons of Ontario. The absence of such a body of opinion- and decision-makers in the U.S. profession was to have far-reaching consequences.

Even in the face of vehement opposition from organized medicine, the Truman proposals might have prevailed as part of a broad agenda of social policy change, as events of the 1960s in both the United States and Canada were later to demonstrate. But the Truman administration could not mobilize sufficient authority or command a broad policy agenda. As in Canada, no window of opportunity for policy change opened. In the United States, however, the failure to consolidate authority occurred not in the arena of relations between federal and state governments but within the federal government itself. Truman could not command the support of conservative Democrats in Congress even before the congressional elections of 1946 which gave control of Congress to the Republicans. There was no bipartisan consensus around which a compromise might have been built in the period in which the White House and Congress were under different partisan control from 1946 to 1948. When the Democrats regained control of both houses of Congress as well as the Presidency in 1948, a window of opportunity might have opened, especially given that national health insurance had been a centerpiece of Truman's presidential campaign. But Truman could not claim a broad popular mandate: he had been elected with just less than a majority (49.8%) of the popular vote in the multiparty presidential election of 1948. Despite attempts to gain support for the administration's national health insurance proposals in each year of Truman's second term, the Democrats still remained divided. Their inability to coalesce around a common coherent proposal was in large part due to the opposition of southern conservative Democrats. It can only be fully understood, however, by appealing to the symbolic dimensions of national health insurance in the United States at the time. In the vehemently anticommunist climate of the day, a broad agenda of social policy change could not be mounted, and national health insurance proposals themselves could not escape the dooming epithet of "socialized medicine" (Starr 1982: 286–89; Skocpol 1993: 538; Maioni 1995: 23–24).

In the wake of these failures, advocates of national health insurance at the national level turned, as in Canada, to what they saw as an incrementalist strategy: an attempt to build coalitions around a number of specific pieces of legislation. Notably, the Hill–Burton Act of 1946, providing for federal subsidization of hospital construction, was the product of a coalition ranging from those who believed that subsidization with relatively few conditions was close to the limit of appropriate federal involvement in the hospital sector to those who saw this support as merely one step toward a comprehensive national health insurance plan (Fox 1986: 124–31). The striking similarity of this strategy to the program of hospital construction grants adopted at the federal level in Canada at the same time was no accident, but was rather another instance of cross-border policy learning and sharing. Participants in the development and implementation of the respective programs consulted with each other and closely observed each other's experience (Agnew 1974: 168). In both countries, advocates of universal national health insurance saw the federal grant program as a step toward that goal. As discussed in the next section, in Canada that expectation was borne out; in the United States it was not.

## The 1950s and 1960s: The Establishment of Governmental Health Insurance in Canada and the United States

In the absence of national health insurance, the American and Canadian systems continued to evolve in the 1950s and 1960s. In a number of respects, that evolution was very similar in both nations. In general, medical services continued to be provided by physicians in private fee-for-service practices; hospital services by nonprofit institutions owned by voluntary societies, religious orders, municipalities, and universities; and extended care in facilities owned by such nonprofit groups or by private independent for-profit operators. The impact of the federal hospital grants programs on the hospital sector, moreover, was similar in the two countries. In each, the for-profit hospital sector, always small, declined further in significance. Between 1948 and 1953, the number of private hospitals in Canada declined by 32%, while the number of public general and special hospitals (including those operated by provincial and municipal authorities and by lay voluntary and religious organizations, but excluding federal hospitals, mental hospitals, and tuberculosis sanatoria) increased by 18% (calculated from Department of National Health and Welfare 1955: 14). In the United States, the comparable changes between 1946 and 1955 were a 5% decline in the number of private hospitals and a 25% increase in the number of public hospitals (as previously defined) (calculated from American Hospital Association 1995: Table 1). In the mid-1950s, more than 80% of all community hospitals, accounting for more than 90% of community hospital beds, were owned by not-for-profit organizations or public authorities, as shown in table 2.1.

The Canadian and American health care delivery systems (and the associated structure of interests) in this period, then, were probably as similar as any two national systems on the globe. Furthermore, the growth and the pattern of private insurance was similar as well. But the two countries differed in one important respect. Whereas Canadian provincial governments became the loci of experimentation with governmental hospital insurance, American state governments did not. Why this should be, given the similar structure of interests in the two nations, deserves some explanation. The answer seems to lie in the realm of institutions and policy legacies.

TABLE 2.1  Community Hospitals and Hospital Beds,
By Ownership Type, United States and Canada,
Mid–1950s

| Ownership | United States, 1955 | | Canada, 1953 | |
|---|---|---|---|---|
| | Hospitals | Beds (000s) | Hospitals | Beds (000s) |
| State/local | 1120 | 142 | 288 | 18 |
| | (21%) | (25%) | (30%) | (23%) |
| Not-for-profit (lay voluntary/ religious) | 3097 | 389 | 522 | 56 |
| | (59%) | (68%) | (55%) | (73%) |
| For-profit, proprietary | 1120 | 37 | 143 | 3 |
| | (19%) | (7%) | (15%) | (4%) |
| Total | 5237 | 568 | 953 | 77 |
| | (100%) | (100%) | (100%) | (100%) |

*Sources:* Department of National Health and Welfare 1955: 14; American Hospital Association 1995: table 1.

In the New Deal era, the resistance of U.S. southern states to welfare-state initiatives, and the inertia of established if limited welfare-state programs in other states, had led reformers to focus on the federal level, and particularly on the area—old-age security—in which state-level initiatives were least well developed. From the watershed developments of the New Deal onward, the federal government was increasingly seen by social reformers as the locus of change in social programs, while states were viewed as politically recalcitrant (Orloff 1988). When national-level initiatives in health care failed in the immediate postwar period, reformers looked not to the states, but rather to the next opportunity at the federal level. On the other hand, supporters of the status quo such as business interests and health care providers tended to focus on state governments, a strategy that "was cheaper and had more certain results than lobbying the United States Congress and the federal executive" (Fox 1996: 103).

Ironically, Canadian reformers, who had no singular example of success at the federal level comparable to the American New Deal (with the limited exception of the adoption of unemployment insurance in 1940) were less likely to see the federal level as the sole route to change and more likely to attempt change at the provincial level. Health care reformers, particularly those associated with regionally based parties, saw provincial governments as legitimate vehicles for the expression of regional preferences.[2] After the failure of national health insurance proposals at the federal level in Canada, windows of opportunity began to open up at the provincial level where, given their exclusive constitutional jurisdiction over health care, governments could function virtually as unitary states in the health care arena. The election of the social–democratic CCF government in Saskatchewan in 1944 had opened one such window; in 1947, as part of its broad social–democratic agenda of social policy change, the

CCF government introduced the first program of governmental hospital insurance in Canada. But it was not only the social–democratic CCF that introduced governmental hospital insurance in the wake of the collapse of the federal proposals. A Liberal–Conservative coalition government in British Columbia introduced comprehensive governmental health insurance in 1947, and in 1950 the Social Credit (a populist party of the right) government of Alberta introduced a more limited program of governmental subsidization of hospital insurance.[3]

With the exception of these governmental hospital insurance plans in four provinces (representing less than one-third of the population), however, the pattern of private health insurance that developed in Canada and the United States in the 1950s was very similar. The system of private, largely employer-based health insurance grew rapidly in both countries in the immediate postwar period. Between 1950 and 1956 in the United States, enrollment in group hospital insurance plans grew at average annual rates of 18% in plans offered by commercial carriers, and 4% in Blue Cross/Blue Shield plans. Enrollment in such plans for inhospital surgical physicians' services grew at an average annual rate of 15% for commercial carriers and 12% for Blue Cross/Blue Shield. Group plan coverage for inhospital nonsurgical physicians' services was less common but even more rapidly growing, with an average rate of enrollment increase of 25% for commercial carriers and 18% for Blue Cross/Blue Shield.[4] Canada evinced a similar pattern: the average rate of increase in enrollment in hospital insurance plans (most of which was in group plans) between 1951 and 1956 was 12% for commercial carriers and 6% for Blue Cross and other not-for-profit plans. The comparable rate of growth for medical care insurance (including "comprehensive" plans covering services both in and outside hospitals as well as plans limited to inhospital services) was 14% for commercial carriers and 20% for the (primarily physician-controlled) not-for-profits (Department of National Health and Welfare 1958: 1).

Despite these similar rates of growth, the development of governmental hospital insurance plans in several provinces in the 1940s and 1950s meant that the extent of enrollment in private hospital insurance plans in Canada was proportionately somewhat less than two-thirds that in the United States.[5] With regard to medical care insurance, however, the pattern was more similar between the two countries, although overall enrollment was proportionately somewhat higher in the United States, and the scope of benefits somewhat broader in Canada. In 1959, an estimated 66% of the U.S. civilian population had some coverage for surgical services, 47% for inhospital nonsurgical physicians' services, and 12% coverage for most medical services in and outside hospital (Somers and Somers 1961: 249–50). In 1961, about 53% of the Canadian civilian population had some form of private medical care insurance, and 44% had some coverage for medical care outside hospital (Berry 1965: 22).

In both countries private health insurance was largely employer-based—a phenomenon that reflects in part the similar levels and patterns of unionization in Canada and the United States in the 1950s and 1960s (Tuohy 1992: 159–63). In the United States in 1958, more than 75% of those with private health insurance were covered by an employer-based plan (Somers and Somers 1961: 228). In Canada in 1961, the comparable proportion was 86% (Berry 1965: 11). Measured another way, prior to the adoption of medical care insurance in Canada about 45% of the Canadian civilian population was covered by employer-based medical insurance—a proportion identical to that in the United States at the same time. In both countries, moreover, the market was divided fairly evenly between commercial and not-for-profit carriers. In both, the not-for-profit sector was dominated by provider-controlled organizations: Blue Cross, controlled by hospital associations, and a number of physician-sponsored medical insurance plans. Although there were tensions between the hospital- and physician-controlled plans in both countries, the two types of plans were linked with varying degrees of formality and competed not against each other but against the commercial carriers (Starr 1982: 306–10; Naylor 1986: 158–60; Agnew 1974: 156–64). Only in their relative degrees of concentration did the two markets significantly vary: in Canada, the largest fifteen firms accounted for more than three-quarters of gross premium income for medical insurance in 1961; in the United States, the largest fifteen firms accounted for only 38% of the gross premium income for health insurance in 1958.[6]

In the late 1950s and early 1960s, then, the institutional mix and the structural balance in the health care arenas of Canada and the United States were remarkably alike. Both accorded a heavy weight to markets and to collegial mechanisms for the delivery and financing of health care. Physicians played central roles as clinical decision-makers and as entrepreneurs in the delivery system. Collectively through physician-controlled and (more or less) allied hospital-controlled insurance carriers, they also played important roles as third-party payers.[7] Private financial interests, through commercial insurance carriers, played potentially important but effectively passive roles in underwriting the costs of a delivery system in which the key decisions were made by physicians. The role of the state lay primarily in financing "public health"-oriented, largely preventive services, in operating public hospitals in which independent physicians carried out a portion of their practices, and in delegating authority for the quality control of professional practice to "self-regulating" professions.

From this common point, however, decisions taken in the late 1950s and 1960s would set these two nations on dramatically different courses. Developments in the broader political arena created rare opportunities for major policy change in the health care arena in both Canada and the United States. Both countries would adopt major programs of state financing of health care services while leaving the existing delivery system essentially untouched. But the scope of the two programs varied greatly, and therein lay the seeds of marked divergence in the future.

*Canada*

In the 1950s, federal–provincial relations in Canada, which had been chilly to initiatives involving federal–provincial cooperation at the end of World War II, began to thaw. A key determinant of this warming climate was a change in leadership at the federal level and in the largest province, Ontario. The change was one of leadership style and personal relations, not partisanship. Within a period of little more than a year in 1948–1949, the federal Liberal Prime Minister Mackenzie King was replaced by his Liberal successor Louis St. Laurent, and the Conservative Premier George Drew by his Conservative successor Leslie Frost. The relationship between St. Laurent and Frost was markedly more cordial that that between their predecessors had been; as a result the general tone of federal–provincial relations began to change (Taylor 1979: 164–66, 183–84; Dyck 1988: 329–30). In the early 1950s, Ontario supported a number of federal–provincial tax- and cost-sharing initiatives. In the mid-1950s, the Ontario government assumed a crucial role in pressing for a cost-shared federal–provincial program of hospital insurance. This, as Malcolm Taylor (1979) has noted, represented a decision "not to go it alone," in contrast to the prior decisions of four other provinces to "go it alone" in introducing their own programs of hospital insurance (105).

The new window of opportunity created by the change in the overall climate of federal–provincial relations opened on a landscape of policy ideas and interests quite different from that which had existed ten years earlier. The rise of private health insurance offered by both not-for-profit and for-profit entities persuaded a number of key participants in the arena of the viability of private-sector mechanisms. The growth of physician- and hospital-sponsored insurance carriers gave the key groups of providers in the system evidence that they themselves could respond to the problems that, a decade earlier, proposals for governmental insurance had addressed. The even more dramatic growth of commercial carriers increased the stakes of private financial interests in the arena. The British NHS was no longer a bold and promising conception: it was a real-life example. And after initial positive assessments it had spawned some disillusionment—reflected in critical commentary in the Canadian medical press and disproportionately represented among those British expatriate doctors who chose to leave the NHS system to take up practice in Canada (Naylor 1986: 159–60, 190). The vitriolic portrayals of the NHS by the American Medical Association in the early 1950s, moreover, "naturally spilled across the border" (Naylor 1986: 160). Medical and hospital groups, favorable to universal governmental health insurance only ten years before, had by the mid-1950s come to favor a program of governmental subsidization of health insurance premiums for low-income individuals (Taylor 1979: 188–94).

Confronted with this changed landscape, governments moved cautiously. A sufficient coalition of support among federal and provincial governments could be assembled only for governmental hospital insurance, not for medical insurance as well—although some provinces (notably British Columbia and Saskatchewan) sought the latter. At federal–provincial conferences in October 1955 and January 1956, the shape of the plan began to be hammered out. The three westernmost provinces indicated their agreement in principle in early 1956. It was not until such an agreement was reached with Ontario in March 1956, however, that the federal health minister could confidently introduce the enabling legislation into Parliament. The legislation passed unanimously in

April 1957. Its implementation easily survived and was indeed accelerated after a change in the federal government with the election of a Conservative government later that year. Between July 1, 1958, and October 1, 1959, all provinces except Quebec entered the plan (Taylor 1979: 211–34). The relationship between the federal government and Quebec did not begin to thaw until after the death of Premier Duplessis in 1959. Quebec adopted its hospital insurance plan under the federal–provincial arrangements on January 1, 1961.

Indeed, if the warming of Ottawa–Ontario relations in the 1950s had a positive effect on the general tenor of federal–provincial relations, the death of Duplessis and the subsequent change in the partisan complexion (from Union Nationale to Liberal) and the policy orientation of the Quebec government ushered in a whole new era. As Gagnon and Garcea (1988) have concisely put it, "In reaction to the philosophy of the Duplessis era, the Lesage administration assumed power with a disposition toward reform, both within Quebec and in its relations with the federal and provincial governments. Its strategy basically entailed an active involvement in intergovernmental relations in an effort to recoup lost political power, prestige, and fiscal resources needed for the development of the Quebec state and society" (305). With the two largest provinces disposed toward constructive engagement with Ottawa and with other provinces in the design of programs, a period of "cooperative federalism" was born—a period in which some of the major pillars of the Canadian welfare state were to be put in place.

This era dawned at a time of economic boom and governmental expansiveness. The Canadian economy grew at an average annual rate of 5% in real terms from 1960 to 1970; and total public expenditure as a proportion of GDP increased from 29% to 35% in the same period (calculated from OECD 1993, vol. 2: 34–35, 40). As the issue of governmental medical insurance rose on the agenda of federal–provincial relations in the 1960s, it was in a context favorable to the design of a generous program. The hospital insurance program had already been designed with open-ended federal cost-sharing provisions and without organizational change in the hospital sector. Medical care insurance would follow and extend this pattern.

As previously noted, health care providers and insurers had abandoned their postwar consensus in support of comprehensive universal health insurance soon after the failure of the federal government's 1945–1946 proposals, and they had come to prefer a system of governmental subsidization of private insurance for low-income individuals. The medical profession's opposition to the adoption of governmental hospital insurance in the 1950s had been grounded not so much in antipathy to the program itself as in the fear that it would be extended over time to include medical services—as indeed had been suggested by some of the key political actors involved (Naylor 1986: 166; Taylor 1979: 190–91). As the possibility of such an extension continued to be raised in the 1960s, the opposition of the profession was redoubled. The general sense of fiscal buoyancy, however, gave governments wide latitude to design the program on generous terms to consolidate support and defray opposition.

Universal comprehensive government-sponsored medical care insurance was first adopted in Saskatchewan under a social–democratic CCF government in 1962. In designing the program, the government explicitly rejected changes in the organization of health care delivery and the mode of medical remuneration, believing that the success of the physician-sponsored medical insurance plans had "irrevocably institutionalized" the fee-for-service system (Taylor 1979: 268). Nonetheless, organized medicine vehemently opposed the program. In introducing the program in July 1962, the government weathered a bitter twenty-three-day doctors' strike. The strike had two important legacies. First, an important feature of the settlement agreement was the provision that physicians' fees for service could exceed those covered by the government plan, with the balance to be paid by the patient. This provision was to be replicated in other provincial plans, and would be a rankling source of conflict until it was removed in the 1980s, as discussed in the next chapter. The second legacy of the strike stemmed from the government strategy of recruiting physicians from Britain to staff community clinics on a salaried basis to provide substitute services—an action that further tainted the community clinic option in the eyes of the profession for years to come.

Once instituted, the Saskatchewan plan had an important "demonstration effect," both positive and negative. Initially, it galvanized several other provincial governments and organized medicine to seek to demonstrate the viability of alternative approaches. In December 1960, as the Saskatchewan plan was being developed, the CMA executive wrote to the Conservative prime minister to request the appointment of a committee to study the issue; nine days later the prime minister responded with the announcement of his intention to appoint a commission. The Royal Commission on Health Services, chaired by Justice Emmett Hall (the Hall Commission), was in place by June 1961 and began a cross-country series of hearings. Throughout, a coalition of medical and insurance interests urged it to recommend a model of governmental subsidization of voluntary private insurance. Meanwhile, several provincial governments adopted their own programs of medical care insurance, supplementary in different ways to private insurance. In 1963, Alberta adopted a program of subsidization of private insurance premiums for low-income individuals, and Ontario and British Columbia subsequently established governmental insurance plans as alternatives to private insurance, with sliding premium scales geared to income.

On the positive side, however, the Saskatchewan plan demonstrated the feasibility of a universal comprehensive governmental plan (Naylor 1986: 233–34). When the Hall Commission reported in June 1964 it astounded the coalition of medical and insurance interests that had urged its establishment, by recommending a Saskatchewan-style universal comprehensive government-sponsored plan as the model to be cost-shared by the federal government. Its recommendations were grounded less in ideology than in pragmatism. It concluded:

> That the number of individuals who would require subsidy to meet total health services costs is so large that no government could impose the means test procedure on so many citizens, or would be justified in establishing a system requiring

so much unnecessary administration. The health services will make enough demands on our resources. We must not waste them. . . .

That the health insurance fund in each province should be administered by
one agency in order to achieve full integration of *all* health services, and thus to
obtain the most efficient administration of all sectors of the proposed health services program. We have recommended that the existing hospital insurance program be administered by the same agency as administers all personal health services. This necessarily means rejection of any proposal that the one phase of
health services, namely payment of physician's [*sic*] services, be administered by a
separate agency. (Royal Commission on Health Services 1964: 743–44, quoted in
Taylor 1979: 346–47)

As for the medical profession, experience with the Saskatchewan plan somewhat tempered its opposition (Naylor 1986: 234). Physician incomes in
Saskatchewan kept pace with those in the rest of Canada in the first years of
the plan (Barer and Evans 1986: 93).

The Hall Commission reported not to the Conservative government that
had established it, but to the successor Liberal minority government. Notwithstanding the fact that conservative governments at the provincial level had
tended to favor a model of subsidization of private insurance, partisanship was
not a bar to consensus at the federal level. All federal parties ultimately supported the model recommended by the Hall Commission. The legislation incorporating this model, the Medical Care Act, was passed in the House of
Commons in December 1966 with only two dissenting votes.

Given this all-party agreement, the consolidation of authority necessary for
the implementation of federal medical care insurance was relatively nonprob-
lematic at the federal level itself, even in the context of a minority government.
In the federal–provincial arena, however, the course to agreement did not run
smooth. Despite the generally positive climate of federal–provincial relations,
some provinces resisted the adoption of the "Saskatchewan model" for the federal medical care insurance program. At a federal–provincial conference in July
1965, the federal government had laid out the broad principles that would
characterize the program—comprehensiveness, universality, accessibility on
"uniform terms and conditions," public administration, and portability. Although these principles were seemingly incompatible with the model of government subsidization of private insurance preferred by several provinces, discussion at the conference had been low-key and opposition muted (Taylor
1979: 354–66). As the federal program took shape over the ensuing months,
provincial opposition mounted. After the passage of federal legislation (particularly after the 1968 federal budget instituted a 2% "social development" surtax
on income tax to finance its contributions to the new cost-shared social
programs adopted over the past decade), a number of provinces (including
Ontario) protested that they were effectively being coerced into participation
in the federal program (Taylor 1979: 375). Nonetheless, over the period
1968–1971, all provinces entered the plan by establishing medical care insurance plans meeting the federal criteria.

The rhetoric and (in the case of Saskatchewan and Quebec physicians) the actions of protest surrounding the introduction of Canadian governmental hospital and medical insurance (referred to generically as medicare) should not be exaggerated in importance. The adoption of medicare was part of a remarkable era in Canadian public policy development, from 1958 to 1971, that also saw the adoption of federal–provincial shared-cost programs for postsecondary education and social assistance, and the establishment of a public pension program involving complex federal–provincial arrangements. These various programs, in effect, constituted a mutually reinforcing momentum of social policy change. The design of the medicare program, moreover, reflects the willingness of governments in buoyant economic times to assuage opposition with generous provisions. Federal contributions to provincial plans were initially open-ended. And the existing delivery system, including fee-for-service modes of remuneration and freedom of choice for both patients and providers, was left intact.

Essentially two structural changes were wrought by medicare in the Canadian health policy arena: the role of private insurers was drastically reduced, and the central structural axis—an accommodation between the medical profession and the state—was redefined. In addition, within the state category, the role of the federal government vis-à-vis the provinces was enhanced. As for the institutional mix, the role of market mechanisms in financing the insurance function was clearly reduced. Similarly, the process of constraining the ability of individual physicians to set the price of their services—already well underway with the rise of the physician-sponsored "prepayment" plans—was accelerated. Otherwise, however, the mix of collegiality, hierarchy, and market in the delivery system remained unchanged. These various changes deserve some elaboration.

*Restriction of the domain of private insurance*   The advent of medicare greatly increased the fiscal role of the state,[8] and effectively shut out private insurers from covering the vast majority of medical and hospital services. Nonetheless, with the adoption of the national hospital insurance program, only one of the provincial Blue Cross plans (in Manitoba) ceased to operate. The others continued to offer coverage for goods and services not covered by the various provincial plans, such as dental care, drugs, and eyeglasses and other prostheses,[9] and various amenities related to hospital care, such as private rooms. With the adoption of medical care insurance, the role of private insurance was further circumscribed. In some provinces the physician-sponsored plans, as well as commercial carriers, continued for a few years to act as carriers for the government plan (as was also the case under the U.S. Medicare program). But in the early 1970s this practice was discontinued: the physician-sponsored plans ceased operations, and the commercial insurers remained confined to coverage of those services not covered by provincial plans.

*The state vis-à-vis the medical profession*   The restriction of the domain of private insurance left two dominant sets of interests in the health care arena—the state, which under medicare became the primary bearer of the costs of hospital and medical services; and health care providers, most centrally the medical profession. The accommodation between these two sets of interests lies at the heart of Canadian medicare.

As will be discussed at greater length in chapters 3 and 7, the particular nature of that accommodation varied across provinces, for it is at the provincial level that health care policy was made, within broad federal guidelines. In some provinces, notably British Columbia and Manitoba, the profession–state relationship was adversarial; in Quebec it was more "statist"; and in other provinces it was more collaborative, albeit marked by episodes of conflict. But as in the British case each of these accommodations revolved around two pivotal trade-offs for the medical profession: one between the entrepreneurial and the clinical discretion of physicians, the other between their individual and their collective autonomy. Essentially, professional associations were willing to negotiate limitations on the entrepreneurial discretion of individual physicians, particularly over the price of their services, in return for a maintenance of professional control over clinical decision-making (Tuohy 1992: 118–20).

Apart from these two fundamental structural changes wrought by the advent of medicare, it is also important to note the implications of medicare for relationships *within* the state, and particularly for federal–provincial relations. The federal government's financial leverage under cost-sharing arrangements gave it a significant steering effect on the system. Initially, by allowing provinces to cover medical and hospital services with "fifty-cent dollars," it favored the provision of such services as opposed to, for example, home care services. Furthermore, although the criteria for eligibility for provincial programs were very generally phrased, the requirement that services must be provided on "uniform terms and conditions" presented a potential—and, as it turned out in the 1980s and 1990s, a real—constraint on the choice of policy instruments by provincial governments.

Such, then, is the story of the introduction of national health insurance in Canada in the 1960s. A window of opportunity was created through the convergence of propitious partisan and federal–provincial climates. The policy that was chosen, made possible by a period of economic boom, fit well with the existing structure of interests in the health care arena: it made no changes to the existing structure of health care delivery, placed physicians at the heart of the decision-making system at all levels, and retained a limited role for private insurance.

### The United States

In the 1960s in the United States, as in Canada, a window of opportunity for major policy change in the health care arena opened. Given the focus of health care reformers on the federal level as just discussed, it was there that the conditions for change had to occur. The landslide election of President Lyndon Johnson in the 1964 elections gave Johnson 61.3% of the popular vote and the Democrats a supermajority of 67% in the Senate as well as control of the House; the stage was set for major reform. This window opened, again as in Canada, in an era of prosperity and expansiveness. The average annual real economic growth rate in the United States from 1960 to 1970 was 4%, and total public expenditures as a proportion of GDP increased from 27% to 32% over that period (calculated from OECD 1993, vol. 2: 34–35, 40). A burst of social policy initiatives, including a number of antipoverty measures under the banner of the War on Poverty, were put in place under the Johnson administration. The passage of the Medicare and Medicaid programs, providing governmental health insurance for the elderly and the indigent, constituted without doubt the hallmark and the pinnacle of these social policy achievements. And yet when the period is viewed in broad historical and cross-national perspective, the question arises: Why did these initiatives not go further? Why did they not yield, as in Canada, a universal health insurance scheme?

The answer to this question lies in the period that led up to the actions of the mid-1960s. Indeed, the line of analysis arguably leads back to the 1930s—to Franklin Roosevelt's decision not to attempt a national health insurance program as part of the major social policy initiatives that constituted the New Deal. Clearly this was a potential window of opportunity for change: Roosevelt had entered office in 1932 with 57.8% of the popular vote, and the Democrats held more than 70% of the seats in the Senate and the House. But Roosevelt did not see health insurance as essential to his agenda of social policy change—indeed, he feared that attempting to achieve it could jeopardize the entire project. When the Committee on Economic Security, appointed by Roosevelt to study policy options for social security, included a discussion of general principles for health insurance, a "storm of protest from the AMA" ensued (Starr 1982: 268). Only a relatively innocuous provision for "further study" of the issue was contained in the bill presented to Congress, and even that was deleted before passage.

The issue was taken up with considerably greater fervor but without success by Roosevelt's successor, President Harry Truman, as already discussed. In the face of successive failures to gain support for national health insurance, advocates of the policy adopted an incrementalist strategy, which allowed for the building of coalitions around a number of limited but significant pieces of legislation. Notably, the Hill–Burton Act of 1946, providing for federal subsidization of hospital construction, previously discussed, was the product of one such coalition (Fox 1986: 124–31). After the Republicans gained control of the White House in 1952, Democratic reformers continued to introduce national health insurance legislation every year for the rest of the decade. Given the very closely divided houses of Congress in this period (in which both parties at different times held bare majorities), this legislation was introduced "not with any hopes for enactment, but to keep alive the idea of health insurance under social security" (Marmor 1973: 30).

In keeping with the strategy of incrementalism, moreover, advocates of national health insurance no longer proposed moving to universal health insurance in a single step. Chastened by the vehemence of the opposition to Truman's proposals, they narrowed their focus to concentrate on the elderly. As James Morone has acerbically put it:

The most important victim of the industry's opposition was the reformers' ideal itself. Liberals slowly whittled away Truman's plan in a vain effort to win political support: from comprehensive national health insurance to national health insurance for the elderly to a partial hospital plan for the elderly. Despite the backpedaling, the terms of the debate never varied. Throughout the 1950s and early 1960s, the industry continued to question the legitimacy and the capacity of American government to implement the reform, regardless of how the liberals defined it. (Morone 1990: 261–62)

Upon his election to the Presidency in 1960, John Kennedy took up the cause of "Medicare" (defined as governmental health insurance for the elderly) with vigor. But although the Democrats held more than 60% of the seats in both the Senate and the House, Kennedy, with his razor-thin margin of victory in the popular vote for president, could not claim a popular mandate for bold social policy changes sufficient to overcome the continuing divisions in the Democratic party. Attempts by administration officials to negotiate compromise positions with key Congressional Democrats (notably Wilbur Mills, Chairman of the House Ways and Means Committee) bore no fruit.

The political context was dramatically changed by the assassination of Kennedy and the subsequent landslide victory of Lyndon Johnson and the Democratic party. Now the Democrats had a congressionally skilled southern president and supermajorities in both houses of Congress. It was the American equivalent of the 1945 Labour landslide in Britain—indeed, in the American two-party contest, Johnson could claim a stronger mandate in terms of popular vote won than could Clement Atlee. Just as in Britain, a dramatic electoral victory followed a period of unsatisfactory search for compromise, and promised to make possible what years of negotiation had not been able to accomplish.

In the face of this historic opportunity, advocates of national health insurance within the Democratic administration appear in historical context to have been fatefully timid. They continued the strategy of incrementalism begun in the 1950s, seeking only passage of a national hospital insurance program for the elderly. The changed political context might have made possible a bolder approach, moving immediately to universal national health insurance, or at least first to universal hospital insurance as in the Canadian case. Instead, the same strategists who had tailored the design of their proposals to fit the narrower political cloth of the 1950s and early 1960s persisted in seeking "Medicare"—that is, hospital insurance for the elderly. Lawrence Jacobs has perceptively drawn the contrast with the British case:

In Britain, the coalition of Labour and Conservative parties was inundated by political division, but on health policy opposing factions agreed on a clear and highly popular objective. In the wake of its landslide victory, Labour used persistent support for this objective to introduce bold new means like the nationalization of hospitals. In stark contrast, the successive defeats of American health insurance schemes convinced reformers that they could build support for their unspoken objective—universal, comprehensive health insurance—only by building on the public's enthusiasm for Social Security. In effect, American policymakers reversed the British approach: the means (Medicare's Social Security approach) was expected to generate support for the unannounced objective. Even after the 1964 election shook Washington's political establishment, longtime reformers like [Assistant Secretary of Health Education and Welfare Wilbur] Cohen steadfastly adhered to their incremental philosophy. But the blinders of incrementalism obscured new political opportunities: instead of pressing for innovative means to move boldly toward their objective, reformers treated Medicare as their objective and simply recycled preelection proposals in framing the administration's bill. (Jacobs 1993: 210–11)

In large part, this cautiousness reflected a mindset shaped by years, indeed decades, of facing the unrelenting opposition of provider groups and their allies to proposals for health care reform. But it also reflected a judgment about what was possible in the context of the broad liberal agenda of the mid-1960s. The coalition support for that agenda within the national government, including not only broad redistributive goals but also sweeping civil rights reforms, was at its peak in 1965 (Orfield 1988). Nonetheless, Democratic reformers feared pressing the limits of their support within the southern wing of the party at a time when historic civil rights legislation was being enacted. Some suggested, indeed, that civil rights reforms and health care reform might come to be explicitly linked. Jacobs (1993) reports that: "The only serious threat to Johnson's leadership in winning congressional approval of Medicare was the divisive issue of race relations. Administrative and congressional officials feared open discussion of the application of the Civil Rights Act of 1964 to Medicare; only this issue had the potential to 'jeopardize the bill' by compelling southern supporters of Medicare to re-examine their position" (198). Such considerations reinforced the strategic judgment that caution was to be the rule.

In the face of what Marmor (1973: 59) has called the "politics of legislative certainty" created by the massive presidential mandate and Congressional majorities enjoyed by the Democrats, opponents of governmental health insurance changed tactics. Instead of the histrionic antigovernment campaigns that had characterized its approach for three decades, the AMA brought forward an alternative proposal: "Eldercare," entailing an expansion of federal aid for state medical assistance for the poor, extending to medical care as well as hospital services.

Democratic reformers were indeed pressed to move beyond their incremental first step of hospital insurance for the elderly to support broader reforms. Ironically, however, much of the pressure came from those who feared that a hospital-only Medicare program would fuel rising public expectations and create a momentum of change that would lead quickly to a universal comprehensive plan. Those who held this view, notably the powerful House Ways and Means chairman, Wilbur Mills, sought to expand the proposal just enough to keep this momentum from developing. And in the end, that is what transpired. The scheme enacted by Congress in 1965 had three components: Medicare Part A, a compulsory hospital insurance plan for the elderly similar to the original administration proposal; Medicare Part B, a government-subsidized voluntary plan to cover medical services to the elderly similar to a Republican proposal; and Medicaid, a program of expanded federal assistance to the states to provide medical and hospital care to the nonelderly poor (defined according to federal criteria), building on the AMA proposal. In another irony, Democratic reformers cooperated fully in this extension of their proposal as a way of achieving gains they had not anticipated so soon. In fact these "[e]rstwhile reformers designed lasting obstacles to achieving their firmly held objective, incremental expansion of Medicare's coverage of services and populations" (Jacobs 1993: 213). With two of the most vulnerable segments of the population—the elderly and the poor—thus protected, momentum toward further change was stalled for long enough for fundamental transformations to occur in the health system—transformations that would greatly complicate future attempts to adopt a comprehensive universal plan. Only one significant extension of Medicare—in 1973, to those qualifying for disability benefits under Social Security—was to occur.

In the design of the Medicare program, American policy-makers made even greater concessions to the interests of providers and private insurers than was the case in Canada. As in Canada, the existing delivery system was left in place.[10] Hospitals and physicians, however, were to be reimbursed by Medicare not according to a negotiated schedule but for "reasonable costs." Hospital charges, moreover, could include costs of capital depreciation and service—a provision firmly resisted by policy-makers in Canada, where hospitals' capital budgets were dealt with separately from operating budgets. Physicians were allowed to bill patients above the amount reimbursed by Medicare.[11] As for insurers, the program allowed hospitals to nominate "fiscal intermediaries," for the administration of their participation in Part A of Medicare; and the "overwhelming majority" nominated Blue Cross plans. Similarly, private insurers were to be appointed by the Secretary of Health, Education and Welfare as "carriers" of Medicare Part B coverage; and in most cases the appointment went to Blue Shield (the not-for-profit counterpart to Blue Cross for the coverage of medical services) (Starr 1982: 375).

The American strategy of incrementalism, culminating in the passage of Medicare and Medicaid, while lacking the full drama of the British and Canadian cases, was of considerable importance for the structuring of both the public and the private sectors, and the relationship between the two. As noted here, the effect of the Hill–Burton hospital construction program, which was targeted at nonprofit and public health care facilities (and primarily at acute care general hospitals), was to enhance the growing significance of not-for-profit facilities in the hospital sector, already favored by various federal and state-level policies of subsidization and favorable tax treatment (Marmor et al. 1994: 57–58).[12] Even more, however, it favored the growth of public facilities—in part because not-for-profits were relatively slow to take advantage of the program, and in part because state funding reduced the need for philanthropic support for hospitals, an important raison d'être of the not-for-profit form (Marmor et al. 1994). These public facilities increasingly became the sites for care of the poor. Similarly, public policy continued to favor the not-for-profit form in the health insurance market, even in the face of growing competitive challenges from commercial providers.

The passage of Medicare and Medicaid in 1965 clearly made for a sharp increase in the fiscal presence of the state in the health care arena. The public share of total health expenditures increased from 24.7% in 1965 to 37.2% in 1970 (calculated from OECD 1993, vol. 1: 108–9). The role of private finance remained dominant, however. Even under Medicare, limitations on coverage and the existence of requirements for deductibles and copayments meant that the government program "came to finance between 40% and 50% of the medical expenses of the aged" (Marmor with Morone 1983: 143). State financing nonetheless had some important (if unintended) consequences for the structure of both health care delivery and health insurance markets. In the delivery system, Medicare and Medicaid gave a boost to the proprietary form by providing an assured source of revenue. At the same time, revenues from public health insurance, as opposed to government grants or private charity, became an increasingly important source of support for nonprofit and public institutions as well. As for the private insurance sector, the fairly consistent direction of public policy from the 1920s through the 1960s to favor the not-for-profit form was continued by Medicare policy on fiscal intermediaries and by the adoption of a cost-based scheme of hospital reimbursement modeled closely on Blue Cross (Marmor et al. 1994: 59–60).

With regard to the institutional mix in the health care arena, little changed. Market mechanisms continued to predominate. The state played a larger role as purchaser; it was not (as in Canada) a monopsonist, however, and was essentially a price-taker. Physicians (and other providers) could continue to function as entrepreneurs in all matters including the price of their services. But the very dynamics of this system were to transform it in ways unanticipated by the participants in the policy arena of the 1960s, not least the profession itself.

The founding moments of the modern British, Canadian, and American "health care states," then, left them very differently positioned to respond to the common challenges that emerged on the cross-national agenda of health policy in the late twentieth century. The next chapter takes up that story.

# The Reforms of 3
# the 1990s

As discussed in chapter 1, the last three decades of the twentieth century saw an evolution of the health policy agenda in which governments became increasingly concerned with controlling the costs of health care, or at least the proportion of those costs borne by public treasuries. The much less buoyant economic and fiscal climates that characterized advanced industrial nations after the oil price shocks of the 1970s and the rise of global competition constrained the ability of governments to meet the level of public expectations for public programs established in more bountiful times—not only in the health care arena, but more generally. Moreover, over the course of this period governments, to varying degrees in different nations, became dissatisfied with blunt budgetary limits as mechanisms of cost control and considered ways in which the incentive structures of public programs, including health insurance programs, could be changed to ensure that public funds were being spent to the greatest effect.

The common themes of this agenda were expressed in quite different ways and with very different results across nations. In Britain, the United States, and Canada, the experience of the 1990s—sweeping policy change in the first, policy stalemate and turbulent market transformation in the second, and relative stability in the third—exemplify the range of this difference. The policy episodes of the 1940s in Britain and the 1960s in the United States and Canada had established systems, each with a different and distinctive inherent logic, that left these three nations differently poised for change at the turn of the last decade of the century.

## Britain

The logic of the decision-making system that developed within the National Health Service can best be described as one of "hierarchical corporatism." This logic will be explored in greater depth in chapter 6. Here, it can be described briefly as a distinctive blend of hierarchical and collegial elements that revolved around a central accommodation between the state and the medical profession. The state confined itself essentially to setting budgets, which flowed from top to bottom down a set of regional hierarchies. The allocation of resources within budgetary limits, however, was largely in the hands of doctors—both as individual practitioners making clinical judgments and as key participants in decision-making panels at each level of the hierarchy.

These basic features of the NHS remained largely inviolable in the postwar period. The structure of the hierarchy itself was redefined over time—notably in a 1974 reorganization that drew the original three pillars of the NHS into a unified structure while reinforcing the corporatist roles of professionals, and in 1982 when the geographic divisions of the unified hierarchy were revised. But the essential terms of the profession–state accommodation persisted. With one exception—the hotly contested policy adopted by the Labour government in 1976 reducing the number of private "pay-beds" in NHS hospitals[1]—there was little change in the structural and institutional characteristics of the British health care system until the 1990s.

### The "Thatcherite project" and the NHS

The election of an ideologically driven Conservative government under Prime Minister Margaret Thatcher in 1979 was an event of world-historical significance, a key marker of the rise in influence of the ideas of the "new right" on the policy agendas of advanced industrial nations. Nowhere, not even in the United States under the Reagan administrations of the 1980s, were these ideas more explicitly proclaimed by the government of the day. As most analysts of the Thatcher period have noted, these ideas constituted a "political project" but not a coherent and well-developed policy agenda. Indeed, in attempting to carry out their "project," the Conservatives under Thatcher were to prove to be decidedly pragmatic, developing and adapting specific policies as circumstances required.

As described by Andrew Gamble, the new right project of Thatcherism "came to have three overriding objectives—the restoration of the political fortunes of the Conservative party, the revival of market liberalism as the dominant public philosophy, and the creation of the conditions for a free economy by limiting the scope of the state while restoring its authority" (Gamble 1990: 336). The commitment of the "Thatcherites" to this project had been forged during the period in which the Conservatives were in opposition in the 1970s.

Thatcher and Sir Keith Joseph founded the Centre for Policy Studies (CPS) in 1975 as a vehicle for the inculcation and dissemination of the ideas of American neoconservatives such as Friederich von Hayek and Milton Friedman in the British context (Sullivan 1992: 150–54). The CPS and related activities resulted not in a detailed policy agenda, but rather in a fierce sense of commitment to an ideological direction: "What makes Thatcherism distinctive as a political project is the scope of its ambitions, and the tenacity with which its leaders pursued them. Thatcherites were convinced that a dramatic break with many existing institutions and policies was necessary if the errors of the past were to be corrected and if Britain was to escape from its long, debilitating decline" (Gamble 1990: 336).

Notable among the characteristics of existing institutions that the Thatcherite project aimed to break were the corporatist elements that had come to pervade the system of industrial relations and the welfare state. British-style corporatism gave institutionally legitimate roles to multiple trade unions and professional and producer groups in both the public and the private sectors (Cawson 1982). The result, according to an influential line of analysis developing as the Conservatives assumed power, had been a paralysis of decision-making capacity, an "institutional sclerosis" that largely accounted for the underperformance of the British economy in the postwar period (Beer 1982; Olson 1982). The British economy grew at only about two-thirds the average rate of growth for the sixteen largest Western nations between 1950 and 1976 (Hall 1986: 25). In part this relative underperformance is an artifact of the time period and reflects the rapid growth of late industrializers "catching up" to early industrializers such as Britain and the United States. But Britain combined slow growth rates with high unemployment and high inflation. After the first international oil price shock, from 1974 to 1979, not only were British economic growth rates well below the OECD average, but British unemployment and inflation rates were well above the OECD average (Hall 1986: 120).

The Conservatives came to power in 1979 determined to cure this "British disease" by dismantling corporatist institutions and adopting monetarist policies including a reduction of public spending (Gamble 1990: 350; Hall 1986: 102; Klein 1995: 137). With a majority government (53.4% of the seats in the House of Commons) in a Westminster parliamentary system, the Conservatives had the consolidated authority to pursue this agenda. But it must be remembered that this authority had been won with less than a majority (43.9%) of the popular vote (Punnett 1994: 63). In two subsequent elections the Conservatives did not improve upon this level of popular support, even while substantially increasing the size of their parliamentary majorities (to 61.1% in 1983 and 57.8% in 1987) (Punnett 1994).

The Conservatives thus pursued their ideological project with due regard to political feasibility (Atkinson and Savage 1994: 10-11). Even their pursuit of monetarist macroeconomic policies has been described as an experiment in "practical monetarism," as the emphasis on five-year money supply and public sector borrowing targets (the Medium Term Financial Strategy) gave way to a greater emphasis on exchange rates and finally, at the end of the decade, to the decision to join the Exchange Rate Mechanism of the European Union (Jackson 1992; see also Hall 1986: 100–7, Dunn and Smith 1994: 78–80). In the welfare-state arena, unemployment insurance was considerably tightened, but attempts to restructure the public pension and social assistance systems were scaled back in response to public opposition (Weale 1990; Sullivan 1992: 199; Pierson 1994: 58–64, 109–15). Some elements of Conservative policy—notably the privatization of publicly owned enterprises—came to assume a greater role than had been originally envisaged, when initial experiments proved promising (Marsh 1991). The "quasimarket" strategy in health and social services, housing, and education began to be seriously considered only in the middle of Thatcher's second term, and did not begin to be implemented until her third term. But despite this pragmatism in developing, learning from, and adapting specific policies, a solid core of conviction—a "strategic sense of direction" (Gamble 1990: 337)—continued to characterize decision-making in the Thatcher governments.

The process leading up to the passage of the NHS and Community Care Act of 1990 needs to be viewed in this context of Conservative conviction and pragmatism. Throughout Thatcher's first and second terms, the NHS was not a target for major restructuring. Early in the first term, the replacement of the NHS by a system of mandatory private insurance was considered by the Central Policy Review Staff (CPRS) (an internal government "think tank" of civil servants and others for the review and assessment of policy options) in a document leaked to the press. This option was, however, roundly rejected by Cabinet.[2] Rather, the emphasis was placed on achieving greater efficiencies without changing the essential features of the NHS. In 1982, the regional hierarchy of the NHS was once again reorganized. Following a rationale of simplification and decentralization, the middle tier of the hierarchy (established in the 1974 reorganization) was abolished: ninety Area Health Authorities, each atop a structure of District Management Teams, were replaced with 192 District Health Authorities (Ham 1992: 29–30). The reorganization also had the effect of reducing the role of Local Authorities in the NHS by removing the "coterminosity" of health districts and Local Authority districts and by reducing the representation of Local Authorities on the District Health Authorities (Ham 1992: 29–30; Klein 1995: 125). It was also consistent with the broader agenda of the Conservatives to shrink local government as "the only form of direct representative government apart from Parliament," and hence a potential platform for partisan opponents (Stoker 1990: 127, 143–44).

The major thrust of the Conservative government toward achieving greater efficiency in the NHS was twofold. First, it attempted to develop a greater managerial capacity within the NHS. In 1982, it commissioned a review of NHS management under Roy Griffiths (later Sir Roy Griffiths), a business executive. The Griffiths inquiry, which reported in October 1983 at the beginning of Thatcher's second term, criticized the corporatist-based "consensus management" of the NHS and the absence of general managers who could be clearly "in charge."[3] It recommended a general management structure with clear performance targets for which general managers were to be accountable—recommendations which were quickly embraced by the government. The review, in fact, represented the emphasis on emulating private-sector "managerialism" that was sweeping the civil service under the Conservatives (Pollitt 1993: 66–71).

The general management structures adopted in accordance with Griffiths's recommendations represented, at least potentially, a strengthening of the hierarchical at the expense of the corporatist dimensions of the NHS. The challenge they presented to established NHS structures was, as we shall see in chapter 6, to a considerable extent absorbed and blunted by the system. The emphasis on managerialism, moreover, was to be replaced by an emphasis on market mechanisms. Nonetheless, the Griffiths reforms paved the way for later developments in at least two respects: they established channels linking politicians and line managers along which reform edicts could flow (Butler 1992: 14), and they began the development of a capacity to measure and assess performance upon which later reforms would depend.

The second prong of the Conservative government's strategy to improve efficiency within the NHS was budgetary. In establishing the NHS budget, it required the NHS to find "cost savings" through greater efficiency without a decrease in service—savings that were to be reinvested in improving service. Moreover, it continued and accelerated the squeezing of the health care budget that had begun under Labour in 1976. The average annual real rate of increase in public health expenditures (deflated by health prices) in Thatcher's first two terms was 1.3%, compared with 2.7% from 1976 through 1979 and 6.6% for the decade of the 1970s as a whole (calculated from OECD 1993: vol. 1, 109, 144). Health services constituted one of the few areas in which public spending continued to increase in real terms in both the last half of the 1970s and the first half of the 1980s (Hall 1986: 116). But the slowing of the average annual rate of increase in budgetary allocations to the NHS yielded what Rudolf Klein has termed an effect of "relative deprivation over time" (Klein 1995: 99). More important, however, the year-to-year level of allocations fluctuated quite dramatically on occasion in both the 1970s and the 1980s, producing ongoing uncertainty in the system. In some years, indeed, NHS spending declined in real terms.

During the first two Thatcher governments, despite the continued real increases in NHS expenditure, the relatively modest policy changes, and Thatcher's assertion during the 1983 election that "the NHS is safe with us" (Klein 1995: 140), anxiety about the future of the NHS continued to grow among providers within the system and in the public at large. From 1983 to 1990, public satisfaction with the NHS as measured by the British Social Attitudes survey steadily declined (Judge and Solomon 1993). This dissatisfaction did not lead to an abandonment of support for the NHS, however. On the contrary, opposition to a "two-tier" health care system increased between 1983 and 1989, as did support for increased public expenditure on health services (Sullivan 1992: 205–7; Butler 1992: 5).

It was not until they had won a third successive majority government in 1987 (a feat unparalleled since 1959) that the Conservatives determined that the political risks of inaction regarding the NHS were greater than the political risks of action. The decision was taken by the prime minister herself. The precipitating event was a public denunciation of governmental "underfunding" of the NHS by the presidents of the three Royal Colleges in an article in the *British Medical Journal* in December 1987, given great attention in the broader public media. The government's first response to the criticism was an emergency allocation of £90 million. But nurses' strikes in January 1988 built media attention to a crescendo (Butler 1992: 3–4). On January 25, 1988, Thatcher "surprised television viewers of [the BBC interview program] *Panorama* (and some of her Cabinet colleagues)" by announcing a review of the NHS (Klein 1995: 176). According to one influential interpretation, Thatcher was roused to this action by her sense of betrayal by the leaders of the medical profession, who were breaching their "implicit concordat" with the state (Klein 1995: 177). The medical profession, indeed, was one of the few groups whose corporatist accommodation with the state the Thatcher governments had not challenged; and this action by its leaders appeared to galvanize her inherent mistrust.

With its consolidated authority, then, the Conservative government had finally formed the will to make major changes to the policy parameters governing the NHS. It was a reluctant decision: this was "the review nobody wanted" (Timmins 1995: 458), and for which the government was ill-prepared in terms of considered policy options. The results of the review, like those of the other decisions taken during the rare windows of opportunity for major change discussed in this book, were nonetheless products of their time. The decisions made during the NHS review of 1988–1989, both substantive and procedural, bear the marks of the broader Conservative agenda of the late 1980s.

*The NHS review*

Procedurally, the review was almost a caricature of the exclusionary decision-making process that marked the Thatcher era, characterized by prime ministerial dominance and Cabinet cliques (Dunleavy 1990: 124–25; Atkinson and Cope 1994). It was conducted by a working group chaired by the prime minister herself, and consisted of four other Cabinet members and two close policy advisors to the prime minister (one of whom was Sir Roy Griffiths). There were no representatives of the NHS itself (other than Griffiths as Deputy Chairman of the NHS Management Board[4]), nor of the medical profession or other professional groups. Consultation was very limited and informal: for example, two meetings were held respectively with selected groups of physicians and NHS managers believed to be sympathetic to the Government's desire for reform (Timmins 1995: 462, Klein 1995: 185). No terms of reference were published, nor were submissions solicited, although unsolicited submissions were received and reviewed (Butler 1992: 5).

With regard to substantive issues, the working group floundered for several months. A broad range of policy options was available for consideration, from proposals for a drastic increase in private finance as favored by the Centre for

Policy Studies (and reminiscent of the discredited CPRS proposals of the early 1980s) to proposals for a "relatively small percentage increase in [public] funding" for the NHS without any radical restructuring as urged by the British Medical Association (Klein 1995: 185; see also Timmins 1995: 460–63, Butler 1992: 5–13). It was not until a Cabinet reorganization changed the membership of the working group that its approach began to gel. The Department of Health and Social Services was split in two. John Moore, who had headed the larger department became Secretary of State for Social Services, and hence was replaced on the working group on NHS reform by the new Secretary of State for Health, Kenneth Clarke. Clarke's arrival sounded the death knell of any further consideration of options based on private finance.

If private finance was rejected as the vehicle of reform, however, market mechanisms were embraced. The broad Conservative ethos of enthusiasm for replacing corporatism with market mechanisms, and group accommodation with competition and entrepreneurship, found expression in proposals for an "internal market" in health care. The embrace of these proposals by the working group needs to be seen in the broader context of British public policy in the late 1980s.

Ideas about the incorporation of market mechanisms into publicly funded systems were clearly in the air. In the education arena, the Education Reform Act of 1988 represented the Conservatives' "first (and still boldest) experiment with quasimarkets" (Challis et al. 1994: 19). Indeed, the case of education reform bears two hallmarks of the Thatcher era: an attack on the power of established professional groups and local authorities, and a mix of pragmatic incremental experimentation and "new right" doctrine. The educational system was the second of the major arenas of British-style corporatism to be attacked by the Conservatives—the first having been the system of industrial relations, which was radically reformed to the particular detriment of trade unions but also to the detriment of peak associations of business in the first Thatcher term (Marsh 1992). Furthermore, "new right" thinking as represented by the Hillgate Group, an education lobby, was clearly influential in the process of education reform. As described by Whitty (1990: 309), the Hillgate Group held that "market forces should ultimately be seen as the most effective way of determining a school's curriculum, but . . . that central government intervention is necessary as an interim strategy to undermine the power of vested interests that threaten educational standards and traditional values." The 1988 act reflected these beliefs. It was less a grand new design than "an amalgam of disparate measures [that] ended up as a more coherent codification of the right's approach to educational policy in the late twentieth century" (Whitty 1990: 311). These "disparate measures" began in 1980 with reforms requiring the Local Education Authorities (LEAs) that managed public schools to accommodate a greater degree of parental choice in selecting the schools their children would attend; the reforms also provided for a number of state-funded "assisted places" in private schools. In 1986, representation of parents on school governing bodies was increased, and LEA representation decreased. In 1988, the role of LEAs (and the role of the teachers' unions with whom they bargained) was significantly reduced and a set of "quasimarket" reforms adopted (Glennerster and Le Grand 1995, Challis et al. 1994, Whitty 1990, McVicar and Robins 1994). The powers of individual school governing bodies were increased under a system of "Local Management of Schools" (LMS). Through parental vote, schools could also elect to be funded directly by the central government rather than through the LEA. Enrollment was to be open, allowing parents to choose (within some limits) the school their child would attend, and funding would be enrollment-based. Schools would, nonetheless, be held to national standards, including, most significantly, a nationally set curriculum.

The education reforms were an important part of the policy climate that shaped the review of the NHS and foreshadowed a number of features of the "internal market" reforms that the review would propose. But there was also another important strand of influence, more specific to the health care arena itself. In 1985, the Nuffield Provincial Hospitals Trust, an influential think tank, published an essay by American economist Alain Enthoven (1985), whose proposals for "managed competition" were to play a centrally important role in the American health care reform debate of the early 1990s. Entitled "Reflections on the National Health Service," Enthoven's essay was a critique of the structure of incentives within the system of hierarchical corporatism (although he did not use those terms), which in his view failed to reward efficiency and innovation. He was particularly critical of the inadequacies of the mechanism for taking into account the flow of patients across District Health Authority boundaries in establishing DHA budgets,[5] which he argued encouraged districts to export patients and did not sufficiently reward the "importing" districts (especially those in inner London, with its concentration of teaching hospitals). Instead he proposed that each DHA be given a needs-based global budget, from which it would fund service to its population, both through its directly managed units and by purchasing services from other DHAs, as well as from private providers. If this model was to work, a method of costing would have to be developed such that costs could be compared across providers. Providers would then, in effect, compete for the business of DHAs. In this sense, the Enthoven model would constitute an "internal market."

If the reform of the industrial relations system represented the first wave of the Thatcherite attack on British corporatist institutions and the educational system the second, then the NHS reforms were the third (Klein 1995: 137). As the NHS review working group sought to find a mechanism for breaking the power of providers and introducing incentives for efficiency into a publicly financed system, "[s]lowly but surely, . . . it became plain that in terms of big ideas for reform of the delivery side of the NHS there was only one idea in town: some version of Enthoven's internal market . . ." (Timmins 1995: 462). The report of the review took the form of a White Paper entitled *Working for Patients,* issued in January 1989 (Secretaries of State for Health, Wales, Northern Ireland, and Scotland 1989), and incorporated in the NHS and Community Care Act of 1990. The White Paper and the subsequent legislation presented a framework for reform (and only a framework, which was to be fleshed out in the process of implementation, as described in chapter 6) that evinced the strong if indirect influence of Enthoven's ideas. Indeed, these ideas were adopted with a greater alacrity than Enthoven himself had recommended. Enthoven had urged experimentation with different pilot projects to test the internal market model; the review, however, recommended the adoption of the framework across the NHS.

The "internal market" reforms set out in the 1989 White Paper and enacted in the 1990 NHS and Community Care Act will be described in more detail in chapter 6, but it can be summarized here. Central to the reforms was the concept of a "purchaser–provider split." Accordingly, District Health Authorities (DHAs) were to become purchasing agencies, which would contract with hospitals for the provision of services. Hospitals and other provider units, for their part, had the option of establishing themselves as independent "trusts" or remaining as "directly managed units" (DMUs) (an option not foreseen by Enthoven, but consistent with reforms in the education arena). Both trusts and DMUs would receive their funding by contracting with DHAs to provide services, but DMUs were more constrained in personnel and financial matters.[6]

The White Paper included another dimension of the purchaser–provider split, which derived from a policy option not contemplated by Enthoven,[7] but mooted by the Office of Health Economics, and particularly by the British health economist Alan Maynard (Butler 1992: 30; Klein 1995: 190). This was the concept of general practitioner "fundholding," under which general practitioners would be given a budget for the purchase of a range of hospital and community services for their patients, as well as for the provision of their own primary care services. This provision was added almost as an afterthought; but, as we shall see in chapter 6, it came to constitute a major feature of the system.

In summary, then, a rare window of opportunity for structural and institutional policy change in the British health care arena opened when a government in its third majority term, with the consolidated authority to make such changes, also formed the will to take the political risks of doing so. That window opened at a time when the dominant set of policy ideas about structural and institutional change in the British health care arena revolved around concepts of an "internal market." Without a specific reform agenda, it was that set of ideas upon which the NHS review seized.

The NHS review developed only a framework for reform. The implementation of its recommendations was very much shaped and incorporated by the characteristics of the existing system. Toward the end of the 1990s, moreover, another major episode of policy change in the British health care arena did not appear to be imminent. The massive Labour victory in the May 1997 election, winning a majority surpassing that of its 1945 landslide,[8] certainly gave the Labour government the consolidated authority to make major policy changes. But a sweeping reversal of the policy parameters of the internal market did not accord well with the broader prudent, centrist, "New Labour" agenda of the government, despite the party's early denunciation of the reforms when in opposition. Instead, Labour moved only to smooth the rough edges of the reforms that most offended its sense of equity. The health care system, having incorporated the internal market reforms, would await another rare confluence of political circumstances before major policy change would occur again.

## The United States

The adoption of Medicare and Medicaid, as discussed in chapter 2, was part of an incremental strategy of policy development. These programs admittedly constituted dramatically large increments of change. But they did not go all the way to universal health insurance; rather they were seen by their Democratic progenitors as major steps in that direction. In the wake of the adoption of these programs, policy development continued to be incremental, but the nature of this incrementalism was, to use Lindblom's (1966) classic phrase, remarkably "disjointed." The sense that incremental policy actions could lead progressively to a comprehensive and coherent program was less and less possible to sustain as attempts to achieve a national health insurance program failed in 1974 and again under the Carter administration in the late 1970s. Rather, coalitions similar in kind to that which had coalesced around the Hill–Burton bill in the 1940s, composed of those who sought progressive increments of change as well as those who would go "this far and no farther," began to form around a variety of policy initiatives. And the ground, meanwhile, was shifting under the feet of policy-makers.

### *The failure of national health insurance proposals in the 1970s and 1980s*

By the mid-1970s, the delivery system in the United States was beginning to be transformed as the logic of the mixed market system played itself out. In the absence of national health insurance, as will be further discussed in chapter 5, public policy elaborated both categorical programs and regulatory constraints. The resulting complexity gave a competitive advantage to providers with the resources to invest in understanding the system and responding strategically. Public policy thus fostered organizational change not only directly (as in the case of Health Maintenance Organizations which were fostered by regulatory legislation enacted in 1973) but also indirectly (as in the case of large multi-institutional chains, many of them for-profit, which sprang up in response to the increasing complexity of the system).

In recognition of this increasing organizational diversity, particularly the role of large corporate entities on the supply and the demand side of the U.S. market, members of the American health care policy community began to turn increasingly to models of reform based on market principles rather than a profession–state accommodation. This meant that the policy landscape on which windows of opportunity for structural and institutional reform might open was quite different in the 1970s than it had been in the 1960s. The incremental expansion of Medicare envisioned in the 1960s fit less well with the changed context of the 1970s.

In 1973–1974, a window appeared about to open. With a Democratically controlled Congress, and a weakened Republican president, consolidated authority might have been mustered around a bipartisan compromise. Key Democratic leaders were strongly committed to achieving universal coverage. By that time, the employer-based system of private insurance had become sufficiently entrenched that any compromise would have had to incorporate a significant role for such a system. Proposals developed by the Nixon administration and by powerful Democrats Senator Ted Kennedy and Representative Wilbur Mills were based on mandated employer-based insurance supplemented by a government plan. But the possibility of compromise was doomed by divisions within the Democratic party regarding the extent of acceptable deviance from a model of expanding Medicare to the population as a whole—especially since it appeared that Democrats might have a "veto-proof" Congress after the 1974 congressional elections (or indeed control the White House as well as Congress after the 1976 presidential and congressional elections) and hence have the consolidated authority to act without engaging in bipartisan compromise (Starr 1982: 403–4).

This expectation appeared to be borne out in 1976. The elections of that year gave the Democrats control of the White House and substantial majorities in both houses of Congress. Jimmy Carter, moreover, had committed himself to national health insurance in his presidential campaign. But again, none of the competing Democratic proposals dominated. By this time, the various regulatory initiatives of the Nixon years, and the responses to them, had spawned further organizational diversity and complexity. A number of "procompetitive" proposals for reform sought to harness this diversity to increase efficiency and expand access. Alain Enthoven, for example, developed the model of a Consumer Choice Health Plan (CCHP) (Enthoven 1978), based on regulated competition among organized health plans such as HMOs, a model that was considered, but not ultimately endorsed, by the Carter administration (Hacker 1997: 47–48). These procompetitive proposals were vulnerable to criticisms that they failed to deal sufficiently with the imperfections of the health care and health insurance markets, particularly with the lack of sophistication on the demand side (Marmor et al. 1983). More telling from a political perspective were the intraparty rivalries to which the competing proposals eventually fell victim (Kingdon 1984: 167–70, 179–80; Starr 1982: 411–14). Once again, as in the early 1970s, no set of political actors had the consolidated authority necessary to weld the various "factions," each convinced that its proposal was most appropriate to the increasingly complex American health care system, into a coherent coalition for reform (Marmor with Goldberg 1994: 8). This was a grim foreboding of what was to unfold in the 1990s.

In the meantime, however, the election of Ronald Reagan as president in 1980 effectively removed the issue of national health insurance from the political agenda for more than a decade. But, as we shall see in chapter 5, the Reagan administration took one of the most consequential decisions in the history of governmental health insurance in the United States when it introduced a system of "prospective payment" for hospitals under Medicare as a

cost-containment measure in 1983. This decision was to have broad reverbera-
tions, as a rising price sensitivity among purchasers and cost-consciousness
among providers swept through the system. While the Republicans may have
ignored the issue of national health insurance throughout most of the 1980s,
their policies in the health care arena fueled fundamental changes in the context in which the issue would next be considered.

The issue of national health insurance emerged briefly again in the presidential election of 1988. The Democratic candidate, Michael Dukakis, had as
governor of Massachusetts introduced a "play or pay" plan for governmental
health insurance, under which employers were required to provide health insurance for their employees or pay a surcharge on their payroll taxes, a plan
which was to take effect in 1992 (but was subsequently delayed indefinitely).
Dukakis touted this accomplishment during his unsuccessful presidential campaign, but polls suggested that it did not resonate strongly with voters (Skocpol
1996: 23). The Medicare Catastrophic Coverage Act, adopted with bipartisan
support in 1988, was similarly ill-fated. Its provisions to increase Medicare coverage for catastrophic illness (and accordingly to increase premiums on a progressive income-related scale) were repealed a year later in a storm of protest
from upper-income beneficiaries. Furthermore, a bipartisan commission established by the act recommended, by a bare majority, a "play-or-pay" approach to
universal health insurance, but the commission was debilitated by internal disagreements that led to dissenting reports from members on both the left and
the right (Skocpol 1996: 34; Hacker 1997: 23).

In the early 1990s, however, the issue of national health insurance began to
reemerge on the political agenda. Health care costs had continued to escalate
through the 1980s: by 1990, total health care expenditure in the United States
amounted to almost 14% of the GDP, the highest in the OECD and far above
the 8% to 10% range in which most other OECD nations clustered. In the
multipayer U.S. system, the diffusion of costs meant that this cost escalation was
not registered politically with the immediacy that might have been the case in
systems in which costs were more concentrated. Nonetheless, over the course
of the 1980s, employer groups began increasingly to mobilize around the issue
of health care reform in response to the rising costs of employee health benefits (Bergthold 1990). Over the same period, moreover, the number of Americans who at least for some period of time found themselves without insurance
coverage relentlessly increased (Starr 1991: 17–19). It was only with the economic downturn of 1990–1991, however, that public concern about the health
care system began to escalate. As Hacker (1997: 19) notes:

> By promoting a sense of economic insecurity, the recession heightened the
> public anxiety about the escalating costs of medical care and the fragility of
> employer-based health insurance. Moreover, the recession was harder on white-
> collar and professional workers than were other recent economic downturns,
> forcing many middle-income Americans who had taken their personal health
> care arrangements for granted to face the prospect of losing their health insur-
> ance or having their coverage cut back.

This growing anxiety was translated onto the political agenda by the "focusing event" of the 1991 senatorial election in Pennsylvania, occasioned by the death of the incumbent.[9] Harris Wofford, a long-shot Democratic candidate, ran against a close associate of President George Bush, Richard Thornburgh, who before contesting the election had been attorney general in the Bush cabinet. Wofford stumbled across the health care issue in the course of his campaign, when a television spot focused on the issue appeared to catch fire with the public (Skocpol 1996: 27; Wofford 1995). Wofford's subsequent surprise victory, by a margin of 10%, was attributed in large part to his embrace of the issue of national health insurance (despite the fact that he had not advocated any particular approach); in Skocpol's phrase it was "an election heard around the nation" (Skocpol 1996: 28). It guaranteed that Democratic aspirants to the party's nomination for president would be attentive to the issue of health care.

### The Clinton campaign and health care reform

The story of the espousal of national health insurance by all Democratic candidates in the 1992 presidential election, most particularly Bill Clinton, and the subsequent development and defeat of President Clinton's proposals for health care reform, has been told by a number of astute observers,[10] and I do not intend to retell it here. What I wish to do is to place the Clinton episode in historical and cross-national perspective, and to make two arguments supportive of the broader thesis of this book: first, that the policy option chosen by Clinton was a product of its historical moment, a moment prepared by previous policy decisions; and, second, that the conditions for creating a window of opportunity for major structural and institutional policy change in the U.S. health care arena of the early 1990s, if they ever truly existed, were extremely precarious and vulnerable to strategic misjudgments.

Let us consider the first of these arguments. At the beginning of the 1990s the range of policy options for health care reform being advocated in the political arena was essentially defined by variants of the alternatives that had been considered since the 1970s, as well as those that had been evolving in response to the rapidly changing health care and health insurance markets. As we shall see in chapter 5, the incentives within a system dominated by private finance, in which the state nonetheless played a large fiscal and regulatory role, had led actors to cost-shifting and risk-shedding strategies that were driving waves of organizational and financial change. The markets for health care and for health insurance were merging as "managed care" entities sprang up to organize risk. Both the demand and the supply sides of these markets were coming increasingly to be characterized by large and sophisticated corporations and corporate networks. The pattern of mobilization for political action was in rapid flux as well.

In this context, at least four types of policy options, each with an associated group of supporters, could be identified in the health policy arena of the early 1990s: (1) a "single-payer" plan (essentially an extension of Medicare); (2) incremental reforms of the health insurance market; (3) a system of "play or pay" employer mandates supplemented in various ways by governmental programs; and (4) some form of "managed competition" on the model suggested by Enthoven in the late 1970s, updated to capitalize upon the growing sophistication and level of organization on the demand side of the health care and health insurance markets. None of these options had been able to command a minimum winning coalition of support, and no durable compromise had been found.

The time was ripe, then, for coalescence around a reform idea that could bridge the prevailing options and be responsive to the economic and political transformation of the health care arena. It would need to provide a path to universal coverage. It would need to be consistent with the rapidly evolving structures of health care delivery and finance. And, because this was the 1990s and not the 1960s, it would have to be both fiscally prudent and responsive to the growing concern among employers about the escalating costs of employee health benefit plans.

Just as the review of the NHS in Britain had gravitated toward the ideas of Alain Enthoven (whose "internal market" model of competition under a budget, tailored to the British context, promised to combine the advantages of the market with those of public finance), so it was Enthoven again whose ideas suggested a bridge to compromise in the early 1990s in the United States. His model of "managed competition," which had been relatively peripheral to the policy debate at the beginning of the 1990s, soon came to assume central importance (Hacker 1997). Not only was it consonant with the evolving organization of the health care arena, but it also resonated with the "New Democrat" approach to policy favored by Clinton: it would "harness market forces to achieve the liberal ideal of universal coverage" (Hacker 1997: 112).

The consonance of the concept of "managed competition" with the evolving economic and political characteristics of the health care arena will become fully apparent only in the context of the description of that evolution in chapter 5. Here, however, the point to be made is that "managed competition" provided a loose rubric under which key actors could seek to reach a compromise. The concept was a loosely defined and evolving one—characteristics that increased its initial appeal but also provided the seeds of potential failure. In the early 1990s it was most closely identified with a group of large insurance and managed-care firms, later joined by the Washington Business Group on Health (a creature of the Business Roundtable, a major big-business lobby), which came to be known as the Jackson Hole Group (JHG). The JHG coalesced around the work of InterStudy, a health policy think tank that had been founded by Paul Ellwood, a physician long active in the HMO arena, in the early 1970s, and took its name from the location of InterStudy's meetings at Jackson Hole, Wyoming. The JHG was formally incorporated as a separate not-for-profit organization in 1992 to pursue policy advocacy as distinct from InterStudy's research focus (Ramsay 1995: 251).

The JHG version of managed competition was based upon Enthoven's work, although the concept changed as it evolved through discussions, and not all participants in the JHG subscribed to its every element. Criticisms of

Enthoven's model in the 1970s had revolved around two concerns: the organized health plans on which it was premised were not prevalent enough to provide a basis for systemwide reform, and the model made unrealistic assumptions
about the level of sophistication and organization among the consumers who
would be selecting among the plans. In the ensuing period, the rapid diffusion
of "managed care" health plans blunted the first criticism, and the rise of purchaser coalitions and Enthoven's own elaboration of his model addressed the
second. Crucially, he developed the concept of an organized purchasing entity
termed a "sponsor." Essentially, then, the managed competition model was
based upon competing health plans and organized sponsors. The JHG assumed
that large employers, alone or in voluntary cooperation with each other, already
possessed sufficient market power on the demand side. For small employers and
individuals, Health Insurance Purchasing Cooperatives would be established.
Employers would be required to offer their employees a choice of plans, and
the employer contribution would be limited to a given percentage of the premium for the average plan in order to give individual employees a price incentive in their selection of plans.[11] Employer contributions above this limit
would not be tax deductible. In the ensuing competition, the JHG believed that
managed-care plans offering comprehensive care to defined populations for a
set annual fee would soon defeat traditional fee-for-service indemnity-based
plans. To prevent insurers from risk-shedding and other destructive behavior,
"The rules of competition must be designed and administered so as not to reward health plans for selecting good risks, segmenting markets, or otherwise defeating the goals of managed competition" (Enthoven 1993).

The JHG proposal was not the only interpretation of "managed competition" on the policy horizon in the early 1990s. A "liberal synthesis"—associated
with liberal Democrats such as California Insurance Commissioner John
Garamedi, Princeton sociologist Paul Starr, and Senators Bob Kerrey, Harris
Wofford, and Tom Daschle—offered a version that incorporated elements of a
"single-payer" model: it would establish purchasing cooperatives that would
cover the entire population of a region (not just those who were not employed
in large firms, as in the JHG proposal) and would operate under a fixed global
budget (Hacker 1997: 76–99). These were major differences from the JHG
model, and at least two elements of the liberal synthesis—the severing of the
link between health insurance and employment status, and the concept of the
global budget—were anathema to the JHG.

The JHG proposal and the "liberal synthesis" did not exhaust the range of
variation in approaches to "managed competition": they might better be
thought of as two modes around which various options clustered. Indeed, as
Marmor and Goldberg said in reviewing various proposals for managed competition, "a lot of suits can go with that tie" (Marmor with Goldberg 1994: 13).
The very malleability of the concept added to its attractiveness as a platform for
compromise. And it was, after all, malleable around a central core that seemed to
catch the wave of the future. "Managed competition" represented an extension
of the model that was increasingly coming to characterize the relationships between large business purchasers and managed care organizations. Indeed, the

federal government, as a very large employer, was a major participant in a managed competition regime. Under the Federal Employees Health Benefits Program (FEHBP), the federal government acted as "sponsor," negotiating coverage with a variety of plans which it then offered as options to its employees. The FEHBP itself was to be held up as a model for reform later in the debate (Peterson 1995: 101).

In August 1992, Democratic presidential candidate Bill Clinton embraced the rubric of managed competition as the framework within which his health care reform package would be developed. The approach appealed strongly to Clinton's "political ideology and political instinct" (Hacker 1997: 112). As governor of Arkansas, Clinton had headed the Democratic Leadership Council, a group of southern Democrats who advocated "centrist" policy positions. Managed competition recommended itself to Clinton as a fresh, forward-looking approach that could appeal to both liberals and conservatives within the Democratic party, and as sufficiently undeveloped that it allowed for a process of compromise and negotiation to flesh it out. With Clinton's electoral victory in November 1992, the road ahead appeared open to just such a process.

### The failure of the Clinton proposal

And yet, two years almost to the day after candidate Clinton had presented his ideas about a managed-competition-based health reform plan, his ambitious attempt to follow through on this promise had been resoundingly defeated.[12] If the idea of managed competition as the way to national health insurance was a product of its time, and was enthusiastically embraced by a newly elected president whose party controlled both houses of Congress, why did the subsequent health reform initiative fail? Various factors—institutional barriers, interest-group mobilization, public opinion, strategic miscalculations—have been adduced to explain this failure, and these explanations will be considered in historical and comparative context in chapter 4. Indeed all of these factors played a role. But they were able to do so precisely because one of the conditions for major policy change in health care—the ability of a set of political actors to mobilize authority on an extraordinary scale—was, if not lacking, at least extremely precarious.

Clinton entered the presidency having been elected in a three-way race with 43% of the popular vote, not a strong popular mandate for an American president. Like Jimmy Carter in the late 1970s, Clinton was the governor of a small southern state who had been elected president as an outsider and had no experience of gaining cooperation with Congress. And his party's control of the Senate fell short of the 60% necessary to prevent procedural delaying tactics by Republicans. These circumstances contrast sharply with those that prevailed in the last episode of structural and institutional reform in the U.S. health care arena in the Johnson era of the 1960s.

These circumstances meant that there were essentially two types of strategies for success in achieving health care reform. One was to build bipartisan support. But such a strategy was dubious for a number of reasons. Clinton had identified himself and his party so strongly with the issue of health care reform—and with the "managed competition" approach—that there was a strong partisan incentive for Republicans to deny him victory. As Allen Schick (1995) has demonstrated, bipartisan initiatives are more prevalent in periods of divided government (when both sides can claim credit) than in periods in which one party controls the presidency and Congress (250–51). Furthermore, the bitter taste of the last acrimonious attempt to reach a bipartisan compromise in health care—the Bipartisan Commission of the late 1980s—still lingered in the capitol.

There was no doubt, however, that a degree of Republican cooperation would be necessary if health care reform were to be achieved. With less than 60% of the Senate, the Democrats could not prevent a Republican filibuster.[13] The second, and more promising, type of strategy would be to create a "bandwagon effect" (Kingdon 1984: 167–70), a sense that the reform was inevitable and that those who sought to have any influence or to claim any credit should climb aboard. For a time, it appeared that just such an effect was building (Skocpol 1996: 55). Consider the following journalistic assessment in February 1993, soon after Clinton's inauguration:

> The momentum behind some kind of federal reform to America's health system now seems unstoppable. The state governors clamored for it just this week in Washington. Sensing change, the country's most implacable health lobbies promise to become more compliant. Doctors joke that, one way or another, their glory days will soon be over. Even insurance companies are starting to sound altruistic: the powerful Health Insurance Association of America recently dropped its knee-jerk opposition to managed competition. Yet so many conflicting interests in health care remain that reform could still founder upon indecision. Cutting through that tangle is what presidents are for. (*The Economist,* February 6, 1993: 26)

Instead of building upon this momentum, however, the Clinton administration held off on health care for a crucial eight-month period. Like the Thatcher government in Britain five years earlier, the Clinton administration needed to develop a more fully fledged proposal to introduce into the legislative process. (Clinton, however, at least had the advantage of having identified the general approach he wished to take.) Like Thatcher, Clinton established a working group to develop a proposal for reform. The president did not chair the group himself, as Thatcher had done, but he did the next best thing—he appointed his wife, Hillary Rodham Clinton, as chair. Like the British working group, the Clinton group worked behind closed doors, adopting a selective and informal (albeit more extensive) approach to consultation. As in the British case, this closely held process confused and alienated a number of interest groups and journalists accustomed to closer involvement and more open access.

It is remarkable that two political leaders with very different styles, in very different partisan and institutional contexts, should have chosen relatively similar processes for developing their health care reform proposals. They were both, however, working within a similar overall universe of ideas (as evidenced by their common intellectual debt to Alain Enthoven). This was a universe of ideas that emphasized the self-interest of the various actors in the system, which could be harnessed through market and quasimarket mechanisms, as opposed to the emphasis on collaboration and accommodation upon which previous systems of public finance had been based.[14] Not surprisingly, that perspective translated into a distrust of the motives of the actors in the political arena, and a sense that the proponents of reform had to sequester themselves to think through the approach to be taken before entering the political fray.

The American group differed from the British in two important respects, however. Around the official twelve-person "task force" of senior administrative officials, chaired by Mrs. Clinton, was an "advisory group" of policy experts, congressional staff members, and administrative officials—a plastic creature that grew at its peak to more than 500 members (Hacker 1997: 122). And its size was matched by the complexity of its product. The NHS review had produced a framework for reform, which would be filled in during the process of implementation. The Clinton task force produced a detailed blueprint. In seeking a proposal that would score well on "goodness of fit" with the American system and hence would have a good chance of being implemented, the task force devised a model that mapped onto the complexity of the existing system. As such, it was itself dauntingly complex and difficult to sell.

Perhaps there was effectively no alternative. Harris Wofford later argued that the administration believed that the details of the plan had to be specified as much as possible at the outset and embedded in statutory legislation so that the implementation of the plan would not be dragged out interminably through the lengthy regulation-making process of the U.S. system. There was also a sense among Democrats that this was a "chance in a lifetime" for comprehensive reform; therefore everything needed to be specified and nothing left to the process of incrementalism that had proved so frustrating to reformers in the past (Wofford 1995). Perhaps an embrace of a different approach to national health insurance, such as the "play or pay" or "single payer" models, would have stood a greater chance of success. These are "hypothetical counterfactual" questions that can never be resolved. What is clear is that Clinton's rejection of these options—each of which would have substantially expanded the fiscal scope of the state—and his embrace of an approach that would harness market forces to public policy goals and that built on the evolving characteristics of the health care and health insurance systems, was an entirely understandable position for an American president with a "New Democrat" agenda in the early 1990s. Just as had been the case in other episodes of major policy change in the health field in the United States and elsewhere, the choice was shaped by the current state of the health care arena and by the broader political agenda of the government of the day.

The task force had essentially completed its work by May 1993, although key questions relating to the financing of the scheme remained to be resolved. An even more closed and tightly held process to deal with these issues was continued through the summer. But further action was delayed by the need for the president to address the mounting crisis over his budgetary proposals (Skocpol 1996: 59–60). Ultimately, the budgetary package squeaked through by the narrowest of majorities—a one-vote margin each in the House and the Senate, with the vice president casting the deciding vote in the Senate. No Republican in either house voted for the legislation (a complete partisan rejection of major legislation unprecedented in postwar American history); and forty-one Democratic Representatives and six Democratic Senators opposed it (National Academy of Social Insurance 1993). It was a dramatic demonstration of Clinton's limited political capital. With such limited capital, he could not invest it simultaneously in two areas as central to his presidency as his first budget and health care reform. The precariousness of the conditions for major health care reform were becoming more apparent.

The delay in introducing health care reform legislation had been costly in terms of lost momentum and lost potential for a bandwagon effect. Nonetheless, some momentum appeared to be recovered when the president announced the outline of his proposals in a joint address to both houses of Congress on September 22, 1993, and subsequently introduced the draft legislation, the Health Security bill, in October. The bill itself, more than 1,000 pages long, defies brief summary. Behind each of its features lay a complex set of technical and political considerations (Hacker 1997: 122–29). If the imperfect health care services and insurance markets were to be tamed but not supplanted, an intricate web of incentives had to be taken into account and the strategic responses of various actors had to be anticipated and channeled through myriad design details.

Central to the plan were two demand-side features: employer mandates and regional purchasing alliances. The requirement that employers provide health insurance to their employees through participation in the plan provided both the major source of finance and much of the regulatory framework. The system was to be financed largely through premiums; employers would be required to contribute an amount per worker equal to 80% of the average premium in their region. Employees would pay 20% of the premium, plus any copayments or deductibles. Employers with more than 5,000 employees could fulfill their mandate independently, by offering their employees a choice of health plans within a federal regulatory framework.

All other employers, as well as individuals, would participate in the plan through regional purchasing alliances, established by each state, which would negotiate with a variety of state-certified health care plans to provide a range of options, each with open enrollment. All insurers and health plans were required to offer a common package of basic benefits, although they were free to supplement the packages on offer as they chose. The system was premised on the ability of large risk pools and the purchasing power of regional alliances to hold down health plan charges. As a backup, however, the entire system was to be overseen by a seven-member National Health Board, appointed by the president, which would monitor the system, establish national and regional budget targets, and impose caps on premiums if costs to purchasers exceeded those targets. While financed largely through premiums, the system also required additional federal subsidies for small businesses and low-income individuals, to be financed through a tax on tobacco and other mechanisms left unresolved. Medicare and Medicaid programs would be articulated with the system: states would have the option of allowing Medicare recipients to transfer their entitlements to obtain equal or better coverage through a regional alliance. Federal and state Medicaid contributions would flow to the alliances, and persons eligible for Medicaid could choose any plan with a premium at or below the regional average.

As Theda Skocpol has demonstrated, public support for Clinton's approach to health care reform, which registered at over 70% in the spring of 1993, still stood at almost 60% immediately after Clinton's September speech. But the complexity of the plan presented an enormous challenge of communication. And Clinton was diverted again by the necessity to garner Congressional support for the North American Free Trade Agreement before a December 31, 1993, deadline—further evidence of his husbanding of his limited political capital. Within three to five months of his September speech, the momentum toward health care reform appeared to be irretrievably lost (Skocpol 1996: 55, 74–75). The bandwagon effect never materialized. Instead of a flurry of attempts to make proposals that would secure their proponents a place at the inevitable table of political compromise around Clinton's proposal (a typical bandwagon effect), what ensued was a competitive frenzy to produce alternatives to the Clinton plan. Indeed, Clinton's own signaling of a willingness to compromise on details of his proposal appeared to be read less as an invitation to join the bandwagon than as an admission of the political weakness of his position.

A strong bandwagon effect would have been essential to counter the "hyperpluralism" of the health care arena (Schick 1995)—a political reflection of the organizational changes that had been driven by the relentless logic of the American mixed-market system (described in chapter 5). In this important sense, the roots of the failure to adopt universal national health insurance in the 1990s go back to the failure to do so in the 1960s. The transformation of the American health care arena since the passage of Medicare and Medicaid in the 1960s was reflected in the pattern of political mobilization. Of the 121 major interest groups active in the health care arena at the federal level in 1992 profiled by Ramsay and his colleagues (1995),[15] 41% were established after 1965 (table 3.1). Proportionately, the greatest expansion in group numbers occurred among groups representing organizations involved in the delivery or private financing of health care [such as the American Association of Preferred Provider Organizations (established in 1983), the American Managed Care and Review Association (established in 1971), and the Federation of American Health Systems (established in 1966)]; among business groups representing health care purchasers [such as the Employers' Council on Flexible Compensation (established in 1981) and the Washington Business Group on Health (established in 1974)]; among consumer advocacy groups [such as Families USA (established in 1981) and the National Women's Health Network (established in 1976)]; and among a variety of think tanks and research institutes occupying various positions among the ideological spectrum [such as the Cato Institute (established in 1977), the Heritage Foundation (established in 1973), the As-

TABLE 3.1 Major Interest Groups Active in Federal Health Care Arena in 1992: Percent Established after 1965, by Category of Interest

| Category | N | % Established after 1965 |
|---|---|---|
| Professionals | 31 | 23 |
| Delivery and/or financing organizations | 26 | 46 |
| Government | 5 | 0 |
| Business | 9 | 56 |
| Consumer[a] | 33 | 45 |
| Research | 17 | 59 |
| Total | 121 | 41 |

*Source:* Compiled from Ramsay (1995). The categorization of groups is my own.

[a] This category includes a variety of disease-specific advocacy groups such as the American Cancer Society and the American Heart Association.

sociation for Health Services Research (established in 1981), and InterStudy (established in 1973)]. In comparison, there were relatively fewer new organizations representing health care professionals and government agencies. New health professional organizations grew up to represent emerging health disciplines [such as the American Academy of Physician Assistants (established in 1968)] or to press a particular set of issues or policy approach [such as Physicians for a National Health Program (established in 1986)]. None of the groups representing government actors, such as the Association of State and Territorial Health Officials (established in 1942), was established after 1965.

The complexity of the pattern of political mobilization in the health care arena was increased not only by the emergence of new groups but also by the fracturing of consensus within and alliances between established groups. Mark Peterson (1993) has described the representational structure of the health care arena as evolving from a "block" structure (a "mutually supportive stakeholder alliance among doctors, hospitals, insurance companies, and business in favor of maintaining the status quo") in the 1940s and 1950s, through a "dyadic" structure in which the dominant alliance was challenged by emerging (largely consumer-oriented) groups in the 1960s and 1970s, to a heterogeneous network of competitive groups with the breakdown of the dominant alliance and the rise of increasing numbers of challengers in the 1980s and 1990s. As noted, Allen Schick (1995) has similarly characterized the arena of the 1990s as marked by "hyperpluralism"—a "fissionlike process [in which] fissures have opened up within broad-based groups that have become transformed into 'federations' of constituencies that no longer see eye to eye on many of the issues that originally united them" (238). This "hyperpluralism," moreover, was reflected not only in partisan differences in Congress but in divisions within the Democratic party itself. Once again, internal divisions hobbled the party in its quest for health care reform—although now the divisions had less to do with the existence of a solid conservative southern bloc than with a mirroring within the party of the fractured interests in the health care arena (Skocpol 1996: 100).

The dynamics of this process of fission and the incentives underlying it are further explored in chapter 5. It is important here, however, to highlight two important groups whose refusal to embrace the Clinton plan at least as a platform for compromise ultimately sealed its fate. One was the group of large health plans and health insurers that had coalesced around the Jackson Hole Group's proposals. Clinton's plan, largely because it attempted to address problems left unresolved by the JHG (notably a mechanism of financing that would yield universal coverage) was more ambitious than that proposed by the JHG. And as the differences between the plans were explored and ambiguous provisions made more explicit, the task of holding a coalition of support together became increasingly difficult.

Central to these difficulties was the issue of an "employer mandate." The JHG never achieved full consensus on it, although some of its publications proposed employer mandates at least as options to be considered. Enthoven himself supported the concept in the 1980s and early 1990s but reversed himself in 1993 on the grounds that "I am now aware of many problems and deficiencies in the employer mandate that I did not see clearly four years ago" (Enthoven 1994: 134). And as already noted, Clinton's proposals for cost containment differed sharply from the JHG's proposal for a "tax cap" on the amount of their health insurance contribution that employers could deduct for tax purposes, as an incentive to seek economical plans. The promising nexus between the JHG plan and the Clinton proposal was broken.

The second major defector from a potential coalition of support for the Clinton plan was the large business community. For a time, it appeared that big business, concerned about the rising costs of employee benefit plans and eager to find mechanisms of cost control and to level the playing field by requiring all employers to bear their share of the burden of health care costs, would be a major ally in the push for national health insurance (Martin 1993; Peterson 1993; Bergthold 1990). But in the end "big business was the big no-show in the health care reform saga" (Martin 1995: 432). This defection reflected a number of factors including internal divisions over the issue of employer mandates and general concern about the scope of the regional purchasing alliances. Big business's hesitation to support the Clinton proposal in the fall of 1993, moreover, meant that over time the proposal became even less attractive as various concessions were made (albeit in vain) to the small business community at the effective expense of large employers (Martin 1995: 433).

Ultimately, then, Clinton could not command the mobilization of authority necessary to enact a program of universal health insurance. His only chance—the possibility that he could act swiftly enough to capitalize on a bandwagon effect—was negated by other crises in his administration. He himself seemed to have recognized the fundamental weakness of his position in an interview in July 1996 with reporters and editors of *The New York Times:*

> I think that [with regard to the health care issue] I overestimated the extent to
> which a person elected with a minority of the votes in an environment that was
> complex, to say the least, could . . . achieve in [sic] a sweeping overhaul of the
> health-care system when no previous President had been able to do it for decades
> and decades, and against the enormous amount of organizational effort and fund-
> ing that was spent to convince the American people of something that was not
> accurate—namely that we wanted to take over the health-care system or that we
> wanted to regulate it with a cumbersome bureaucracy. . . . (*The New York Times,*
> July 30, 1996: A8)

As the momentum behind the Clinton proposal slowed to a halt, a gaggle of
competing proposals was elaborated, each attempting to develop the impetus to
break from the pack. But all had their weaknesses. The "single-payer" proposals
were born out of time: they fit ill with the fiscal conservatism of the 1990s—
even if they seemed to promise cost control overall, they would dramatically
increase the public share. The proposals, like those of the Jackson Hole Group,
that attempted to work within the complexity of the existing system, fell victim to the same dynamic that defeated the Clinton proposal: a dynamic of escalating complexity arising from the need to anticipate behavior within a web of
incentives. As each was modeled by the Congressional Budget Office, none was
able to demonstrate the effects that it purported to be able to achieve.[16]

On September 26, 1994, Senate Majority Leader George Mitchell announced that he was unable to find the sixty Senate votes necessary to prevent
a Republican filibuster of Democratic reform initiatives, and that health care
reform was therefore effectively dead for the current Congressional session.
With this demise, and with the subsequent Republican capture of both houses
of Congress in November 1994, the issue of comprehensive universal health
insurance was swept from the political agenda, to be replaced by a return to incrementalism. At the very end of the 104th Congress (1995–1996), a flurry
of bipartisan activity included the passage of a health care bill sponsored by
Democratic Senator Ted Kennedy and Republican Senator Nancy Kassebaum,
adopting regulatory measures to require health insurers to cover workers who
changed jobs, or who had exhausted their already existing entitlements under
federal legislation to coverage for a specified period upon leaving a job.[17]
(Regulation of premiums for this coverage, however, was left to occur under
state authority, if at all.) To ensure Republican support, the Kennedy–
Kassebaum bill also provided for pilot projects to test the feasibility of Retirement Savings Accounts as a private alternative to Medicare. With the reelection
of Clinton and the retention of Republican control of Congress in the November 1996 elections, the period of divided government was extended. In the
ensuing 105th Congress, attention to health care issues focused on incremental
reforms to Medicare, proposals for federal subsidies for health insurance coverage for poor children, and increased regulation of managed care plans (Iglehart
1997). Budget legislation in 1997 provided for a modest increase in Medicare
premiums and a few additions to covered services, as well as $20.3 billion over
five years in federal transfers to the states to provide coverage for currently
uninsured children, to be financed largely through increased tobacco taxes.

Meanwhile, the turbulent transformation of the U.S. health care services and insurance market continued apace, as will be further discussed in chapter 5. If and when a future window of opportunity for major change in health policy opens, it will open on a landscape shaped by this process, and the policy options considered will be shaped accordingly. The fate of those options will depend primarily on factors not within the health care arena itself, but in the broader political arena. Major structural and institutional change in health care policy will have to await the advent either of an era of broad bipartisan cooperation or of a massive partisan mandate that gives a party committed to such reform control of the White House and supermajorities in Congress.[18]

### Developments at the state level

The American states themselves were also the sites of considerable policy activity in the early 1990s (Leichter 1992; Rogal and Helms 1993; Chisman et al. 1994; Holahan et al. 1995b).[19] Although some of this activity preceded the Clinton reform effort, much of it was shaped by the anticipation of reform at the federal level. As the attempt to adopt comprehensive health care reform at the federal level from 1992 to 1994 focused attention on the issue, and then failed spectacularly, state-level attempts at reform were thrown into increasing prominence. Numerous commentators debated whether the political systems or the capacity of the states would allow them to play a classic "laboratory" role within the federation in developing innovative approaches to health care reform (Rich and White 1996; Leichter 1997; Sparer 1998).[20]

State-level experimentation occurred, however, within a fairly tight range of variation. Essentially, state-level health care reforms involved (1) different types and degrees of insurance regulation; (2) various extensions of the scope of coverage for low-income individuals, including expansions of Medicaid; and (3) various mechanisms of cost control within these structures, with a strong emphasis on the use of managed care. No state, through any method, achieved universal coverage.[21] And even in those states that pushed the envelope of American-style health care reform within these parameters, initial proposals were "rolled back" as a result of political change or implementation difficulties.

*Insurance reform*   In the late 1980s and early 1990s numerous states enacted a variety of measures of insurance reform, such as restraints on the use of preexisting conditions limitations, provisions for portability across employers, and various types of community rating. The populations to which these reforms applied varied from the small-group market to the overall insured market (Curtis and Haugh 1994). A number of these reforms were highly contentious, and in several cases proposals for insurance reform were scaled backed or not implemented. In the state of Washington, for example, legislation in 1995 omitted a number of measures set out in 1993 framework legislation but not implemented, including community rating (Crittenden 1995).

*Expansion of coverage to low-income beneficiaries*   Perhaps the most significant dimension of state-level reform was the expansion of coverage for Medicaid recipients and other low-income groups. Various expansions of Medicaid coverage were undertaken, a number of which required various forms of waivers from the federal agency which administered Medicaid, the Health Care Financing Administration (HCFA). The most comprehensive of these reforms were conducted under federal "1115" Medicaid waivers[22] through which the HCFA waived federal eligibility requirements in state Medicaid programs to allow for experimentation with programs that would further the goals of the Medicaid program. As of 1996, demonstration projects were underway in ten states (Rowland and Hanson 1996). One of the requirements for the issuing of a waiver was that the program be revenue-neutral to the federal government. Typically, these programs extended state-subsidized coverage to "low-income" individuals not eligible for Medicaid and relied heavily on managed care mechanisms to control costs. The definition of the "low-income" threshold varied from 100% of the federal poverty level (FPL) in Ohio to 300% of the FPL in Hawaii. Programs also varied in the extent to which other eligibility restrictions applied, and in the income-related sliding scale of premium subsidization (Holahan et al. 1995b). In one case, Oregon, expansion of the population covered was coupled with limitation of benefits, as discussed in chapter 1.

In a number of cases, initial plans for expansion of coverage to low-income beneficiaries were scaled back. In Minnesota, the implementation of the expansion of low-income coverage, like other aspects of the state's plans to achieve universal coverage, was delayed and staged on a more incremental basis than had been envisaged in framework legislation enacted in 1992 (Blewett 1994; HCFA 1995b). In Kentucky, plans to extend state-subsidized coverage to all residents below the FPL under a 1115 waiver approved in 1993 were not implemented (HCFA 1995c). Tennessee, which in 1994 introduced the most dramatic expansion of coverage under a 1115 waiver—offering state-subsidized insurance through managed care to all uninsured residents—encountered severe implementation difficulties and announced a temporary closure of enrollment in the program in 1995 (Gottlieb 1995).

Various proposals advanced in the U.S. Congress in the late 1990s as part of the return to incrementalism in health policy reform promised to provide greater flexibility for states in covering low-income individuals. Most of these proposals also entailed decreased federal contributions. Federal budget legislation in 1997, however, provided $20.3 billion over five years for federal transfers to the states to extend coverage of children under Medicaid and other state programs. Medicaid reform per se remained on the agenda.

Expansions and extensions of Medicaid were not the only measures that states used to increase coverage for low-income beneficiaries. The state of Washington's 1993 legislation, for example, provided for state subsidization of private insurance for low-income beneficiaries under a Basic Health Plan financed through taxes on tobacco, alcohol, insurers, and hospitals—and this provision, unlike some others, was retained in legislation passed in 1995 (Crittenden 1995). Hawaii's 1991 State Health Insurance Plan (SHIP) offered state-subsidized coverage for low-income uninsured and was rolled together with Medicaid under the Health QUEST program under a Section 1115 waiver in 1994.

*Cost control*   The most common instrument of cost control in state health care reform measures was a heavy reliance on managed care. As noted, this was an important instrument for expanding coverage to Medicaid recipients and other low-income beneficiaries. Managed care was also an important component of broader reform plans. The comprehensive plan set out in Minnesota's 1992 framework legislation, for example, centered around the development of managed care entities—Integrated Service Networks (ISNs)—that would provide a benchmark for the regulation of other providers (Blewett 1994). Tennessee offered coverage to all uninsured residents, with a sliding scale of income-related premium subsidization, through its TennCare program of managed care. The state of Washington's 1993 framework legislation included provisions for cost control through a structure of regulated managed care (Crittenden 1995). Each of these attempts at establishing regulated systems of managed care suffered reversals. The implementation of the Minnesota plan was delayed, the managed care framework proposed in Washington was abandoned, and Tennessee encountered major implementation problems.

States also attempted to control costs through other means, such as various forms of rate regulation. Perhaps the most ambitious of these attempts was yet another component of the Minnesota plan: the establishment of annual limits on total health care expenditures, to be accomplished through regulation of health insurance premiums, physician fee schedules, hospital payment rates, and utilization review. These aspects of the Minnesota plan raised enormous information problems, exacerbated by the shielding of self-insuring employers from the reach of state regulators under the federal Employee Retirement Income Security Act (ERISA), to be discussed later. Their implementation was delayed along with other parts of the Minnesota plan (Blewett 1994).

Beyond these three dimensions of reform—insurance reform, expansion of coverage to low-income beneficiaries, and cost control mechanisms—a few states flirted with more sweeping changes, notably employer mandates and single-payer models. Versions of the single-payer model reached various stages of formal consideration in Ohio, Michigan, Oregon, and Vermont, but none was adopted. Proposals for various types of employer mandates did not survive change in the partisan complexion of legislatures or state houses in Massachusetts, Washington, and Minnesota. Only Hawaii, as noted later, pushed the boundaries of the American employer-based insurance system by instituting and maintaining an employer mandate. Otherwise, the pattern of employer-based coverage, in which offer rates and the scope and breadth of benefits declines with the size of business, appeared to be very similar across states (Cantor et al. 1995).

State-level experimentation, in short, involved various permutations and combinations of the common elements of an American model—insurance reform, state supplementation and subsidization of private insurance, and cost control largely through managed care. The range of variation in reforms actually achieved, moreover, was even narrower than the range of variation in reform proposals.

In part, the limited range of variation of state policies was attributable to the constraints of federalism. Perhaps the most notable example was the constraint established by ERISA, which shielded employers that chose to self-insure from the reach of state regulation of health benefits. This provision thwarted New Jersey's attempts to develop an all-payer rating system (Volpp and Siegel 1993), as well as Minnesota's attempts to gather information essential to its proposed system of all-payer regulation (Blewett 1994). The ERISA constraint faced states wishing to institute employer mandates with the choice of attempting to craft a policy that would be proof against an ERISA challenge (as in the case of Massachusetts's 1988 plan and a 1992 proposal by the state of Washington, neither of which was implemented) or seeking an exemption from or amendment to ERISA itself (as in the case of the 1993 Washington proposal and the Oregon proposals of 1989 and 1991). The failure to gain exemption from ERISA doomed attempts to institute employer mandates in Washington and Oregon, and in Washington this failure marked a "turning point" at which support for the broad package of health care reform began markedly to decline (Crittenden 1995). Only in Hawaii had this constraint been at least partially obviated. There, the institution of an employer mandate predated the enactment of ERISA in 1974. Hawaii's employer mandate was successfully challenged in the courts as contravening ERISA in 1983, but state officials were able to persuade Congress to grant Hawaii an exemption from ERISA on the grounds that its employer mandate had predated the federal legislation. Any change to the mandate, however, would require a further exemption (Neubauer 1993). Exemptions from federal legislation were also needed, as already discussed, to allow for state experimentation with some forms of extension or restructuring of Medicaid programs. Such waivers were more forthcoming than was the case under ERISA, but they nonetheless involved lengthy negotiations between federal and state officials.

There is no doubt that such federal legislative provisions constrained state action. But it is worth noting that there was relatively little experimentation at the state level even before the ERISA constraint came into effect. Even in Hawaii, whose employer mandate just predated ERISA, the expectation of the proponents of reform was that the federal government would soon be adopting a national health insurance scheme. According to Neubauer, "Advocates of the bill saw themselves not so much as bold innovators but as anxious to join in what they viewed as an impending national development" (Neubauer 1992: 156). Furthermore, the federal constraints affected only certain policy instruments—most particularly those related to insurance reform. They did not prevent states from adopting, for example, tax-based approaches to reform.

Why did windows of opportunity for sweeping policy change not open up in the 1990s in at least some of the fifty possible locales offered by the American states? We addressed this same question in chapter 2 concerning the immediate postwar period. And just as the failure of broad health policy reform at the federal level in the 1990s has its roots in the incrementalism of the 1960s, so the failure of the states to enact broad policy reforms in the 1990s stems in part from their failure to do so in an earlier era. In chapter 2 I argued that policy legacies had predisposed health care reformers to focus their activities at the federal, not the state, level. When federal action failed or was limited, reformers kept looking for the next federal chance. Because of this, the states fell victim to the same dynamic that increasingly constrained policy action at the federal level, as the logic of the existing system led to a "hyperpluralism" of interests. As at the federal level, the complexities of negotiation among these various interests were exacerbated by the difficulties of holding together the diverse constituencies of some of the negotiators, notably those representing large businesses and the medical profession. Divisions within as well as between these constituencies over a period of protracted negotiation led to the fraying of support for health care reform not only at the federal level, but also to various degrees in states such as Massachusetts (Bergthold 1990: 917), Oregon (Fox and Leichter 1993: 93), Washington (Crittenden 1995: 303), and even Hawaii (Neubauer 1993: 37).[23]

Nonetheless, it did appear in the early 1990s that the political will had been formed and the authority had been mobilized in a number of states to take sweeping reform initiatives—extending in some cases to the proposed adoption of a single-payer model. These initiatives fell victim to two interrelated factors: strategic decisions at the state level, and developments at the federal level. A common strategy at the state level was to focus initially on gaining legislative agreement to a framework of reform, leaving the details to be worked out by a commission, often with a regulatory as well as a policy development mandate. The makeup of these commissions, and the modes of consultation that they adopted, were highlighted by some observers as important factors in determining the subsequent fate of their recommendations. Generally speaking, however, the effect of this methodical strategy, in a context of complex and fragile coalitions of support for health care reform, was to allow time for these coalitions to unravel.[24] And in the 1990s time was the enemy of reform, as the tide of partisan politics turned rapidly against large-scale reform after the failure of the Clinton initiative at the federal level.

Skocpol (1996) has argued that the Clinton initiative was not only defeated by mobilization on the right, but that it actually catalyzed that mobilization by providing an ideal target—a Democratic initiative that could be portrayed as a threatening, complex, "big government" intervention. Undoubtedly the health care reform debate did fuel the "turn against government" that swept the Republicans to their historic Congressional victories in November 1994. And that same tide changed the complexions of state legislatures and, in some cases, governorships—and with them the chances of enacting large-scale health care reform at the state level.

## Canada

In the three decades after the establishment of the federal medicare program (which was fully in place by 1971), the Canadian health care system showed a remarkable structural and institutional stability. No major policy change on the order of the NHS internal market reforms occurred, nor was there even an unsuccessful attempt at major change as occurred in the United States. (And whereas, in the absence of major policy change, the United States saw a market transformation in the health care arena, the organization and finance of health care delivery in Canada was much the same in the 1990s as it was in the 1970s—the most marked difference being a degree of state-led horizontal restructuring in the hospital sector.) The most significant policy episode, the passage of the Canada Health Act in 1984, involved a reinforcement of the principles of medicare. It was an assertion of the role of the state, and within the state the federal government, to further constrain the role of private finance and the entrepreneurial discretion of individual physicians. Despite its high symbolic significance, however, its tangible effects on the operation of the health care system were marginal.

The rest of this section will trace out this policy history in somewhat more detail. And it will begin to develop an argument to explain this relative stability, an argument that will be continued in chapter 7. The stability of the system was in large part the result of the internal logic of the Canadian version single-payer system of national health insurance—central to which was a long-term accommodation between the state and the medical profession. This accommodation was established on terms even more favorable to the medical profession than those of the "implicit bargain" underlying the British NHS. Canadian medicare, as a product of the 1960s and not the 1940s, was established at a more generous funding level and without the organizational changes that accompanied the establishment of the NHS—private, fee-for-service practice continued to be the norm for both specialists and general practitioners.

The logic of the profession–state accommodation that underlies Canadian medicare will be explored at some length in chapter 7. The task of this section is somewhat different: it is to explain why no set of political actors, at either the federal or the provincial level, determined to intervene in the health care arena to make major changes in the policy parameters governing the system. After all, the decision to establish medicare in the first place was not generated by the internal logic of the health care arena; rather, it was part of a broad agenda of social policy change in the arena of federal–provincial relations. But in the three decades after the adoption of medicare, political forces at federal and provincial levels, and in the federal–provincial arena, operated to reinforce the structural and institutional status quo in health care.

### Federal–provincial financial arrangements

The policy of the federal government after the late 1970s was essentially to reduce, on a gradual and unilateral basis, its share of the financing of provincial health insurance programs, while retaining sufficient fiscal leverage to ensure provincial compliance with the five "principles" of medicare: universality, comprehensiveness, access of "uniform terms and conditions," portability, and public administration. The reduction of the federal share occurred over time through the operation of a highly arcane formula, modified over time either through federal–provincial negotiations or unilaterally by the federal government. The reader must bear with some of this arcana to understand the "stealthy" and incremental nature of the reduction in the federal fiscal role.

The process began in 1977 when the Established Programs Financing (EPF) arrangements were adopted through federal–provincial negotiations conducted in the shadow of a threat by the federal government to act unilaterally. The EPF arrangements moved from a shared-cost basis of funding to a block grant system. Federal transfers for health care (and postsecondary education) were divided into two roughly equal components. One was in the form of a cash transfer conditional on the provinces continuing to meet the federal conditions of eligibility. This cash transfer was to be calculated on the basis of one-half of the per capita transfer to the province in 1975–1976, escalated by the rate of increase in nominal GNP and population (not at the rate of actual health care costs). The other "half" of the transfer was unconditional; it took the form of "tax points," essentially the revenue generated by a specified number of percentage points of the income tax yield of the federal basic tax in a given province.[25] This shift to tax points made provinces whose economies grew at a rate less than the GNP less well off in the short term, and transitional payments were provided to ensure that no province was worse off than it would have been had the entire transfer been a cash grant indexed to GNP and population growth.[26] (In addition, in response to concerns that the terms of the federal program provided incentives for the overutilization of hospital services, a per capita grant—initially C$20 to be escalated essentially at the same rate as the total transfer for health insurance—was made for "extended care services" such as home care. No conditions other than the reporting of data were attached to this transfer.)

In the event, the economic downturn of the late 1970s and early 1980s meant that tax points were not as lucrative as had been expected, and "transitional adjustment payments" threatened to become a fixture of the arrangements. In the early 1980s, a change to the transfer formula was made that, while technical and little remarked upon, marked the beginning of a set of structural amendments to the federal–provincial relationship in the health care arena. The change was simply to calculate the *entire transfer* to a given province on the basis of the per capita transfer in the base year, escalated by nominal GNP and population growth. The conditional cash component of this transfer was calculated as the difference between the yield of the tax points and the total provincial entitlement. The conditional component of the transfer, the basis of the federal government's policy leverage, hence became the residual once tax points had done their work, and over time this conditional component could potentially dwindle to the vanishing point.

The federal government still retained considerable financial leverage in the early years of this arrangement. This was nowhere better demonstrated than with the passage of the Canada Health Act in 1984, to be discussed in the next section. Shortly after the passage of the Canada Health Act, however, with the coming to power of the Progressive Conservatives at the federal level in 1984, the change in the federal–provincial balance implicit in the EPF formula revisions was accelerated. The Conservatives constrained the escalation of the total EPF transfers to the provinces—holding them below the rate of increase in nominal GNP from 1986 to 1990 and freezing them from 1990 onward. Since the tax point portion of the transfer continued to grow more or less in line with nominal GNP, the conditional cash transfer portion became correspondingly smaller. It was estimated that in the first decade of the twenty-first century the conditional portion of the federal transfer would disappear entirely (at different rates in different provinces), and with it the federal government's policy leverage over medicare.[27]

On returning to power in 1993, the Liberals continued the process of adjusting transfers to the provinces. In the 1995 budget, driven entirely by a deficit-reduction agenda, the Liberal government consolidated transfers for social assistance with EPF transfers to create a new "Canada Health and Social Transfer" (CHST) and set out a new schedule for the reduction of those transfers over time. Like the former EPF transfer, the CHST was made up of cash and tax point components, and the cash component was conditional on provincial compliance with the Canada Health Act and on the province providing social assistance without a minimum residency requirement (no conditions relating to postsecondary education were specified). The budget set out a schedule of reductions until 1997–1998, and federal–provincial negotiations were to follow on the formula for allocating the transfer across provinces and on a set of national principles regarding the programs covered by the CHST (Courchene 1995: 92–93). Federal–provincial negotiations fell apart almost as soon as they were attempted, however, and the federal government continued to act unilaterally (McCracken 1996). In 1996, the federal government announced that a "cash floor" for CHST transfers would be established at C$11 billion annually for five years beginning in 1998–1999. Then in the course of the 1997 federal election campaign, the prime minister announced that this floor would in fact be established at C$12.5 billion and would be guaranteed at that level indefinitely.

Calculating the effects of these various changes on the fiscal balance between the federal government and the provinces in health care is not straightforward. Perhaps the most clear-cut comparison is the following: total federal transfers for health care (including more than transfers for health insurance) as a proportion of total provincial health spending (including more than health insurance) declined from 40% in 1975 to 33% in 1994. But in 1975, the entire federal contribution was in the form of conditional cash payments. In 1994, about one-half of the federal contribution was in the form of unconditional tax points, which provinces by then considered to be their own-source revenue. Furthermore, about one-quarter of the conditional transfer was for extended care programs, for which the only condition was the reporting of data. From the mid-1970s to the mid-1990s, then, federal fiscal leverage over provincial compliance with the terms of medicare declined from 40% to 12% of total provincial health care expenditures (calculated from Health Canada 1996: tables 2A, 8A). The shift to the CHST secured C$12.5 billion—a total amount equivalent to about one-quarter of total provincial health expenditures (projected as of 1998–1999)—as available for the federal government to enforce the principles of medicare. This in effect increased federal fiscal leverage in the health field while reducing overall federal contributions to provincial budgets for social programs: it represented a decrease by one-third of the federal government's cash transfers for health, postsecondary education, and social assistance over the latter half of the 1990s (Department of Finance 1995: table 4.4).

### The Canada Health Act

Even while reducing its fiscal presence in the health care field over the course of the 1980s and 1990s, then, the federal government maintained its fiscal leverage. And on occasion it used that leverage, largely to defend the boundary between the public and private sectors. The primary example of this defense was the passage of the Canada Health Act in 1984.

As part of their respective accommodations with the medical profession, a number of provinces (six of the ten by the late 1970s) allowed physicians the option of "extra billing" their patients—that is, billing patients over and above what the government plan would pay. (As noted in chapter 2, such an option was a key provision of the agreement that ended the Saskatchewan physicians' strike in 1962.) Only about 10% of physicians in Canada exercised this option, and the amount of extra billing was estimated at only about 1.3% of total physician billings under medicare. In no province did this amount exceed 3% (Tuohy 1988). The economic and political significance of extra billing was increased, however, by the fact that it was "clustered" in certain specialties and localities. Even more important in political terms, extra billing flew in the face of one of the fundamental principles underlying Canadian medicare—the removal of financial barriers to access to medical and hospital care.

The symbolic significance of the extra-billing issue, then, far outweighed its fiscal implications, or even its economic impact on the vast majority of physicians. In the early 1980s, a federal Liberal government declining in popularity and facing non-Liberal governments in each of the provinces, seized upon the issue of extra billing as a way of symbolizing its commitment to preserving the universality of the nation's most popular social program—and, by extension, of other programs. It portrayed non-Liberal governments in the provinces as allowing the principle of universality to be eroded by condoning extra billing, and introduced legislation, the Canada Health Act, penalizing those provinces by providing for federal transfer payments to be reduced by an amount equal to the estimated amount of extra billing in any given province—a dollar-for-dollar penalty.

If the issue had symbolic significance for the federal Liberals, it was symbolically important for the medical profession as well. It had come to symbolize the preservation and legitimization of private, individualistic, entrepreneurial medical practice even in the context of a largely state-funded system. An Ontario study showed that about one-half of physicians who had chosen "opted-out" status had done so largely for ideological reasons and did not charge fees greatly in excess of the government plan (Wolfson and Tuohy 1980). Further-more, attitudinal support for extra billing within the profession was not con-fined to those who actually practiced it (Tuohy 1988: 285–86). The CMA mo-bilized strongly against the proposed legislation, arguing that Canada had "one of the better and more cost-efficient health care systems in the world" which suffered only from underfunding. The CMA asserted that extra billing rep-resented a source of badly needed funding and re-affirmed the status of phy-sicians as "independent, patient-employed professionals responsible to our patients" (Baltzan 1983: 347).

In one sense at least, the federal strategy backfired. The federal Conserva-tives, whom the Liberals had hoped to tar with the same brush as their siblings in power in several provinces, supported the legislation, and, like its predecessors the Hospital Insurance and Diagnostic Services Act of 1958 and the Medical Care Act of 1966, the Canada Health Act passed with the support of all parties in Parliament. It incorporated and clarified the principles of universality, acces-sibility, comprehensiveness, public administration, and portability; in addition, by prescribing "dollar-for-dollar" penalties for extra billing and other user charges, it specified sanctions under the EPF arrangements for violating the cri-teria of universality and accessibility.

With the passage of the federal legislation, policy action shifted to the provincial level. Within the three-year deadline imposed by the Canada Health Act, all provinces came into compliance. They did so, with one exception, by elaborating their respective accommodations with organized medicine (as will be further discussed in chapter 7), to compensate the profession for the loss of the extra-billing option. Hence, although the passage of the Canada Health Act constituted an undeniable symbolic defeat for the medical profession, there were significant tangible and structural gains for the profession as a result of the legislation. (The exceptional case was Ontario, where for reasons that will be more fully elaborated in chapter 7 the profession became locked in a losing bat-tle of wills with the provincial government.)

In the period of Conservative majority government from 1983 to 1993, federal action in health care was limited to the progressive constraint of federal financial contributions to provincial health insurance plans under the medicare program. Upon returning to power in 1993, the Liberals moved once again to reinforce the structural and institutional policy parameters of the system. First, they invoked the provisions of the Canada Health Act to challenge the practice in four provinces of allowing private health clinics variously offering ophthal-mologic, abortion, and specialized surgical services to charge "facility fees" to patients while receiving reimbursement from the provincial plan for providing insured health services. The bulk of this activity involved clinics offering ophthalmologic services (particularly cataract surgery) in Alberta. Federal–provincial negotiation over the issue were held without result between June 1994 and September 1995. In January 1995, the federal minister of health wrote to all provincial and territorial governments indicating that these "facility fees" would be interpreted as user charges in contravention of the Canada Health Act, and establishing a deadline of October 15, 1995, for provinces to come into compliance. The deadline passed, and federal penalties were invoked; in May 1996, however, the Alberta government announced that private clinics would no longer be allowed to bill patients as well as receiving reimbursement from the public plan. Instead, the provincial plan would pay facility fees related to insured services.[28] Federal policy thus guarded against the development of a British-style system of private alternatives to publicly funded services in niche areas.[29]

### The National Forum on Health

The principles of the existing system were also publicly reinforced through a second initiative taken by the federal Liberal government: the appointment of the National Forum on Health Care. In October 1994, the prime minister announced that he would chair a National Forum on Health to "develop a new vision for Canada's health system for the 21st century."[30] As in the case of Britain and the United States, a working group closely associated with the head of government was established to flesh out the agenda of health care reform for the 1990s. The National Forum was distinctively Canadian in a number of respects, however. Its birth was preceded by federal–provincial wrangling. The forum was initially conceived as a "neutral" body made up of members without governmental affiliations, who could consider the future of medicare outside the context of federal–provincial negotiation. The provincial governments, however, saw it as an attempt by the federal government to set the terms of debate. Several months of argument over what role the provinces should play ended in stalemate after the prime minister rejected the suggestion that the forum be cochaired by the prime minister and a provincial premier, and the forum went ahead as a solely federal initiative. In his opening remarks to the first meeting of the forum, the prime minister took care to make it clear that the Forum would not preempt or replace federal–provincial negotiations: "This Forum is not an intergovernmental body. It does not replace the Conference of Health Ministers. It has a very different function—one of leadership in promoting dialogue and debate about longer term health issues that are neither federal nor provincial" (Chrétien 1994: 1). The provinces officially boycotted the forum, although several of the forum members were also officials or members of provincial government advisory bodies. Provincial governments sent "observers" to some meetings on an informal basis.

The forum was also distinctively Canadian in the finely tuned regional, and, to a somewhat lesser extent, functional balance of its membership. Of the twenty-two members (not including the prime minister as chair or the health minister as vice chair), six were from the Atlantic provinces, six from Quebec, four from Ontario, and seven from the western provinces. Eleven of the members, including all five physician members, had academic affiliations. Three members were drawn from hospital administration or governance, six from consumer or other advocacy organizations, and one from organized labor.

The forum's report, issued in February 1997, was a solid endorsement of Canadian medicare. It argued that the "key features" of the system—"public funding for medically necessary services, the 'single payer' model, the five principles of the Canada Health Act, and a strong federal/provincial/territorial partnership"—must be preserved and protected (National Forum on Health 1997, vol. 1: 20). And while the report argued that the current level of public funding was sufficient given the existing scope of the program, it also argued for an expansion of that scope to include home care, pharmaceuticals, and potentially other goods and services currently offered in the private sector. It argued that all "medically necessary" services must be fully publicly funded, without resort to user charges, extra billing, or other sources of private finance. The report recommended some reorganization of health care delivery, particularly with regard to primary care, although it did not specify these changes beyond reference to the need for other than fee-for-service mechanisms of funding and remuneration, and it recommended a federal "transition fund" to support pilot projects that would test various organizational innovations.[31] As for the federal–provincial balance, the forum argued for "predictable, stable federal transfers" and suggested a cash floor of C$12.5 billion (National Forum on Health 1997, vol. 1: 13)—a suggestion which, as already noted, the prime minister embraced a few months later. And finally, the forum went beyond the health care field to embrace a line of analysis growing in influence in the cross-national social policy arena—a focus on the "social determinants of health." It argued, among, other things, for "a broad, integrated child and family strategy consisting of both programs and income support" (National Forum on Health 1997, vol. 1: 24).

In short, the National Forum on Health, unlike the review of the NHS in Britain or the Clinton task force in the United States, solidly endorsed the structural balance and the institutional mix of the existing system. Its recommendations, if followed, would shift the balance of state and private finance somewhat in favor of the former. Depending on the interpretation of its cryptic recommendations regarding organizational change, the recommendations might imply some change in institutional mix in the direction of an increase in hierarchical dimensions. But the changes implied were marginal; essentially the forum reaffirmed the prevailing model.

In the wake of the forum's report, the federal Liberal government seized upon two of its recommendations—for a national "pharmacare" program and for a national home care program—as possible candidates for action by the government as it began to experience the fiscal dividend of balanced budgets in the late 1990s. Of the two proposals, home care had the greater resonance. It was seen as an essential complement to the downsizing of hospitals (to be discussed in the next section); it offered the opportunity for the federal government to gain considerable leverage for a relatively marginal increase in expenditure; and in an era of incremental change it entailed only modest changes to the structural balance of the system and particularly the public–private mix, while forestalling a likely shift in that balance under the logic of the existing system. In the mid-1990s an estimated 80% to 90% of home care services was provided under publicly funded provincial programs, although problems of definition mean these figures should be treated with caution. Provinces had received per capita grants in support of "extended care services" including home care as part of the cash transfer under EPF arrangements until they were rolled into the CHST, but the federal government had never attached conditions to these grants other than reporting of data. The result was a patchwork of programs across provinces; the programs varied greatly, for example, in the extent to which they imposed user charges or provided services through public sector direct service workers or through contracts with private not-for-profit and for-profit providers (Shapiro 1994). Establishing a conditional transfer program in this area would allow the federal government to influence, if not to dictate, the principles under which such programs would be organized on a more consistent basis across provinces. Depending upon the content of those principles, it could also forestall, constrain, or regulate the greater incursion of investor-owned providers of home care services that appeared likely in the late 1990s.

The provinces, however, still chafing at the progressive reductions in federal funding for medicare, were decidedly cool to the prospect of another federal program of conditional transfers before those cuts had been redressed. The prospects of intergovernmental agreement on a national home care program, while not negligible, pressed the limits of the possible in the federal–provincial climate of the late 1990s.

### The provincial level: regionalization and hospital restructuring

Throughout several changes in government, then, the federal government either actively or passively supported the model of Canadian medicare, even while reducing the level of its own fiscal contribution. The level of complacency among provincial governments was, not surprisingly, somewhat less. None, however, called for or embarked upon major structural or institutional change to its health care system. Provincial policies will be more fully discussed in chapter 7, in the context of discussing the provincial-level accommodations between the medical profession and the state that characterize the logic of Canadian medicare. But it is important to note that the relative stability of the Canadian system is a function of provincial as well as federal policy.

In the late 1980s and early 1990s every province established a task force or commission of inquiry to give policy advice on issues of health policy. Although their emphases varied, the reports of these bodies exhibited a number of common themes, including a shift from institutionally based to community-based care, a reallocation of functions among health care personnel, a decentralization of decision-making to regional councils representing a variety of interests in the health field, and a broadening of focus to develop policies based on an understanding of determinants of health beyond the health care delivery system (Tuohy 1992: 139). These themes seemed to represent the lineaments of an emerging consensus—and indeed as we have seen they were generally echoed in the federal National Forum on Health report in 1997. But all these recommendations were made at a level of generality that left much to the process of implementation.

In practice, by far the predominant focus of public policy in the health care arena at the provincial level was on restructuring in the hospital sector, primarily through increasing horizontal integration, reducing the number of acute care beds, and to some extent building up capacity for community-based care.

The mechanisms through which these changes were accomplished varied across provinces. In all provinces except Ontario, regional structures for the management of the hospital sector were established, although the organization and the mandate of regional boards varied widely. All of the boards had the authority to allocate budgets across institutions and agencies in their region. No province, however, granted the boards revenue-raising authority; all received global budgets from the province. These global budgets were initially determined on a historical basis, although in each province the development of a needs-based allocation formula was on the agenda. (Again, Saskatchewan led the other provinces in this regard. Saskatchewan was the first to implement a needs-based global budget for each regional authority, comprising a per capita allocation adjusted for measures of predicted utilization of health care services. Initially these weighting factors were based on standardized mortality rates, while further refinements to the formula were under development [Lewis 1996: 11].) In two provinces the scope of the boards' authority was restricted to institutional services; others embraced some community-based services as well. In Quebec, local community centers offering health and social services were established in the 1970s, and were included, along with hospitals, long-term care facilities, and other agencies, within the mandate of the regional boards. And tiny Prince Edward Island, which with a total population of 130,000 might seem an unlikely locus for regionalization at all, established regional boards with a mandate embracing a broader range of social as well as health services than in any other province. In no case, significantly, did the mandate of regional boards extend to physicians' services, although some maintained various types of medical liaison committees.

In some cases, the mandate of regional boards extended to the direct management and operation of the institutions under their purview. In British Columbia, Alberta, and Saskatchewan, the regional boards replaced the boards of individual institutions, and the assets of the institutions were transferred to the regional boards.

The composition of the regional boards also varied. In Saskatchewan, from 1995 onward, two-thirds of the membership of each board was directly elected on a geographic ward system.[32] In other provinces, members were appointed by the provincial governments, although most other provinces intended to introduce direct election at some point in the future. In a survey of members of boards in five provinces, Lomas and his colleagues found that only a minority of members were employees of health care or social service agencies (18% on average, with a range from 6% to 36% by province), but 70% on average had experience in serving on a health care board, and one-third had previously held government appointments on health care or other boards (Lomas et al. 1996a: 11; 1996b: 16).

The different mechanisms for determining board membership reflected the different political traditions of various provinces, which in turn shaped the agendas of incumbent governments. Saskatchewan's "populist" approach, for example—including the direct election of regional boards and broadly consultative processes—contrasted with the "corporatist" approach characteristic of Quebec, where regional boards were elected by regional assemblies whose members were drawn from four "electoral colleges"—municipalities, community health and social service organizations, socioeconomic groups including business and labor organizations, and health care institutions. How durable these various structures would prove to be was unclear as of the late 1990s: in other related arenas such as occupational health and safety, Quebec's corporatist structures had proved to be more durable through partisan change in government than had multipartite bodies based on different models in other provinces. Signs of tension between regional bodies and provincial governments began to emerge in some provinces shortly after the bodies were created (Lomas 1996: 15).

In contrast to the 1970s and 1980s, when it had appeared that the combination of the local economic and symbolic significance of hospitals, combined with an area-based legislative system, made it practically impossible for a provincial government to close a hospital, in the 1990s provincial governments of all partisan complexions showed a remarkable determination to stay the course. Different strategies for hospital restructuring through regional boards were pursued in different provinces. In Saskatchewan, a substantial amount of "downsizing"—the closing of fifty-two small rural hospitals (representing about 200 beds in total)—was accomplished by the provincial government before regional boards were established, so as to avoid encumbering the boards with such politically difficult tasks at their inception (Lewis 1996). The boards were nonetheless expected to continue restructuring over time. Newfoundland and Manitoba followed similar strategies. In Alberta and New Brunswick, in contrast, an important part of the mandate of the newly created regional boards themselves was to accomplish a significant reduction of the system. And in Quebec, the task of allocating budget cuts to institutions was implemented through a regional board structure that was established in the 1970s and revitalized in the 1990s.

Ontario was the exception to this strategy of regionalization. In Ontario regional bodies—the district health councils—remained advisory only and had no budgetary authority. In the early 1990s, each council was charged by the New Democratic Party (NDP) government of Ontario with developing a hospital restructuring plan for its region. In keeping with the managerialist tradition of the provincial government, the Conservative government that succeeded the NDP in 1995 established a Health Services Restructuring Commission (HSRC) and turned the recommendations of the various district health councils over to that body for review and decision, announcing that the government would abide by the decisions of the HSRC.[33] This dramatic attempt to depoliticize decisions about hospital closures was put to the test when the HSRC indicated its intention to direct the closure of the sites of the sole francophone-only teaching hospital in Ottawa (the Montfort Hospital) and two teaching hospitals in Toronto, one of which had a long history of providing a professional venue for women physicians and a focus on "women's health" (Women's College Hospital) and the other having a more recent history of service to the gay community and the homeless in a downtown area of the city (Wellesley Central Hospital). The institutions themselves were to be acquired by or merged with other hospitals in the respective cities.

In only one case did the HSRC appear to have bowed to political pressure in revising its decisions. This being Canada, it was the case that raised a threat to "national unity." In February 1997 the HSRC issued a notice of intention to direct the closing of the Montfort Hospital site and the amalgamation of Montfort as an institution with three other Ottawa hospitals on a single site. The process allowed for a comment period before the issuance of the commission's final recommendations. The Montfort notice was the subject of a furious lobbying campaign, and provoked unprecedented public interventions from the prime minister, Jean Chrétien, and the Quebec premier, Lucien Bouchard, in support of maintaining the hospital. In its response to the HSRC report, the ministry of health (represented by the deputy minister, not the minister, in keeping with the depoliticization of the process), stated only that it wished to see the francophone services offered by the Monfort survive. Subsequent to the notice three new members, including one francophone, were added to the commission. In its final report for Ottawa, the HSRC relented to allow the Montfort to continue to exist on a substantially reduced scale. Intense lobbying campaigns on behalf of Women's College and Wellesley Central did not bear similar fruit: the commission's final report for Toronto directed the closure of their sites, although it provided for the new merged or amalgamated institutions to operate ambulatory care centers in those locations. Several hospitals took the HSRC directives to judicial review, but the legislation under which the commission had been established left few grounds for challenging its decisions.

All this activity regarding hospital restructuring, however, amounted to marginal change in the overall structural balance or institutional mix of the system. Horizontal integration of hospitals changed their organizational configuration, but did not significantly change the weight of hierarchy in the system. The process of restructuring nonetheless involved a greater degree of state activism in the exercise of the state's regulatory authority and monopsony power than had been typical in the relationship between provincial governments and hospitals. In those provinces in which provincially appointed (or directly elected) regional boards replaced the governing structures of individual institutions and took over their assets, there was a permanent expansion of the scope of formal state authority in the hospital sector. The effective degree of expansion was open to question. The provincial government had previously had effective control of the hospital sector through its budgetary and regulatory authority; provincial appointment of boards with managerial authority promised to give the provincial government access to finer levers of control. By the late 1990s, the systems were not mature enough to judge the extent to which they would in fact lead to increased provincial government intervention, or would function in effect as local institutional boards on a larger scale. In this regard, Lomas's survey of board members is enlightening. Most expressed attitudes consistent with roles as local representatives jealous of the independence of their boards. Of the five provinces surveyed, only in Alberta did an appreciable proportion of board members (13%) feel accountable to the minister of health. On average across the five provinces, 13% felt accountable to "provincial taxpayers," but for large majorities of board members the lines of accountability ran to the local citizenry (Lomas et al. 1996b: 13). Large majorities also expressed confidence that their board would "make better decisions than those previously made by the province," but about one-half of board members, on average, felt "restricted by rules laid down by the provincial government"—and that sentiment was stronger in those provinces in which regional boards had replaced the boards of individual institutions (Lomas et al. 1996b: 11, 15).

In Ontario, the formal expansion of state authority necessary to achieve restructuring was purported to be temporary. There, the HSRC was established for a four-year period under an extremely controversial piece of omnibus legislation passed in 1996 empowering the Cabinet (and in some cases individual ministers) with a set of "tools" to achieve reductions in spending—tools that in some cases involved unprecedented levels of discretion. Prior to the passage of that legislation, there had been no legislative head of authority under which the Cabinet or a minister could order the closing or merger of hospitals, although the legislature could of course do so through the passage of specific legislation. By adopting the HSRC mechanism, the state effectively enhanced its capacity to act expeditiously,[34] and by acting it expanded the scope of state authority. It must be noted, however, that in Ontario and elsewhere the restructuring process, while often extremely controversial at the local level, was carried out with the cautious endorsement and collaboration of provincial hospital associations (further discussed in chapter 7).

Furthermore, the ongoing result in Ontario was not to change the relationship between the state and the hospital sector. Hospitals continued as self-governing bodies receiving global budgets from the provincial government, although the determination of those budgets began to move away from its traditional historical base toward formulas designed to reward efficiency. And in those other provinces in which individual institutions continued to exist under the jurisdiction of regional boards, regionalization amounted in effect to a reorganization within the state (as regional bodies took on functions previously performed at the center), rather than a redefinition of the state–hospital relationship. In Quebec, for example, regional boards were given mandates to establish priorities and service plans and to allocate budgets, all within a policy framework established by the provincial government or subject to the approval of the minister (Duplantie 1996: 3).

All this restructuring, then, took place well within the structural and institutional parameters of Canadian medicare, although it pushed the boundaries of the understandings between provincial governments and hospital providers that had grown up within the system. Indeed, with few exceptions the provinces operated their health insurance systems under the model of Canadian medicare enshrined in the Canada Health Act. (The major exception, Alberta's attempt to allow private clinics to charge above the government benefit for insured services, disappeared when the issue was resolved, as previously discussed.) Why was there no frontal challenge to the medicare model in any province, at a time when governments in most advanced industrial nations were at least questioning the structural and institutional premises of their systems?

The answer to this question is threefold. First, provincial governments continued to believe that they could achieve their fiscal targets without structural or institutional change to the system, by elaborating their accommodations with providers and particularly with the medical profession. Second, the great popularity of the program meant that there were great political risks to any government that moved unilaterally to challenge it. Third, even if a number of provincial governments were to seek to negotiate changes to the program, there were substantial barriers to the mobilization of authority in the federal–provincial arena.

The first of these reasons will be explored in chapter 7. Here I will anticipate that discussion only by noting that profession–state accommodations had proved resilient throughout the 1970s and 1980s, although they had come under increasing strain by the mid-1990s as the rate of real increase on public spending in health care leveled off. A similar phenomenon had preceded the rupturing of the accommodation between medicine and the state in Britain in the late 1980s, a rupture that finally persuaded Prime Minister Thatcher that the political risks of intervening strongly in the health care arena were outweighed by the risks of inaction.

The political risks of tampering with Canadian medicare, however, were particularly high—hence the second reason that no government chose to challenge the model. A widely cited 1988 cross-national poll showed that Canadians were more satisfied with their health care system than were either American or British respondents, and that they overwhelmingly preferred the Canadian system to the British or the American. A large majority of American respondents, on the other hand, preferred a Canadian-style system to their own (Blendon 1989). Subsequent polls reinforced these results (Gallup Canada 1991). As individual consumers, Canadians were at least as satisfied with the hospital and medical services available to them as were consumers in other advanced industrial nations. For example, 73% of Canadian respondents in a 1994 cross-national poll rated the quality of health care services available in their community as "excellent" or "good," compared with 72% in Germany and 65% in the United States. Only 8% of Canadian respondents reported being unable to get needed medical care in the previous year, and 16% reported having to wait more than one week to see a doctor.[35] Furthermore, Canadians' levels of expectation about what constituted appropriate medical care appeared to be roughly similar to those of Americans and Germans (Blendon et al. 1995).

The Canadian public's support for medicare, however, went well beyond its benefits to them as individual consumers. Indeed, medicare became virtually a defining element of the Canadian identity. During the heated and wrenching public debate over the Free Trade Agreement (FTA) with the United States in 1988, for example, politicians opposing the agreement repeatedly invoked medicare as one of the things that distinguished Canada from the United

States, and alleged that it was threatened by the agreement. Public opinion polls showed that this allegation was the most effective way of galvanizing opposition to the FTA (Johnston and Blais 1988).

By the mid-1990's, however, there appeared to be a growing public concern that medicare was in jeopardy. Cross-national polling by Blendon and his colleagues (1995) found that the proportion of Canadian respondents who believed that "on the whole, the system works well and only minor changes are necessary to make it work better" had fallen from 56% to 29% between 1988 and 1994. Canadian levels of satisfaction, in effect, converged with those of Germans, but remained higher than those of Americans. Support for the five principles of medicare remained very high, but signs of erosion began to be apparent. Almost 90% of respondents in a 1995 poll held the principle of universality to be very important, and majorities of more than 80% similarly rated the principles of accessibility, comprehensiveness, and portability. Each of these levels represented a 3 to 4 percentage point drop in support since 1991. The principle of public administration, however, was rated as very important by only 64%—a 13 percentage point drop since 1991 (Coutts 1995). In 1996, an Ontario poll indicated that 46% believed that the quality of care at their local hospital had worsened over the previous year—the highest level of deterioration reported across a range of public services including education, physicians' services, municipal services, and public transit (Walker 1996). Support for private sources of funding, however, remained low, and most polls indicated majorities in support of increased public spending on health care (Coutts 1995; Greenspon and Winsor 1997).

In this context it is not surprising that no provincial government was prepared to take the risk of unilaterally challenging the medicare model. The banning of extra billing by all provinces after the passage of the Canada Health Act, and later Alberta's capitulation to Ottawa's demands that it cease allowing private clinics to charge facility fees, are cases in point. In none of these cases did the financial penalties to be imposed by Ottawa amount to significant proportions of the provincial budgets for health care, at the existing level of noncompliance.[36] Rather, the political stigma of noncompliance with principles of medicare registering supermajorities of public support was one that provincial governments were not prepared to bear.

One solution for provincial governments might appear to have been a renegotiation of the interpretation of the principles of medicare to allow them greater flexibility. The federal–provincial climate of the 1980s and 1990s, however, was distinctly inhospitable to such negotiations. The incubus of constitutional discord could not be shed throughout this period, and it cast a pall over almost all federal–provincial discussions. The protracted negotiations that had led up to the passage of The Constitution Act, 1982, which finally accomplished the formal "patriation" of Canada's constitution from Britain, left a multiple legacy. In the first place, the negotiations left a sense of "unfinished business." The constitutional changes of 1982 dealt almost entirely with the design of an amending formula and the entrenchment of a Charter of Rights and Freedoms. Despite prolonged discussion, no consensus could be reached on changes to the federal–provincial division of powers, and almost no changes were made.[37] This might not have been a problem: the Canadian constitution had proven remarkably flexible in accommodating changes in the federal–provincial balance in different areas over time, and might have been expected to do so in the future (Tuohy 1992). But there was another major perception of unfinished business after the passage of the 1982 constitutional legislation: it had been passed over the objections of the Quebec government (albeit with the support of federal members of Parliament from Quebec, including the prime minister). Over the next decade, there were two major but ultimately abortive attempts to negotiate a package of constitutional reforms acceptable to all provinces and the federal government. Among their provisions was an explicit constitutional recognition of the federal government's authority to establish shared-cost programs (such as medicare) in areas of exclusive provincial jurisiction, and a concomitant recognition of a provincial government's entitlement to "reasonable compensation" should it choose to opt out of such a program to offer its own program "compatible with the national objectives" (Tuohy 1992: 76–77). This might have allowed provinces greater flexibility in programs such as medicare, subject to judicial interpretation of the degree of "compatibility" of provincial programs and the "reasonableness" of compensation. Neither of these initiatives succeeded, however; the first (the "Meech Lake Accord") failed as the result of the defection of certain provincial governments, the second (the "Charlottetown Agreement") when it was submitted to a national referendum at which it was rejected.

Over all of this constitutional conflict hung the specter of Quebec separatism. A referendum in Quebec in 1980 on an ambiguous question about support for "sovereignty-association" for Quebec failed, with a 60% vote for the "No" side. Fifteen years later, in October 1995, a second referendum failed by a razor-thin margin to approve the proposal that Quebec become sovereign after seeking to negotiate an "economic and political partnership" with Canada. Between these landmarks, and afterwards, the "national unity" issue kept the federal–provincial arena one of heightened sensitivity.

In this context, the likelihood that sufficient federal–provincial authority could be mobilized to renegotiate the terms of medicare was very slight, as developments in federal–provincial relations in the health care arena in the 1990s demonstrated. As the federal government continued to assert its role as guardian of the principles of the Canada Health Act even while continuing to reduce its financial contribution, provincial governments became increasingly resentful. This resentment was further piqued by the Liberal government's announcement of the Canada Health and Social Transfer in its 1995 budget. At their annual meeting in August 1995 (to which the separatist premier of Quebec paid only a brief visit), the exasperation of the premiers was fully aired: as one premier colorfully put it, the federal government could not be both "gate-keeper and purse-snatcher" (Sheppard 1995). But when it came to taking collective action to resolve the issue, ideological divisions among the parties in power at the provincial level, differences in the interests of "have" and "have-not" provinces, and the rankling issue of Quebec all frustrated any common agreement. The premiers (minus Quebec) could agree only on continued attempts to define national standards for social programs, including what core of essential services should be covered under medicare, through a Ministerial Council on Social Policy Reform and Renewal.

The Ministerial Council, made up of provincial cabinet ministers but not the premiers, produced a Report to the Premiers several months later, which proposed, among other things, exclusive provincial responsibility for the design and delivery of health programs under the terms of an accord to be negotiated among federal and provincial governments; however, the report proposed no mechanism of enforcement. The document remained simply a report to the premiers.

Over the next three years, negotiations continued on both an interprovincial and a federal-provincial basis. In this process negotiations over health care were bound up with negotiations over what came to be called a "social union" framework—essentially a framework to define the federal government's role in social policy areas that lay within the constitutional jurisdiction of the provinces. Finally, in February 1999, a resolution of a sort was reached. The federal government agreed to a phased restoration of its transfers to the provinces for health care, to approximately what they had been in 1995, before the institution of the Canada Health and Social Transfer. The restored amount was equivalent to about 5 percent of total provincial spending on health care, but it also had an important symbolic effect in signaling a loosening of fiscal constraints. For their part, all of the provinces agreed to allocate the restored funding entirely to "core" health care services and programs and expressed their commitment to the principles of the Canada Health Act.

The federal government and all of the provinces except Quebec also signed a separate agreement on a "social union framework." Included among its provisions were the following: a reiteration of commitment to the principles of the CHA; an agreement to refer disputes about provincial compliance with the conditions of shared-cost programs (including the CHA principles) to an undefined dispute resolution mechanism (although ultimate authority to determine compliance remained with the federal government), and an undertaking by the federal government not to introduce any new shared-cost program without the consent of six of the ten provinces. The agreement was to be reviewed after three years.

Taken together, these developments could be seen as establishing the conditions for progress toward an elaboration of the Canadian medicare model to include, for example, national home care or pharmacare programs. The commitment to the CHA model had been reaffirmed. The restoration of the federal transfer met the provinces' necessary condition for discussing any new programs. The requirement for agreement by six provinces before a new shared-cost program could be established was in practical terms a low hurdle: it could be met by six "have-not" provinces representing about 15 percent of the population. And the federal government's new fiscal latitude heightened the prospect of some new program spending in the future.

Other factors, however, gave less reason to expect such policy changes. Most important, the Quebec government had refused to endorse the social union agreement, insisting among other things upon an "opting out" clause that would allow a province to choose not to participate in a shared cost program but to receive equivalent compensation targeted to the same "priority area." In that context, federal-provincial negotiations over new social programs were likely to take the form of a three-dimensional chess game in which each negotiating move had implications not only on the plane of social policy but on the "national unity" plane as well.

Furthermore, the restoration of federal funding did not substantially change the environment in which provincial-level accommodations between the state and the medical profession had to be worked out, although it promised to bolster somewhat the mood of the negotiations. Federal transfers, after all, were returned to their nominal 1995 levels—levels at which real per capita spending on health care had already begun to decline—and were not adjusted for inflation or population change. In effect, the federal fiscal changes and the associated federal-provincial agreements amounted to a return, with modest changes, to the status quo ante—to the way things were before the institution of the CHST.

In summary, the relative lack of major policy change in Canada in the 1980s and 1990s was attributable in part to the unwillingness of any government to take the political risk of taking unilateral action to alter a program with broad public support. But it was also in part a default option, given the inability of federal and provincial governments to come to any agreement regarding acceptable change. As the 1990s drew to a close, however, there were some signs that at least the first of these factors might be changing. Growing levels of public anxiety raised the risks of inaction as well. Provincial governments continued to respond to this dilemma by elaborating their accommodations with providers in their own jurisdictions, placing these accommodations under increasing pressure. The future of the Canadian system, indeed, seemed to depend on the resilience of those accommodations—a theme to which we will return in chapter 7.

The contrasting experiences of Britain, the United States, and Canada in health care policy in the 1980s and 1990s demonstrate the importance of factors in the broader political arena that either favor or frustrate the development of the conditions for major policy change. The Thatcher government in its third successive term had both the will and the mobilization of authority to take action in the context of its broad policy agenda: the Clinton administration had the will but not the ability to mobilize authority; and Canadian federal and provincial governments had neither. That is the argument of this chapter in its starkest terms. The next chapter, however, takes account of explanations of the experience of these three nations that have been offered by other scholars and relates them to the framework of this argument.

# Institutions, Ideas, Interests, Actors, and the Accidents of Policy Episodes | 4

Readers of the literature of comparative public policy will recognize the argument of the previous two chapters as a version of "historical institutionalism." This approach emphasizes the importance of decisions taken at crucial points in time, decisions that become crystallized in the formal and informal rules governing behavior, and that establish the context in which subsequent decisions will be made. Historical institutionalism, however, is a house with many mansions: it allows for a variety of emphases regarding the factors that bring about critical moments of decision-making and that shape decisions at those moments.

In this book, I have emphasized the critical importance of the *timing* of intersections between developments in the health care arena and developments in the broader political arena. In chapters 2 and 3, I argued that episodes of policy change in the health care arena were brought about by the opening of "windows of opportunity" as a result of events in the broader political arena, and that as a result, the timing of those episodes was, from the perspective of the health care arena, virtually "accidental." The resultant policy decisions were then the product of a complex interaction between ideas and constellations of interest then current in the health care arena, and the agenda of the dominant political actors of the day. In this chapter, I relate this argument to a number of other attempts to explain differences in health policy outcomes across nations.

## Political Institutions

One version of historical institutionalism emphasizes the importance of the institutional structure of government in explaining policy outcomes. Institutional structures, on this argument, vary in their capacity to facilitate or to frustrate policy action. The structure of American government, in particular, is held up as the quintessential example of institutional constraint on policy action (Steinmo and Watts 1995). All institutions, moreover, have organizational biases that channel the representation of interests. For example, just as tax policies in the United States, Britain, and Sweden can be understood as the product of institutions that differ in the ways they channel the influence of business and labor (Steinmo 1989), so health policies in Sweden, Switzerland, and France can be understood as the outcome of institutions that channel the influence of the medical profession to different points in the policy process (Immergut 1991).

A fairly straightforward argument can be made linking differences in health policy in Britain, Canada, and the United States to differences in their respective political institutions. In Britain, as a unitary state with the Westminster system of parliamentary government, the party that commands a majority of the House of Commons faces relatively few institutional constraints on the policy action it can take. Canadian governmental institutions, with a Westminster parliamentary system but a decentralized federal structure, provides more platforms for political contest and compromise, at least among federal and provincial government executives. And the United States, with its congressional system of checks and balances and the localized party structure that has grown up around it, provides myriad opportunities for influence (or veto) of policy action. Hence it should not surprise us to find that British governments have been able to make major policy changes in the health care arena on not one but two occasions: establishing the state-hierarchical system of the NHS in the 1940s, and reforming it along "internal market" lines in the 1990s. Nor is it surprising that Canada's federal system should have tempered the degree and pace of change, yielding less dramatic change in the health care delivery system as a result of state action, and fewer episodes of change over time. Finally, the inability of the United States to adopt comprehensive universal health insurance despite numerous attempts at both federal and state levels is evidence of the institutional paralysis of the American system.

This neat explanation bears further examination. In Canada, after all, medicare was adopted at the federal level during a period of minority government, when institutionally afforded opportunities for veto were unusually high. More generally, if broad political institutions are the culprits, we should find a similar pattern of variation across these three countries in other policy areas. But in another area of social policy—public pensions—we find a somewhat different story. The British and Canadian public pension systems developed in increments over time. Britain introduced flat-rate public pensions in 1908, but through a process of incremental change over the twentieth century the benefit continued to be so low as to require a substantial portion of the elderly population to rely on means-tested assistance. It was not until 1975, after a decade and a half of competing partisan promises, that an earnings-related contributory tier, the State Earnings-Related Pension Scheme (SERPS) was added (Pierson 1994: 54–55). Canada began with a means-tested pension, cost-shared between federal and provincial governments, in 1927, then added a universal flat-rate pension, Old Age Security (OAS) in 1951, and a contributory earnings-related scheme, the Canada Pension Plan (CPP) and an income-tested Guaranteed Income Supplement (GIS) in 1966. Constitutional amendments were required in 1951 and again in 1964 to give the federal government the authority to act unilaterally in this field—although the provincial governments retained "paramountcy."[1] This provision for provincial paramountcy meant that the establishment of the CPP in practice required complex federal–provincial negotiations, as would any subsequent change to the program (Banting 1987: 49–50).

In contrast to this incremental pattern of development in Britain and Canada, the public pension system of the United States was substantially put in place by the "big bang" of the Social Security Act of 1935, which established a contributory, earnings-related public pension plan (Leman 1977), although benefits were enhanced and eligibility extended over time (Quadagno 1988: 153). In 1969, as part of a package of public assistance legislation, a means-tested component, Supplemental Security Income (SSI) was added, but SSI was to continue to be a modest component of the public pension system, reaching a small and declining proportion the elderly population (well below 10%) in the 1980s (Banting 1992: 29; Pierson 1994: 55). The U.S. scheme, unlike those in Canada and Britain, lacked a universal tier, but its scope and level of generosity was such that "[f]or the overwhelming majority of Americans, public-retirement provision meant a single program, Social Security. Regardless of age or income (except for those well below the poverty line), Americans expected to turn in their retirement to the same source of public benefits" (Pierson 1994: 55).

The British and Canadian programs provided an income floor for the lowest income groups but were more fragmented and less generous to upper income categories. The rate of replacement of preretirement income by public pension income was substantially higher in the United States than in either Britain or, for much of the postwar period, Canada—although Canadian replacement rates overtook those in the United States in the 1980s for lower and average income groups as the Canadian system matured (Aldrich 1982; Banting 1992: 29).

In the 1980s, changes in public policy relating to pensions were attempted in all three countries, with varying results (Pierson and Weaver 1993). In all three countries, governments were forced to back away from proposed pension reforms and to make more modest changes than they had intended. The Reagan administration in the United States, after having had to retrench significantly from its proposed benefit reductions in 1981, did in 1983 achieve a short-term reduction in the form of a delay in indexation, and a long-term reduction in the form of an extension of the retirement age from 65 to 67. In Britain, the Thatcher government suffered a major public reversal when it backed away from a 1983 proposal to abolish SERPS and instead adopted technical changes that would reduce benefits from SERPS in the long term (having also made changes to the indexation of the basic pension that would reduce payout in the long term). In Canada, an attempt to reduce benefits across the board by partially deindexing the basic OAS pension was abandoned, even by a majority Conservative federal government with jurisdictional authority, to be replaced by a reduction and eventually an elimination of basic pension benefits for upper income earners.

In summary, then, the above stereotypes of British, Canadian, and American governments—Britain the decisive unitary Westminster model, Canada the elite accommodationist model of Westminster-based federalism, and the United States the paralyzed complexity of a congressional model overlain with federalism—do not seem to hold in the pension arena. Canada's plan, it is true, does reflect a number of federal–provincial compromises over time. But Britain's plan hardly reflects decisive state action: niggardly and fragmented, it was put in place in increments over time. The U.S. scheme, in contrast, was the product of a founding moment—comprehensive (though not universal) in its scope and increasingly generous through subsequent modifications. In the 1980s, moreover, the American, British, and Canadian governments were all driven to make "technical" changes that would reduce pension benefits over time. Institutional factors can explain some of the *detail* of these policy choices—the absence of a universal tier in the U.S. model reflects the veto power of southern conservatives in Congress (Quadagno 1988), and the focus on the basic pension as the object of change in the 1980s in Canada reflects the fact that the federal government could make these changes unilaterally, while changes to the contributory CPP required negotiations with the provinces (Tuohy 1993).[2] But if differences in political institutions could explain *broad patterns of difference* in policy outcomes and in the dynamics of policy change, we would expect those broad patterns to hold across policy arenas—and we do not observe in the pension arena the pattern of difference that we see in the health care arena.

In fact, the depiction of unitary-Westminster, Westminster–federal, and congressional–federal systems sketched here is more a caricature than a characterization of British, Canadian, and American governmental institutions. In particular, the depiction of the American system as beset with insurmountable obstacles needs to be tempered. There is no doubt that the institutional bar for success is set higher in the United States than in Britain. There is possibly no better illustration of that fact than a comparison of the political and institutional resources that could be brought to bear by Margaret Thatcher and Bill Clinton in seeking health care reform. Clinton entered the presidency with a 43% plurality of the popular vote; the Conservatives formed a majority government in Britain in 1987 with a virtually identical 43% of the popular vote. Similarly, the 57% majority enjoyed by the Democrats in the Senate compares closely to the Conservatives' 58% majority in the House of Commons. Yet this level of support was insufficient to ensure success in the American system, and sufficient for success in Britain.

This is, nonetheless, a difference in degree but not in kind. Major change can be accomplished in the U.S. system, whether through partisan supermajorities as was the case in the 1960s when the Medicare and Medicaid programs were put in place, or through a consolidation of authority in a bipartisan coalition as occurred in the case of tax reform in 1986 (White 1995). We need to look further to discover what has stymied major policy change in the health arena since the 1960s. Nor should the institutional prowess of the British system be exaggerated. It was not until her third successive majority victory, it must be remembered, that Margaret Thatcher was willing to take on the reform of the NHS. As Pierson and Weaver (1993) remind us, the Westminster system may concentrate authority, but it also concentrates accountability. Major policy change under such circumstances requires the firming of political will.

A somewhat more modest version of the institutionalist argument still needs to be considered: the argument that institutions shape policy by establishing the channels through which various interests can exercise their influence—that institutions, willy-nilly, "bias" the policy process. Certainly the disproportionate influence of southern conservatives on U.S. social policy through much of the twentieth century, given the strategic location of their representatives in the congressional committee system, is an example of such institutional bias. More generally, however, institutions can be seen to shape both the form and the content of policy by affecting the *stage* of the policy process in which influence is brought to bear by various interests.

A contrast among the three countries under review here is relevant in this regard. The legislative process of the congressional system provides veto points for strategically placed interests; it is the threat of such vetoes by key participants in the health care arena that has created complex and extensive legislative packages on a number of occasions, as compromises are struck and various opponents are placated by particular provisions. In Britain, a majority government can pass legislation in the teeth of strong opposition from central actors in the health care arena, as was the case with the passage of the NHS and Community Care Act of 1990. But those actors must still be accommodated in the process of implementing the legislation. The NHS and Community Care Act, indeed, was little more than a framework document whose details, as we shall see, remained very much to be defined. That process of definition occurred on an ongoing basis in a context peopled largely by health care providers and state actors, and yielded policies in practice that accommodated the interests of the medical profession. Similarly, in Canada, the Medical Care Act of 1966, passed with multiparty support in the Canadian federal parliament against considerable medical opposition, provided essentially a framework of "principles" with which provincial medical insurance plans would have to comply in order to qualify for federal cost-sharing. With the passage of that legislation, action shifted to the provincial level, where organized medicine and provincial governments reached particular accommodations, as will be described in a later chapter.

British and Canadian institutions, then, allowed essential features of the policy framework to be established before that framework was fully fleshed out through the accommodation of interests. American institutions, in contrast, required the policy framework to be jerry-built from the outset through the participation of interests in the legislative process. And sometimes, as in the case of the various health care reform proposals developed in 1993 and 1994, the results are too unattractive to garner a winning coalition of support. (It is worth noting, however, that one approach that does not appear to work, on the basis of experience in some American states, is the passage of rough framework legislation and the creation of a new body to work out the implementation details. Such an approach sends a signal of unfinished business and indeterminacy that encourages the reopening of issues and allows coalitions of support to unravel.)

## Policy Legacies and Path Dependency

Another version of historical institutionalism looks not to the broad institutional structure of government for policy explanations, but rather to the extent to which particular modes of policy action become institutionalized in a given policy arena. This is a version of the scholarly interest in "path dependency" discussed in chapter 1. In such an argument, for example, the Clinton initiative in the 1990s failed at least in part because it did not fall within a "policy legacy" on which it could build. Specifically, it did not build on the legacy of Social Security, as had the Medicare program (which, by the 1990s, had itself become part of that legacy) (Skocpol 1995). Lawrence Jacobs has argued that the design adopted for U.S. Medicare in the 1960s was much influenced by the policy legacy of Social Security. "The public not only consistently identified the elderly's health care as a major concern but also continued to favor a particular policy direction, a reform of existing health care arrangements which enlarged the state's role via the Social Security system" (Jacobs 1993: 138).

Commentaries on the establishment of Britain's NHS have emphasized the continuity between features of the NHS and features of the preexisting system, particularly the role of local authorities in the health care arena (Ham 1992: 15–17). The Canadian federal medicare program also built upon policy initiatives at the provincial level. A "policy legacy" argument, moreover, can be invoked to explain not only what did happen but what did not. The absence of policy initiatives at the state level in the United States after the failure of national health insurance proposals in the immediate postwar period can be attributed at least in part to a policy legacy that accustomed reformers to look to the federal, not the state, level for policy action, as argued in chapter 2.

A "policy legacy" approach can yield important insights. But it needs to be elaborated in several important ways. In the first place, it should be noted that at any given time a number of "policy legacies" may be available to be pursued. At the time of the founding of the NHS, for example, policy-makers could have chosen to build upon the model of the existing national health insurance scheme adapted from Germany in 1911, rather than establishing a new system of state delivery incorporating the role of local authorities and nationalizing the hospitals. For President Clinton, in the development of his health insurance proposals in the early 1990s, there were at least three relevant policy legacies: one the Medicare program, another the complex system of federal and state regulation of the insurance market, and a third the massive Federal Employees Health Benefits Program. In the event, Clinton's proposals drew some elements from the latter two legacies, abjured the first, and added some elements that were entirely new. An argument focusing on policy legacies needs to be able to explain why some legacies are followed and others not.

Taking this question further, we need to be able to explain what brings about dramatic shifts in the course of public policy—what are the circumstances under which the constraints of policy legacies are, if not broken, at least relaxed sufficiently to allow significant innovation to occur. As David Wilsford has argued, the general observation that policy development tends to be "path dependent" makes it all the more important to understand the conditions—the particular conjunctions of events—under which *deviations* from the path occur. Some political institutional systems, as already argued, make such major policy change more unlikely than others. In Wilsford's words:

> Across all systems, big reform is not the norm; it is usually quite difficult, although not impossible. Comparing systems, those that are leveraged from the center or the top (Germany, France, Britain), in combination with propitious conjunctural conditions (Germany, Britain) enjoy a greater likelihood of big reform than do weak, fragmented counterparts (the United States) requiring huge, unlikely conjunctures to accomplish big change. (Wilsford 1994: 252)

Wilsford's perspective is very similar to the one taken in this book, and I return to it later. First, however, other explanatory emphases need to be taken into account.

## Public Opinion and Cultural Understandings

In seeking to understand the conditions under which major changes in health care policy have occurred, as well as the content of those policies, some observers have attributed such change to broad currents of public opinion. Developments in public opinion over time and differences across nations, it is argued, account for the timing of episodes of policy change within a given nation and for broad patterns of difference in policy content across nations.

Lawrence Jacobs, for example, argues that in the process of developing health care policy in Britain and America in the postwar period, policy-makers were broadly constrained by public expectations or "socially shared understandings" that were shaped in part by experience with established policy frameworks. In wartime Britain, a public dissatisfied with the existing organization of health service delivery and financing was galvanized by the publication of the Beveridge report to imagine a comprehensive and universal state-sponsored system. Those expectations, however inchoate, established the context in which policy would be developed. In the early 1960s in the United States, public opinion polls consistently measured health care for the elderly as one of the dominant issues of public concern and also indicated support for "a particular policy direction, a reform of existing health care arrangements which enlarged the state's role via the Social Security system" (Jacobs 1993: 138).

This type of argument implies that the case I have made so far in this book—namely that the opening of "windows of opportunity" for major changes requires a confluence of factors that allows a set of political actors to mobilize sufficient political authority to take action, and that places health care policy in a prominent position within the broad agenda for action—ignores an important antecedent variable. It is the development of a broad current of public opinion that sweeps majority governments or Congressional supermajorities into power and that establishes the broad outlines of the agenda for change.

Those who argue for the fundamental importance of public opinion must, however, confront the issue of the direction of causality. Public opinion is shaped as policy options are developed and presented by policy-makers. It was, after all, the publication of the Beveridge report in Britain in 1942 that defined the possibilities to which public opinion, as measured in polls, responded. The Harris polls in the United States which found public support for an expansion of Social Security to provide health care coverage for the elderly in the 1960s were, after all, posing questions in which the policy options had already been framed and did not include comprehensive universal health insurance (Jacobs 1993: 92–94, 137–40, 191–93). In any event, they did not indicate a "public clamor" for the program—they reflected rather the determination of President Kennedy to "keep the spotlight of national media on Medicare" (Jacobs 1993: 144). In the 1990s, intense media coverage of the health care reform debate and the development of a blizzard of competing proposals in Congress in 1993 and 1994 in the United States paralleled, and arguably contributed to, an increase in uncertainty and an erosion of public support for any major change in health care policy (Brodie and Blendon 1995; White 1995).

At most, public opinion may pressure policy-makers that "something must be done," and establish broad parameters as to acceptable policy responses. High levels of public dissatisfaction with the health care system preceded the establishment of the NHS in the 1940s (Jacobs 1993: 113–17, 169–71); mounting public concern about the future of the NHS preceded the NHS reforms of the 1990s (Blendon and Donelan 1989; Judge and Solomon 1993); and public dissatisfaction with the U.S. health care system (the highest levels of dissatisfaction among ten advanced industrial nations) preceded the failed attempts to make major policy change in the 1990s (Blendon et al. 1990). Conversely, high levels of public satisfaction with Canadian medicare throughout the 1970s and 1980s and into the 1990s meant that any attempt at major policy change would carry great political risk. But if it establishes general pressures and constraints, public opinion gives very little direction as to specific policy responses. Consistently, the levels of support for policy change decline as one moves from broad calls for action to specific policy recommendations—a pattern that holds true across time and nations from the 1940s in Britain to the 1990s in the United States (Jacobs 1993: 113–17; Brodie and Blendon 1995; Jacobs and Shapiro 1995).

Public opinion may be a factor contributing to the opening of windows of opportunity for major policy change, then, but it is neither necessary nor sufficient to explain the timing of their opening or the policy changes that occur as a result. The adoption of Canadian medicare was not preceded by a groundswell of public concern about health care coverage or public pressure for policy action. Public support for a governmental program of universal comprehensive health insurance was considerably lower in the 1960s, when Canadian medicare was adopted, than it had been in the 1940s, when the attempt by the federal government to negotiate a national health insurance program with the provinces failed (Naylor 1986: 122, 158, 236; Taylor 1979: 367). In the late 1980s and early 1990s, the policy direction taken by the Conservative government in Britain flew in the face of public opinion, which polls showed to be opposed to key features of the "internal market" reforms by substantial majorities (Blendon and Donelan 1989). And high levels of public dissatisfaction with the American system did not, in the end, provide sufficient momentum to carry any major policy change through to adoption in the 1990s.

## Political Culture and Parties

Another version of the argument that public opinion creates the conditions for policy change and establishes the parameters for policy options looks to broad strains in national political cultures, and in particular their manifestation in party systems, to explain cross-national differences in health care policy. Notably, the absence of a social–democratic party in the United States is invoked to explain the absence of a program of national health insurance.

A historical-institutionalist version of this argument has been made by Antonia Maioni (1995), who argues that the structure of Canadian political institutions provided a foothold for social democratic forces in Canada that was lacking in the United States. Several institutional features—the Westminster parliamentary model coupled with the exercise of party discipline, the lack of mechanisms of "intrastate" federalism (that is, mechanisms for the representation of regions per se within the structures of the federal government), and the decentralized nature of Canadian federalism—worked together to channel the expression of regionally based protest into third parties and to provide platforms for those parties at the level of provincial governments. Over time, the Canadian system generated regionally based parties of both the left and the right, who came to power at the provincial level and who, from a strong provincial base, were also able to play a key third-party role at the federal level. In the United States, the decentralized nature of the party system and the existence of regional platforms in the U.S. Senate channeled regionally based factions into the major parties, where they were driven to compromise with other ideological elements. The existence of an independent voice on the left played a key role in the development of Canadian health policy: the social–democratic Cooperative Commonwealth Federation (CCF), later the CCF/NDP (New Democratic Party) government of Saskatchewan led in the introduction of both governmental hospital insurance in 1947 and governmental medical care insurance in 1962. Furthermore, the electoral threat from the CCF at the federal level nudged the federal Liberals toward support for national health insurance in both the 1940s and the 1960s.

The role of the CCF/NDP in the history of Canadian health policy (or, for that matter, of the Labour party in the history of British health policy) cannot, of course, be ignored. But the presence of a party of the left is not sufficient to explain the differences in health care policy across the United States, Canada, and Britain. As noted in chapter 2, governmental hospital insurance was introduced by a number of provincial governments in Canada in advance of the federal program, and in only one of those provinces did social democrats form the government or even constitute an electoral threat at the time.

More tellingly, the presence of a party of the left has not led to differences across these three nations in other areas of the welfare state, similar to those that we observe in health care. In general, all three nations can be characterized as having "liberal" welfare states—that is, welfare states which, in contrast to the universalistic social–democratic model, provide limited benefits primarily to those most disadvantaged in the market. Means-tested programs predominate, universalism is limited, and the middle and upper classes turn to the market, not the state, for insurance against income disruption and illness (Esping-Andersen 1990). Canada and Britain diverge from this model in the health care arena; the United States, as noted, diverges from the model with its relative generosity to middle- and upper-income earners under its public pension scheme. The difference in the strengths of parties of the left cannot alone explain this cross-national and intranational variation.

Another, less institutionally oriented version of the argument regarding the importance of the strength of the left identifies a solidaristic strain in the political culture, an organic view of society that links both "tories" and social democrats (Lipset 1990). On this argument, Canada and Britain are both distinguished from the United States by the presence of such a strain:

> Both toryism and socialism view society as a community, an organic entity in which all parts function for the good of the whole. Toryism justifies an inequality of condition in the interests of the collective good: the positions of various "estates" are grounded in a comprehensive framework of social values prescribing their functional responsibilities, their social obligations and, to a large extent, the just rewards attached to the fulfillment of those responsibilities and obligations. The bourgeois reaction to this inequality of condition is to attack ascribed privilege and to emphasize equality of individual opportunity, first in the ownership of property and then in access to the franchise and the largesse of the state. Socialism, in turn, extends this egalitarianism to embrace equality of condition, emphasizing common (at first class and then community) interests over individual interests. In a culture with no vestigial memory of the organic concepts of toryism, such an appeal has less resonance.
>
> Hartz [1955] and McRae [1964], and later Horowitz [1966], have applied this approach in discussing the differences between Canadian and US political culture. Both English Canada and the US are bourgeois "fragments" thrown off from England, and hence both cultures are dominated by liberal individualism. Through a war of independence, moreover, the American republic renounced any vestigial toryism and founded a society explicitly dedicated to principles of Lockean liberalism. "Loyalists" in English Canada, on the other hand, while basically bourgeois liberals, retained and defiantly preserved what Hartz has called a tory "streak" or

"touch." French Canada, moreover, dominated by the hierarchical Roman Catholic Church, preserved its "feudal fragment" faithfully into the mid-twentieth century. (Tuohy 1986: 395–96)

This argument about differences in political culture, if broadly applied, suffers from the same weakness as that relating to parties of the left: why, if these differences have yielded more social–democratic outcomes in the health care arena in Canada and Britain than in the United States, do we not observe similarly stark differences in other areas of the welfare state in these three nations? The answer requires giving the argument more focus, within the framework presented in this book. One of the key manifestations of the "tory streak" in the health care arena in Canada, and arguably in Britain as well, has been in patterns of *medical* opinion, and in positions taken by organized medicine at critical junctures and in the ongoing playing out of the logic of the respective systems.

As noted in chapter 2, the medical professions of both Canada and Britain, in contrast to their American counterparts, were fundamentally supportive of state action to achieve universal health care coverage in the 1940s (although they were internally divided over issues of medical remuneration), and they participated actively in discussions to shape the proposed systems. The Canadian profession had become more hostile to the notion of governmental health insurance by the 1960s, and Saskatchewan doctors went on strike in opposition to the introduction of medicare in that province in 1962. Like the American Medical Association (but with considerably less vehemence), the Canadian Medical Association sought to promote a model of governmental subsidization of low-income subscribers to insurance plans offered by multiple carriers. But once that battle was lost, the Canadian profession soon moved to establish accommodations with provincial governments that, as in the British case, traded off entrepreneurial discretion for collective professional autonomy. It was, indeed, a "red tory" response—an acceptance of some social responsibility for the mitigation of costs in return for the maintenance of a privileged position in the decision-making structure (Tuohy 1992: 118–19). And it contrasted with the overwhelming identification of American physicians with the entrepreneurial ethos in American political culture (Rothman 1993: 278–80).

As we shall see in part II of this book, this accommodation between the profession and the state in Britain and Canada was central to the playing out of the logics of those systems. While such accommodations would not, perhaps, be impossible in the entrepreneurial and individualistic medical culture of the United States once appropriate incentives were in place, they were facilitated in Canada and Britain by solidaristic strains within medical political culture at important periods in the evolution of those systems.

## Interests

This discussion of the role of organized medicine brings us to another category of explanations of the variation in health policy outcomes across nations: the differential role of various organized interests. Explanations of the failure of attempts to adopt comprehensive universal health insurance in the United States in the 1930s through the 1960s have given substantial weight to the power of a constellation of interests, revolving around organized medicine and its allies in the insurance industry and the broader business community, albeit mediated through the institutional structures of the U.S. congressional system and bolstered by the ideological complexion of the political culture (Starr 1982: 279, 369; Morone 1990: 255–56; Skocpol 1993: 536–39; Marmor 1973). But the adoption of national health insurance succeeded in other countries, such as Canada, against the opposition of the medical profession and the insurance industry. As noted in chapter 2, not only the organization of health care delivery but also the extent of private employer-based medical care insurance was very similar in the United States and Canada at the beginning of the 1960s, yet Canada adopted a comprehensive universal medicare scheme and the United States did not. Even in the relatively propitious climate of medical opinion in which the NHS was established in Britain, opposition from medical specialists and especially from general practitioners had to be placated through government concessions in the design of the system.

It is true that the force of medical opposition to national health insurance in the 1930s through the 1960s in the United States is probably unmatched in any other case. But the Clinton proposals for health care reform failed in the 1990s even when they were endorsed in principle by substantial components of organized medicine and received ambivalent and wavering support from the American Medical Association. By the 1990s, indeed, the formerly united phalanx of interests opposing national health insurance had fractured into "hyperpluralistic" complexity (Schick 1995; Jacobs 1997). That national health insurance proposals should fail in the face of united and of divided opposition for medical and business interests suggests that the explanatory force of organized interests as a variable needs to be qualified.[3]

What needs to be explained in the U.S. case (that is, the singular case of the alleged "success" of organized interests in entirely defeating rather than shaping proposals for comprehensive universal health insurance) is why a comprehensive universal plan was not adopted *in the 1960s*—particularly when, under similar conditions in the health care arena, such a plan was adopted in Canada. As will be demonstrated at length in chapter 5, all else flows from this critical moment. If the United States had a health care arena like no other in the 1990s, that was the result of the logic of the system left in place by the decision not to adopt comprehensive universal health insurance in the 1960s. And it was in the 1960s that the institutional constraints of the U.S. system were least confining, with the Democrats in control of the White House and both houses of Congress, with supermajorities. If there was an unexcelled "window of opportunity" for the adoption of national health insurance in the United States, this was it. Why was this opportunity missed? That question leads us to the final category of explanatory factors to be explored here—the role of strategic judgment.

## Strategic Judgment

The role of strategic judgment is typically given more attention in single-case studies than in comparative analysis. This is not surprising: it is hard to imagine an argument that the ability of political actors to "read" a political situation and to respond accordingly varies systematically across nations. And yet, at critical moments, the judgments of human beings have had enormously important consequences—indeed, they became part of the history of institutional development that shaped the context in which subsequent judgments would have to be made.

Accounts of decision-making in each of the episodes of major policy change in Britain, the United States, and Canada in the 1940s through the 1990s are replete with descriptions of individuals and groups of actors forming judgments about which policy directions to pursue, based on their assessment of the array of political forces they faced. These judgments were formed within the constraints established by all of the factors outlined here—the institutional context, the prevailing climate of ideas, and the constellation of interests. But rarely if ever could it be argued that those constraints determined a specific policy outcome; and the role of judgments made by individuals and groups of political actors needs to be taken into account in any explanation of policy development.

In the 1940s, for example, the British Labour Party had a number of options as to the design of a program of comprehensive universal health care coverage. As Lawrence Jacobs concluded on the basis of his extensive review of the documentary evidence, "The Labour government's attempt to fulfill its popular mandate was . . . neither automatic nor consensual. Rather, cabinet ministers had significant misgivings and disagreements over how to weigh the benefits of bold reform against the risks of significant controversy" (Jacobs 1993: 171). The massive Labour majority permitted bold action and allowed of the interpretation that there was a public mandate for a broad agenda of social policy change. But the parliamentary majority had been won, after all, with less than a majority of the popular vote. Furthermore, as Pierson and Weaver (1993) remind us, concentrated authority carries with it concentrated accountability—and a number of influential Labour cabinet ministers were wary of expending the political capital necessary to achieve bold reform (Jacobs 1993: 172–76). Ultimately, however, the arguments of Aneuran Bevan and other ministers on the left of the party won the day, and the judgment was made to proceed with a "bold" initiative, the boldest dimension of which was the nationalization of the hospitals.

In Canada, the scope for strategic judgment was more constrained by the nature of federal–provincial relations. Nonetheless, an important judgment was made by the federal cabinet in 1956 and 1957—in the face of Quebec's general opposition to shared-cost programs and Ontario's opposition to including medical services in any governmental health insurance program—not to press beyond the nine-province "lowest common denominator" of consensus on governmental *hospital* insurance. A decade later, a different judgment was made: the federal government chose to risk the ire of the Ontario and Quebec governments by instituting a "social development" tax in support of a national medical care insurance program over the opposition of those two largest provinces.

In the 1950s the federal government was aware of the potential steering effects of such a staging of hospital and medical care insurance—the potential to foster hospital-based forms of treatment (Taylor 1979: 200). But it chose to capture an emerging consensus as federal–provincial relations began to thaw for the first time in the postwar period. In retrospect, this appears as a wise decision. The climate of federal–provincial relations continued to improve with the unfolding of the "quiet revolution" in Quebec; that climate, together with the "demonstration effects" of the national hospital insurance program and of the introduction of governmental medical care insurance in Saskatchewan, reduced the political risks of introducing the federal medical care insurance legislation in 1966, even in the face of the expressed opposition of the governments of Ontario and Quebec.

But at the time, no group of political actors has the benefit of hindsight. If this gift were given, it would have been of great benefit to those who made health policy in the United States in the 1960s. There, the decision was made not to attempt to adopt comprehensive universal health care insurance, but rather to take the politically less risky course of seeking governmental health insurance for the elderly and the poor, and later the disabled. This approach was consistent with the strategy of incrementalism that advocates of universal health insurance had adopted since the late 1940s, and it built upon the popular policy legacy of Social Security. But, again in retrospect (as discussed at greater length in chapter 2), this judgment appears to have squandered a historic opportunity. As Starr has put it, "At a time of expansive reform [Democratic strategists] continued to back a measure framed in the more conservative 1950s" (Starr 1982: 369). The hesitation of Democratic reformers related not only to their sense of the power of health care providers but also to the ongoing fear of "losing the South" in a period in which the Democrats had also pressed historic civil rights reforms. It is possible, however, that providers could have been faced down and at least a minimum level of support gained with sufficiently generous provisions, as was the case in other nations (notably Canada). The tempering of ambitions in health care so as not to alienate southern support, already judged to have been pressed close to its limit by civil rights reforms, demonstrates how changes in health care are shaped by the broader political agenda at critical moments of major change. Whether that support could have been pressed further by a congressionally skilled southern president remains one of history's tantalizing "hypothetical counterfactuals."

We will, indeed, never know whether in 1965, with a strong president, a united government, and a sweeping popular mandate, the Democrats could have pressed forward to a universal plan. But it is quite conceivable that had a different strategic judgment been made and the introduction of universal national health insurance been attempted, the subsequent history of American health policy would have been very different. In reality, much of the momentum for universal health insurance was lost once the most vulnerable segments of the population—the elderly, the disabled and the poor—were protected.[4] And as discussed in chapters 3 and 5, the playing out of the logic of the private market-dominated system left in place as a result of this strategic judgment made it much more difficult for subsequent attempts at the introduction of a universal plan to succeed.

The decision of Democratic policy-makers not to seek a universal plan in the 1960s in the United States may stand as the most dramatic example of the impact of strategic judgment on policy outcomes within a window of opportunity for change. But strategic judgment also played a role in the development of the "internal market" reforms in Britain in the late 1980s and early 1990s and in the failed policy initiatives in United States in the 1990s. In the British case, as discussed in chapter 3, the Conservative government did not form the will to make major policy changes to the NHS until it had won its third successive majority, and did so only when the prime minister came to the view that the political risks of inaction outweighed the political risks of action. In contrast to the political circumstances under which the NHS was founded, NHS reform did not, in the late 1980s, flow from the government's broad agenda. Rather, it was drawn into that agenda by a reluctant set of policy-makers who had no clear idea of what was to be done. The governmental agenda hence established the parameters for NHS reform, but did not specify a particular policy direction. As Klein puts it, "There was certainly an ideological *bias* among many of those taking part [in the review], in that they tended to share a belief in markets and competition. But there was nothing like an ideological *programme*" (Klein 1995: 188, emphasis in original).

Two key strategic judgments were made regarding the NHS reforms. The first related to process: the decision to have a very closely held review by a small group of Cabinet members, chaired by the prime minister herself. The second related to substance: after the review committee floundered for months in search of a policy direction, the prime minister decided that it should focus on "changing the structure of the NHS rather than its finance" (Klein 1995: 189). These two decisions yielded the White Paper of 1989, a framework for radical change in the structure of the NHS—but only a framework, whose details would need to be worked out by those who had been excluded from its conception.

Finally, we need to consider the role of strategic judgment in the outstanding case of policy failure covered in this book: the Clinton proposal of 1993 in the United States. A number of journalistic and academic interpretations of this episode place heavy emphasis on the role of strategic misjudgment in explaining the demise of this attempt at achieving universal health insurance after an apparently promising start. As in the case of the British internal market reforms, two key strategic judgments were made, one relating to substance and the other to process. But in this case the substantive judgment was made first. This was the portentous decision in 1992 by then-candidate Clinton to embrace the concept of "managed competition" as the framework for his reform initiative. At the time, as discussed in chapter 3, the concept promised to offer a compromise among competing principles and proposals, and to build upon trends already developing within the American health care system. It was, moreover, consistent with Clinton's "New Democrat" agenda. At the same time, however, it was an innovation that differed significantly enough from any of the proposals on the table in the early 1990s that it did not carry with it any congressionally powerful nucleus of supporters. And it lacked a gestation period sufficient to bring a coalition of support to fruition (Morone 1995: 396). In the end, it became a "road to nowhere" (Hacker 1997). Working out the details of the proposal involved an escalating dynamic of complexity, and the resulting scheme was vulnerable to caricature by opponents as a bureaucratic monstrosity (Johnson and Broder 1996; Rovner 1995: 193–94). Nor was there a readily available analogy in the experience of most Americans to provide a communications hook (Skocpol 1995: 74).[5]

The second strategic judgment of the Clinton administration was to adopt an exclusionary process for the development of the "managed competition" model. The establishment of the task force headed by Ira Magaziner and Hillary Clinton closed out members of Congress and in particular represented the foreclosing of the possibility of a bipartisan initiative. A bipartisan approach was probably doomed in any event: as Allen Schick points out, bipartisanship has typically been a more effective strategy in periods of divided government than in periods of united government. In the 1990s, in particular, "By the time health reform was on the agenda, the parties had become so polarized that their differences could not be bridged by normal legislative interaction" (Schick 1995: 255). But the task force approach did have several other important consequences. It submerged the president's agenda from view during a critical period in which the momentum for reform should have been building. This problem was compounded when, just as the task force was close to reaching a conclusion in June 1993, the congressional battle over the president's budget proposals intervened—and action on health care reform was postponed until the fall. Momentum still appeared to be with the president when he unveiled his proposals in September 1993. But the delay had given opponents of the plan time to develop counterstrategies and alternatives (Rovner 1995: 188–91).

In choosing a complex and unfamiliar model of health care reform, and a secretive, exclusionary, and lengthy process for developing the details of that model, President Clinton may well have made strategic errors. But it is not at all clear that different judgments would have yielded a different outcome. Clinton's greatest strategic error may have been in overestimating his own strength as president. The hurdles he faced as a president elected with less than a majority of the popular vote and a Senate majority short of the sixty seats necessary to prevent filibusters and other procedural maneuvers greatly reduced the probability of success. Reviewing previous attempts to enact change in health policy in the United States, Hugh Heclo concurs with Thomas Jefferson that "great innovations should not be forced on slender majorities," and notes that "Clinton's major reform effort was launched from an extremely narrow base of presidential political capital" (Heclo 1995: 90, 94). Allen Schick agrees: "A weak president should not make strong demands: . . . In making demands, Bill Clinton acted like a strong president who had the resources to get what he wanted. In fact Clinton was only strong enough to block the alternatives he did not want" (Schick 1995: 266). In the end, the timing was wrong—if the Democratic president had the political will to bring about major policy change in the health care arena, he did not have the consolidated political authority. To have accomplished change in that context would have required an extraordinarily dexterous political strategist—indeed, if it could have been accomplished at all. If the failure to adopt national health insurance in the 1960s in the United States was a missed opportunity of historic proportions, the failure in the 1990s was the ineluctable outcome of an illusory opportunity.

## Understanding Policy Episodes

Clearly all these factors—political institutions, policy legacies, political culture and parties, public opinion, organized interests, and strategic judgment—play a role in explaining policy outcomes in the health care arena. Having recognized that truism, the more difficult task is to define a framework within which the intersection of these factors can be understood. This book presents such a framework—one that focuses on the timing of episodes of policy change that occur when a set of political actors has the ability to consolidate the political authority necessary to accomplish change and the political will to focus those resources on change in the health care arena. Differences in political institutions establish different degrees of constraint on the ability of any given set of actors to consolidate authority—hence major episodes of policy change are more rare in some nations than in others. Once these opportunities arise, what happens is shaped by a number of factors—the partisan complexion of the dominant set of political actors; the prevailing climate of policy ideas, both broadly and within the health care arena itself; the constellation of interests in the arena; and the strategic judgments made by both the proponents and the opponents of change. Because all these factors are in a state of flux, what matters critically is the timing of the opening of windows of opportunity for change.

This focus on "windows of opportunity" provides an explanation of how, under extraordinary circumstances, policy legacies are established and particular policy paths are embarked upon. It demonstrates how rare are the conjunctions of factors that lead to such major policy change. The first part of this book has explored those conjunctions that have (or have not) created the conditions for major policy change in the health care arena, in particular episodes in the postwar histories of three Anglo-American countries. In so doing, it has made the argument that the timing of these episodes, determined largely by factors beyond the health care arena in the broader political system, has been critically important in affecting the content of the health care policies adopted. But this explanation of foundational policy episodes deals with only part of the puzzle of "path dependency" in policy arenas. It still remains to answer the question as to why policies, once established, are so difficult to change? What is the mechanism through which they become self-reinforcing (Pierson 1997)? Part II of this book examines *how* the policies established in those episodes have their "legatory" effect—not simply by habit or accustomation, but rather through the logics that they establish, logics with their own dynamics that over time can either reinforce or transform the structural and institutional characteristics of the health care system.

# The Distinctive Logics of National Systems

II

# The United States | 5

## The Logic of the Mixed Market

The hallmark of American health policy, as noted in part I, has been its incrementalism. In contrast to the cases of Britain and Canada, in which major episodes of policy change established enduring organizational frameworks for the delivery and financing of health care, U.S. public policy both directly and indirectly fostered continuous organizational change in the health care arena, as private actors responded and adjusted to the incentives and constraints established by incremental policy changes.

American public policies maintained private markets as the predominant mechanism for the provision of health insurance and for health care delivery. Efficiency and equity improvements were sought through regulating and supplementing markets, not, by and large, through supplanting them. The majority of Americans, about 62% in 1993, continued to be covered by health insurance purchased on private markets, subject to both federal and state regulations that fluctuated over time in focus and stringency. Nonmarket mechanisms for the financing of health care (taxes and social security contributions) remained confined to a minority of the population, about 23%, who were insured under the Medicare and Medicaid programs for the elderly, the disabled, and the indigent. And a substantial and slowly growing minority of Americans (15%, up from 13.7% in 1980) had no health insurance coverage at all (HCFA 1995a: 322).

Within this market-oriented system, purchasing decisions nonetheless became increasingly collectivized. In the first place, although the public share of health expenditures [about 44% in 1991 (OECD 1993, vol. 1: 252)] was low relative to other OECD nations, it nonetheless made federal and state governments a substantial presence in the health care market.[1] Second, private health insurance was largely employer-based. Of Americans with private health insurance in 1993, 86% acquired it through their employers (calculated from Holahan et al. 1995a: 255). The employer-based character of the system was facilitated by a key feature of the policy framework, which allowed employers to deduct the full cost of providing insurance coverage to their workers for tax purposes. Employers who chose to self-insure for the purpose of providing health care coverage for their workers were, moreover, shielded by federal legislation from state regulation of their health care plans. Large employers were hence major purchasers of health insurance, and self-insuring large employers were major purchasers of health care.

The health care delivery system, like the system of health care financing, was also organized on market principles: it was composed of independently organized providers of care who offered their services on the market, subject to various forms of regulation by governmental and professional bodies. Governmentally owned facilities, primarily public hospitals, constituted a small and declining proportion of the total.

In the terms used in this book, then, the institutional mix of the U.S. system in the 1970s and 1980s was one in which market elements had a heavy weight, tempered by various forms of hierarchical and collegial controls. As for its structural balance, it accorded a more dominant role for private finance than did any other OECD nation except Turkey. The policy parameters that governed this mix and balance did not change significantly between the 1960s and the 1990s. But within those parameters, the system was transformed through the working out of its own internal logic. It was a logic of entrepreneurialism, which generated a cycle of increasingly complex market strategies and regulatory responses, encouraged the rise of for-profit entities in an arena once dominated by professional practices and not-for-profit insurers and providers, and perhaps ironically led to an increasing reliance on hierarchical mechanisms on the part of both state and private financial actors. In the process, reliance on mechanisms of collegial control—and the power of the medical profession—were dramatically reduced.

This chapter first traces the development through the 1970s and 1980s of incremental changes to the policy parameters established in the 1960s. It then examines the central features of the system that developed within these parameters: the rise of managed care, the regionalization and nationalization of markets, and the growing role of for-profit enterprises. Next it traces out the implications of these developments in reducing the historical medical dominance of the politics and economics of health care, and more generally demonstrates how the logic of the system transformed the political terrain on which the next major attempt at policy change—the Clinton initiative of the 1990s as discussed in chapter 3—had to be contested.

## Regulation in the 1970s

The 1970s saw a number of regulatory initiatives at the federal level. Through that decade, health care expenditures continued to rise as a proportion of GDP—a not surprising outcome given, as Marmor and his colleagues point out, "the inflationary forces at work in medicine—principally broad health insurance coverage, pluralistic financing, and weak countervailing regulatory authorities" (Marmor et al. 1994: 60). Unable or unwilling to adopt a broad-based fiscal strategy in the form of national health insurance, U.S. federal policymakers turned instead to a piecemeal variety of regulatory controls to channel but not to supplant market forces.

These incremental measures did not require the marshaling of political authority and will on the scale that would have been necessary for a comprehensive restructuring of the health care arena. They required, rather, the building of specific and pragmatic coalitions. That strategy was, in turn, even more vulnerable to the need for various concessions to members of the coalition than a massive mobilization around a central defining agenda would have been. The result was a set of programs that was "dispersed bureaucratically, disconnected from the major financing of care, and celebrated with visions of success that no reasonable analyst should have accepted" (Marmor et al. 1994: 22).

The regulatory strategy of the 1970s was essentially three-pronged. One policy thrust was generated by the desire to encourage more efficient modalities of health care delivery. Prepaid plans for hospital and medical care had been pioneered by the Kaiser Permanente group in the 1930s and 1940s, and were receiving increasing attention from leading health policy analysts such as Paul Ellwood, who coined the term "health maintenance organization" (HMO) to describe the type. For a set annual fee, these plans enrolled members who were then entitled to receive a more or less comprehensive package of services as required. This approach thus linked the insurance function to the delivery function, and decoupled, at least at the corporate level, the link between the level of service provision and the level of reimbursement. Presumably, then, it eliminated the incentive to "overservice."

Enthusiasm for this mode of delivery led the Nixon administration to propose legislation providing for federal start-up grants for HMOs and requiring employers offering health insurance benefits to include an HMO option, where available. The subsequent legislative maneuvering then revolved around the definition of the category of "HMOs" to be eligible for such treatment—the range of benefits that eligible HMOs had to offer, and the ratings policies that they had to adopt. In response to pressure from organized medicine (which had opposed the development of prepaid group practice as a fundamental threat to the fee-for-service mode which it equated with professional autonomy) as well as from competitive insurers, these eligibility requirements were defined quite stringently: HMOs were required to offer a comprehensive benefit package and to practice "community rating"—setting a single premium for all enrollees in a given community (Mueller 1993: 22, 50–51). This program was mixed in its effects: it subsidized the development of HMOs but placed them at a competitive disadvantage in the market. Later, however, in response to countervailing pressures from both business and labor groups as well as from HMOs themselves, and to the rise of a "procompetitive" policy strategy in the 1980s (as discussed later), the criteria for "federal qualification" as an HMO (as well as preferential treatment of "federally qualified" HMOs) diminished to the vanishing point (Mueller 1993: 51; Ramsay 1995: 220).[2] A variety of state-level policies, however, continued to establish the regulatory context in which HMOs functioned.

These public policies clearly had an impact on the momentum of HMO development, and on the directions in which that momentum was channeled. The number of federally qualified HMOs rose from 42 in 1977 to more than 300 by the mid-1980s (Mueller 1993: 51). As these organizations were cut loose both from federal funding and from the constraints that such funding imposed, the diversity of the HMO universe multiplied accordingly. In the mid-1980s, however, a public policy change was adopted that was to have a more substantial, albeit indirect, effect upon the development of HMOs: the shift to prospective payment under Medicare to be discussed below.

The second policy development in the 1970s was also directed at taming the unruly growth of the health care industry. Much academic attention has been paid to the checkered history of "health planning" agencies in the United States. Federal legislative involvement in this area began as early as 1963, with an amendment to the Hill–Burton Act that authorized federal matching funds for geographically based health planning agencies (Ramsay 1995: 73). It was in the mid-1970s, however, that "health planning attained its short-lived zenith, at least in organizational terms" (Ramsay 1995: 73). In 1974, the National Health Planning and Resources Act established a network of geographically based Health Systems Agencies (HSAs), autonomous from state governments. The legislation was supported by a coalition including those whose primary concern was with improving access to health services and those concerned with cost containment, and again ranging from those who saw the program as laying the groundwork for the development of a comprehensive national health insurance system to those whose view of the agencies' role was much more modest (Mueller 1993: 22–24, 69). It also reflected the growing strength of the consumer movement in the 1970s: at least 50% of the membership of each agency had to be representative of "consumers."

As in the case of the HMO legislation, numerous compromises necessary to secure legislative passage blunted the thrust of the initiative: the mandate of HSAs was effectively restricted to approving the construction of new facilities, subject to appeal to the respective state governor. Recommendations regarding existing facilities were to be advisory only, and proposals to give the agencies power to review and approve hospital and physician prices were dropped early in the process.

The program actually came to be focused much more on cost containment than on ensuring equitable access. Evidence for the success of HSAs in braking the growth of health care facilities was, however, mixed and contested. The emergence of the "procompetitive" agenda of the 1980s, together with the defection of a key member of the coalition supporting HSAs—the American Hospital Association—sounded the death knell of the program, which was terminated when Congress refused to reauthorize it in 1986 (Mueller 1993: 71–75). It nonetheless left a legacy: it laid the groundwork for a number of state-level planning initiatives, and it had an important symbolic effect in reducing the legitimacy of the medical profession as the dominant force in the health care policy arena (Morone 1990).

The third prong of the regulatory agenda of the 1970s was the attempt to enlist the medical profession to develop collegial mechanisms of quality as well as cost control, in the form of peer review organizations charged with reviewing the utilization of health care services. The first generation of these organizations comprised the Professional Standards Review Organizations (PSROs) established in 1972 to review hospital-based medical services provided under Medicare, with a mandate to reduce overutilization and ensure quality and effectiveness of care through a process of "concurrent review." PSROs were voluntary, not-for-profit, locally based physician organizations funded by the federal government for that purpose. Despite their medical aegis, however, PSROs foundered under the growing opposition of physicians and the pressure of conflicting expectations in Congress and the federal executive as to the relative emphasis to be placed on cost control and quality assurance (Wareham 1994).

A second generation of peer review agencies, termed Peer Review Organizations (PROs), was introduced to replace PSROs under the Tax Equity and Fiscal Responsibility Act (TEFRA) enacted in 1982. In keeping with the procompetitive spirit of the time, these second-generation PROs were financed through contracts awarded through a process of competitive bidding, rather than the former grant-based system. A delay in implementing the PRO program, however, meant that it was introduced into a cost-control context that was dramatically reshaped by the advent of the Medicare Prospective Payment System (to be discussed shortly). Like the PSROs before them, however, the PROs suffered from conflicting expectations and medical opposition. Numerous amendments to the program were made by Congress in the late 1980s; appropriations for it began to decline in the 1990s, and by the mid-1990s it remained only tenuously in existence in the face of proposals to terminate it, including one in the Clinton health care reform proposal of 1994 (Wareham 1994: 98; Weissenstein 1994).

## Prospective Payment in the 1980s

The federal regulatory initiatives of the 1970s, then, with their mixed records of political support and policy success, underwent substantial change or termination in the 1980s. They were, indeed, ill-suited to the deregulatory and decentralist thrust of the Reagan administrations. Ironically, however, the policy change with the most dramatic impact on the structure of health care delivery and the health care market in the post-Medicare period was a product of the first Reagan administration. It was not a regulatory policy per se, but rather a more aggressive use of the major fiscal instrument in the federal government's arsenal—payments to hospitals under Medicare.

In 1983, the federal government shifted the basis of hospital reimbursement from a cost-based system to the Prospective Payment System (PPS). This change dramatically altered the incentives facing health care providers and set in motion a chain of responses that continued to reshape the industry.

Under PPS, hospitals were paid on the basis of national average costs per admission, weighted by the diagnostic categories into which patients were classified at the point of admission, as well as a number of other factors.[3] For each of more than 400 of these "diagnosis-related groups" (DRGs), weights were calculated based on national average lengths of stay and service intensity. The level of reimbursement, then, was established *at the point of admission,* and did not relate to the costs actually incurred in treating a given case. Under PPS, the financial risk involved by case (though not the risk of incidence of particular types of cases) was shifted from the payer to the provider of care.

The shift to PPS radically changed the financial incentives facing hospital providers. As Shortell and his colleagues have noted, any system of "up-front" calculation of payment, including the DRG-based system, means that the various components of the delivery system become "cost centers," not "revenue centers" as they are under cost-reimbursement or fee-for-service payment schemes (Shortell et al. 1994: 48). Hence under PPS, providers had a greater incentive to manage the hospital system to reduce costs per case. This incentive was magnified as successive congressional votes "ratcheted down" (i.e., reduced the rate of escalation of) reimbursement rates under the DRG-based formula (Mueller 1993: 82).

In response, hospital providers sought to control costs, as will be discussed shortly, but they also sought to *shift* costs. Cost-shifting had been a central feature of the economics of health care delivery system for decades, as providers sought to take advantage the different levels of price sensitivity of multiple private and public payers. Indeed, the shifting of the costs of "uncompensated" care (essentially charity care and bad debts) onto Medicare charges was explicitly recognized and condoned, but also limited, in the PPS reimbursement formula. With the tightening of controls under PPS, hospitals had an increased incentive to shift costs to less price-sensitive private payers.

The evidence for such shifts in practice has been a matter of considerable academic debate. Broad aggregate trends support the cost-shifting hypothesis. The ratio of hospital transaction prices to average costs was consistently higher for private than for public payers, and the divergence between the two grew consistently between 1985 and 1992. In 1985, Medicare payments to hospitals just covered average costs, having risen slightly over the previous five years. By 1993, Medicare payments amounted to 89% of average cost. Medicaid ratios dropped fairly steadily over the 1980s, from about 90% of average cost in 1980 to under 80% by the end of the decade. In the early 1990s Medicaid rates began to rise, and by 1993 they covered 93% of average cost. Meanwhile, however, rates paid to hospitals by private payers were well above average costs and increasing. In 1980, private payers paid on average 110% of average costs; by 1992 this ratio had risen to 131%. After 1992, however, the ratio for private payers began to decline (Weissenstein 1995b: 3; see also Morrisey 1994: 37–41). Using a different measure, Thorpe reported that hospital profits from private health insurance (defined as private insurance payments minus costs of treating privately insured patients, as a proportion of total costs) declined from 12.1% in 1991 to 10.7% in 1994. Losses from Medicare and Medicaid declined from –4.6% to –2.7% and from –2.0% to –1.6%, respectively, between 1991 and 1994 (Thorpe 1997: 354–55). These aggregate trends are consistent with the hypothesis that charges to privately insured patients were raised to compensate for the tightening of reimbursement policies under Medicare and Medicaid in the mid-1980s, until the resistance of private payers forced a tempering of this strategy in the early 1990s.[4]

As private payers were faced with increasing hospital prices, then, their price-sensitivity appears to have increased as well. Indeed, what has been referred to as the "competition revolution" in health care was driven not by the supply side but by the demand side, by the rise of activist and sophisticated purchasers (Fuchs 1993: 169). The emergence of intermediate entities to play the role of "organizing and managing the consumption of care" (Chernichovsky 1995) as discussed in chapter 1 was the most significant organizational development of the 1980s and 1990s.

## The Rise of "Managed Care"

These intermediate "managed care" entities took a bewildering variety of forms. A number of different types of HMOs, having been fostered by federal financial support in the 1970s and freed from federal regulatory constraints in the 1980s, offered comprehensive prepaid packages of care, including hospital care provided by hospitals either owned by or contracted with the HMO. Classic "staff-model" HMOs employed physicians in large multispecialty settings within a unified management structure. Closely related "group" model HMOs, of which Kaiser Permanente is the quintessential example, maintained a separately organized medical staff. A "network" or "independent practice association" (IPA) variant of the HMO concept, which accounted for a relatively small proportion of total HMO enrollment at the beginning of the 1980s, expanded rapidly over the course of that decade. The IPA model comprised physicians practicing in solo or small group practices which remained organizationally distinct while being linked together through contractual or ownership arrangements. Preferred Provider Organizations (PPOs)—organizations of independent providers who contracted to provide services for discounted rates in return for guaranteed patient volumes—emerged as an alternative to HMOs. Physician–Hospital Organizations (PHOs)—organizations attempting to integrate independent physicians and hospitals for the purpose of contracting with insurers, employers, or indeed with HMOs and PPOs—developed as yet another variation, although it has been suggested that PHOs might represent merely a transitional form of organization (Jaklevic 1995). Meanwhile, traditional indemnity-oriented insurers adopted a variety of utilization review and "managed care" strategies.

This brief overview does not exhaust the variety of organizational forms, which defy categorization. Indeed, the rapid proliferation of different versions of HMOs, PPOs, PHOs, etc. outpaced the development of public policies regulating the insurance function—a matter of political conflict between, for example, HMOs which faced a variety of state-level regulation and PHOs which generally did not. Attempts to bring some definitional order to this diversity identified several dimensions along which managed care entities vary: the underwriting mechanism (for example, prepayment or indemnity), which determined the degree to which financial risk was borne by the payer, the intermediary, or the provider; the extent to which consumer selection of provider was restricted; the degree to which and manner in which utilization controls were placed on physicians' practice; and the range of care for which the entity undertook to arrange provision (Weiner and de Lissovoy 1993; Robinson 1993).

"Staff model" HMOs lay at one end of these spectra; prepaid coverage meant that the HMO assumed all financial risk, consumer choice of provider was restricted to physicians employed by the HMO, medical practice was subject to various forms of utilization control, and the HMO undertook to provide a comprehensive range of care. At the other extreme were managed care indemnity plans, which differed from traditional indemnity plans only in placing utilization controls on providers. Between these extremes lay an almost infinite number of possible permutations and combinations of organizational and contractual arrangements. As Weiner and de Lissovoy noted, the typical health insurance plan was in fact "an interwoven lattice of numerous corporate entities" involving both hierarchical and contractual connections. And each of the entities making up this lattice was likely to be involved in numerous other lattices as well (Weiner and de Lissovoy 1993: 79).

The variety of these organizational forms and the blurring of lines between them make consistent definitions and the tracking of trends over time difficult. What is clear, however, is that managed care came, within a decade, to characterize most forms of employer-based coverage in the United States. In 1988, about 29% of all those with employer-based coverage were in some form of managed care plan; by 1995, this proportion had risen to 71% (Davis et al. 1995a; Thorpe 1997: 341). As we shall see, moreover, state governments adopted various forms of managed care in their Medicaid programs. In 1995, HMO enrollment stood at almost 70 million and PPO enrollment at more than 90 million (Peterson 1998).

For both providers and recipients of care, these developments made for a complex and turbulent environment. According to a 1995 survey, 87% of practicing physicians participated in at least one managed care plan, 61% had at least three managed-care contracts, and 26% contracted with ten or more plans. Entry and exit from plans showed considerable fluidity: more than 60% of physicians reported joining a plan in the previous three years; about one-quarter attempted to join a plan but were denied; and about 20% reported leaving a plan either voluntarily or involuntarily (Schoen and Collins 1996). A 1994 study of employment-based health plan enrollees in three major cities found that 54% of those in managed care plans had changed plans in the previous three years; and in three-quarters of these cases the change was involuntary, as the result of an employer decision or a job change. Forty-one percent of the managed-care enrollees who changed plans reported that the change required them to change physicians, as opposed to only 12% of those who changed traditional indemnity plans (Davis et al. 1995a: 103–4). From the physician's perspective, 86% of a 1995 national sample reported losing patients because the patient's plan changed (Schoen and Collins 1996).

The plethora of organizational and contractual arrangements was driven by essentially two imperatives in the American health care marketplace of the 1990s, both emanating from the demand side. First, the demand (primarily from employers, but also from state Medicaid agencies) for plans offering comprehensive benefit packages for defined populations required the management of a broad continuum of care. Second, the increasing price-consciousness of both public and private payers required that care be provided in the least costly setting feasible (and particularly that hospital utilization be kept to a minimum). As the intermediaries who sought to "organize and manage the consumption of care" confronted these imperatives, they were faced with classic "make or buy" trade-offs: that is, they had to weigh the costs of writing, executing, and monitoring contracts with separately organized providers against the costs of building their own organizations. Responses to these trade-offs drove an endless wave of restructuring.

Contracting remained the most common mechanism for integrating health care delivery, but the trend toward vertical integration of health care facilities, already apparent in the 1970s, escalated over the 1980s and 1990s. By 1993, for example, substantial numbers of community hospitals were contracting with HMOs, PPOs, group practices, and other nonhospital entities, while smaller but significant numbers were more directly integrated with such entities (table 5.1).

Horizontally, hospital mergers resulted in fewer and larger hospitals. From 1965 to 1993, the number of community hospitals declined by 8% while the number of community hospital beds increased by 24% (calculated from American Hospital Association 1995: table 1). In 1994 and 1995, merger activity exploded. *Modern Healthcare* magazine recorded 184 hospital mergers in 1994 and 230 mergers in 1995, although there is some overlap in these figures (Lutz 1995a: 43). Prior to 1993, the AHA reported fewer than twenty mergers per year. Hospitals were also drawn into multi-institutional chains and alliances spanning large geographic areas. In 1995 a merger of American Healthcare Systems and Premier Health Alliance created the largest of these entities, an alliance comprising 25% of U.S. community hospitals, with revenues three times larger than the largest hospital chain, Columbia/HCA (Scott 1995). Columbia/HCA also took a major vertically integrative step, moving into the insurance industry through a joint venture with Blue Cross/Blue Shield of Ohio.

Managed care organizations as well as hospitals were involved in horizontal and vertical integration. *Managed Healthcare* magazine reported forty-two HMO

TABLE 5.1 Community Hospital Vertical Integration and Contracting, 1993; Percent of Hospitals Reporting Types of Arrangements[a]

| Health Care Entity | Owned by Hospital | Provided by Hospital's System | Provided through Joint Venture | Provided through Formal Contractual Arrangement |
|---|---|---|---|---|
| Independent Physician Association | 4.6 | 2.3 | 1.7 | 12.0 |
| Group Practice | 11.2 | 3.3 | 0.9 | 12.2 |
| Physician–Hospital Organization | 7.9 | 3.1 | 4.3 | 3.5 |
| HMO | 5.6 | 4.4 | 3.0 | 21.2 |
| PPO | 11.4 | 5.7 | 4.0 | 24.5 |
| Indemnity/Fee-for-Service Insurer | 8.4 | 2.2 | 0.7 | 17.2 |

Source: American Hospital Association 1995.

[a] Hospitals could report more than one type of arrangement.

mergers and acquisitions from the second quarter of 1994 to the first quarter of 1995 (Troy 1995). In 1996, the Aetna insurance firm expanded the HMO side of its business dramatically with the acquisition of the large managed care organization US Healthcare—a deal that drew widespread attention not only because of its size (Aetna paid $8.9 billion for US Healthcare, and became the largest medical benefits firm in the United States) but also because of US Healthcare's profitability and reputation for innovativeness. The Aetna/US Healthcare acquisition was a major development in the continuing trend toward increasing concentration in the managed care industry. Based on 1995 enrollment data and taking account of the Aetna/US Healthcare acquisition, it was estimated that by mid-1996 the four largest HMOs in the United States accounted for more than 50% of total HMO enrollment (Thorpe 1997: 343–44).

Some of the enthusiasm for vertical integration nonetheless appeared to be cooling in the late 1990s, as some of the most high-profile examples encountered economic and legal difficulties (Marmor 1998). While various versions of vertically and horizontally integrated firms continued to be formed, it appeared likely that even more varied types of "virtual" integration through contracting would continue to be the dominant mode of organization within a highly complex mix (Robinson and Casalino 1996).

## Regional versus National Markets

The developments discussed in the previous section were highly regionalized phenomena. The extent and type of managed care "penetration" varied greatly across regions. In 1994, the percentage of households with either an HMO or a PPO plan as primary coverage ranged from 66% in the Pacific region (as defined by U.S. census divisions) to 46% in the West South Central region. The

Pacific region ranked highest in HMO penetration, at 35%, while the East South Central region ranked lowest in HMO penetration (at 14%) but highest in PPO penetration (at 34%). Among smaller geographic units, the variation is considerably more stark. At the state level, combined HMO–PPO penetration ranged from more than 70% to less than 30%. The variation in HMO penetration was somewhat greater than was the case for the more loosely organized PPO form. HMO penetration ranged from about 40% in Massachusetts and California to less than 10% in Wyoming, South Dakota, North Dakota, Arkansas, and Mississippi. Only one state, Maine, had less than 20% PPO penetration; and two, Utah and Alabama, had more than 40% (*Managed Healthcare* 1995). At substate levels, the character of local markets shows a similar range of variation. Using a different measure of HMO penetration (HMO enrollment as a proportion of all private health insurance enrollment) to compare fifteen selected communities, Ginsburg and his colleagues found a variation from about 38% in Minneapolis/St. Paul, Minnesota to just more than 10% in Houston, Texas (Ginsburg 1996: 12).

This regional variation reflected the essentially locally based economics of health care delivery discussed in chapter 1, which has historically concentrated power in the hands of local hospitals and physicians. The development of HMOs, and then PPOs and other alternative models, has been variously facilitated or constrained by the culture and organizational configuration of local provider communities (Ginsburg 1996: 15–17). Increasingly, it was also driven by the emergence of locally based business coalitions or even large single employers as sophisticated and aggressive purchasers.

Regional variation in the degree of organization and market power of purchasers was even greater than was the variation on the supply side. In some cases, such as the Buyers' Health Care Action Group (BHCAG) in Minneapolis/St. Paul, the Massachusetts Healthcare Purchasing Group, and the Pacific Business Group on Health, coalitions of firms were established to enhance their market power. In most cases, the primary strategy of these coalitions was to bargain aggressively over price. Some, such as BHCAG, however, also began to implement clinical guidelines focused on cost-effectiveness (Christianson et al. 1995: 124; Lipson and De Sa 1996). In other communities, the major market power on the demand side was exerted not by coalitions but by large employers playing a leading role in bargaining down price increases. Self-insurance by employers also rose in the 1990s,[5] giving rise to demand for third-party administration, but this phenomenon also varied widely across regions. In some cases, such as the Self Insurers' Association in South Carolina, such firms banded together to increase their bargaining power. In addition, a number of states began in the 1990s to sponsor purchasing alliance for small employers, but there was wide variation in the mandate and effectiveness of these bodies (Lipson and De Sa 1996).

Purchasing coalitions varied in their degree of cohesion and in their aggressiveness in dealing with providers and intermediaries. In some cases, they dissolved as key members broke away to negotiate independently. In others, their aggressiveness was tempered by cross-membership with the boards of provider organizations such as hospitals (Lipson and De Sa 1996: 73).

Regional variation thus continued to be a dominant characteristic of the American health care arena. But it existed in tension with a number of nationalizing forces, as is apparent in the history of the merger activity discussed in the previous section. At first this activity reflected the regionalized nature of health care markets. One study of eleven organized delivery systems found that the extent of clinical integration diminished when units were more than fifty miles apart on average (Shortell et al. 1996: 162). Early HMO mergers also tended to occur between organizations in relatively close geographic proximity.

But broader forces in the political economy of American health care gave rise to organizations spanning large, even nationwide, geographic areas. Multistate delivery organizations can benefit from system-level learning about the complex web of federal regulatory and fiscal provisions—not only Medicare and Medicaid requirements, but other programs such as the Civilian Health and Medical Program of the Uniformed Services (CHAMPUS) and the Federal Employees Health Benefits Program. They may also have an advantage in negotiating with multistate corporate employers, by reducing the transaction costs of developing consistent benefit packages. The huge purchasing power of nationwide organizations gives them great leverage in dealing with suppliers, with a resultant reduction in costs that may give them a price advantage over locally based competitors. Finally, providers with a large geographic span may be able to develop a base of experience from which to countervail the influence of the local professional networks that have yielded wide local variations in practice patterns.

In summary, the historic localism of health care markets was reflected in the 1980s and 1990s in the emergence of bargaining relationships among sophisticated purchasers, providers, and intermediaries at local and regional levels, and of distinctively regional patterns of organizational and contractual arrangements. That regionalism was nonetheless being eroded by the rise of horizontally and vertically integrated firms with broad geographic spread. These firms represented a significant and powerful new element in the American health care arena, with both economic and political implications.

## The Growing Role of For-Profits

Another powerful element in the American health care arena in the 1980s and 1990s, which was not new but grew dramatically in importance, was the role of for-profit organizations. Arguably the incentive to maximize "profit"—broadly defined to include rents accruing to the "labor-managed firm" of the medical practice and the surpluses of not-for-profit organizations as well as the profits of for-profit enterprises—has always played a central role in decision-making in the U.S. system. Both for-profit and not-for-profit entities face incentives to maximize profit/surplus. The essential difference between them lies in how the proceeds are treated: in the case of for-profit corporations, they are distributed to investors in the form of dividends or increased equity; in the case of not-for-profit entities they are reinvested in the organization according to its mission or mandate. This is not a trivial difference, as we shall see, but it should not obscure the profit-maximizing calculus common to both (Institute of Medicine 1986: 184–85; M. Morrisey 1994: 18–19).

Until the mid-1980s, profit maximization essentially meant revenue maximization; under an open-ended fee-for-service system with indemnity insurance, the provision of more services meant more revenue and more profit. In such circumstances all incentives in the system drove toward expansion: the professional objective of employing skill and technology to the fullest, and not-for-profit mandates of community service, as well as profit maximization. The advent of cost-conscious purchasers in the mid-1980s, however, broke this "alignment of incentives." In the changing market, profit maximization came increasingly to depend upon cost-minimization strategies that came into potential or actual conflict with professional or community objectives. In general, these strategies were adopted first in the growing for-profit sector of the health care industry.

The for-profit form has a long and somewhat checkered history in U.S. health care. In the late nineteenth and early twentieth centuries, the for-profit proprietary hospital was the predominant model of ownership in the U.S. hospital sector (Marmor et al. 1994: 54–55). Over the course of the twentieth century, however, public policies favored the development and expansion of not-for-profit private and governmental ownership of hospitals, through beneficial tax treatment and direct subsidization. By 1965, 60% of community hospitals (with 70% of all community hospital beds) were owned by not-for-profit corporations, while 15% of hospitals (with 6% of beds) were owned by for-profit corporations. In the next three decades, however, growth in the for-profit sector outpaced both not-for-profit and public sectors. Between 1965 and 1993, the number of beds in for-profit community hospitals increased by 111%, compared with a 27% increase in not-for-profit hospital beds and a 5% decrease in public hospital beds. In 1993, the share of community hospital beds accounted for by for-profit institutions was still only 11% (calculated from American Hospital Association 1995: table 1). But the for-profit sector was highly concentrated—in 1993 the five largest for-profit systems owned more than three-quarters of all for-profit hospitals and 95% of all for-profit beds.

These data predate the wave of mergers and acquisitions that picked up momentum in 1994, in which for-profit entities made major gains. As a result of this activity, publicly traded for-profit firms made a net gain of almost 22,000 hospital beds from not-for-profit or privately owned organizations between the first quarter of 1994 and the third quarter of 1995 (Fubini 1996). In response to this formidable competitive challenge, not-for-profit hospitals as well became increasingly linked in national and regional systems. Peterson reports that "Nationally, only a fifth or fewer hospitals expect to be free-standing institutions by the end of the [1990s], neither bought nor part of an alliance or network" (Peterson 1997: 298).

With regard to managed care organizations, the rise of the for-profit form was much more dramatic. By the mid-1990s for-profit firms accounted for the majority of managed care enrollment; and the momentum of growth continued. Indeed, between 1981 and 1997 the for-profit share of managed care enrollment rose from 12% to 62% (Srinivasan et al. 1998). The further expansion of HMOs thus appeared almost certain to increase the span of the for-profit model.

The growth of for-profit institutions reflects the declining advantages conveyed by the traditional instruments of public policy support for not-for-profits. Conditions attached to tax-exempt financial instruments limited the flexibility of not-for-profits to adapt to the rapidly changing marketplace. Substantial start-up capital was necessary for the development of HMOs, PHOs, and other types of integrated health care organizations. With the decline of government and philanthropy as sources of capital,[6] not-for-profit firms were essentially limited to operating surpluses and borrowing to obtain capital. For-profit organizations, with their access to equity markets, had a clear advantage in this regard.

The need to appeal to investors also gave for-profit organizations a strong incentive to expand their market share, fueling the movement toward horizontal and vertical integration. As the Institute of Medicine presciently put it in 1986:

> Investor-owned companies have powerful motives for expansion. The price of their stock—and, therefore, their continued access to equity capital, as well as the value of the assets of their stockholders—depends heavily on growth in earnings, particularly for companies that represent themselves to investors as growth companies. In a field such as acute hospital care, in which the market is maturing, achieving increased earnings may require increasing market share or moving into new markets. Growth can often be achieved more easily through acquisitions than through internal operations. Hence, some observers believe that the growth imperative of the investor-owned sector could change the overall for-profit/not-for-profit/public composition of health care even more in the future than it has in the past. (Institute of Medicine 1986: 184–85)

The impact of for-profit institutions on strategic decision-making within the health care industry, moreover, was disproportionate to their market share. According to Marmor and his colleagues, for-profit institutions were more sensitive than their non-profit counterparts to the changing incentives facing health care providers (Marmor et al. 1994: 63–79). In particular, for-profit facilities were less likely to offer services used disproportionately by the indigent and more likely to screen patients on the basis of insurance coverage or other measures of ability to pay. Prior to the adoption of prospective payment, when revenue maximization was the primary driver of profits, there was some evidence that for-profits had higher margins on and greater utilization of ancillary services.[7] With the introduction of prospective payment, it was argued that for-profits would be most likely to respond to the incentive to screen out the more costly cases within any particular DRG category (Feder et al. 1984). There is little if any direct evidence of such behavior, but as we shall see later the growing differences in the financial circumstances of various types of hospitals were consistent with this hypothesis. The insurance rating practices of for-profit firms, furthermore, forced not-for-profit plans such as Kaiser Permanente and Blue Cross/Blue Shield to abandon their practices of "community rating" (that is, charging the same premium to all members of a community risk pool). By offering lower premiums to cover lower-risk persons, the for-profits threatened to "cream-skim" the community risk pools, leaving the not-for-profits with only the higher risks.

The behavior of for-profit providers presented a substantial market challenge to not-for-profit providers, and threatened the very financial viability of public institutions. The shedding of uninsured and indigent patients by the for-profits, at a time when the proportion of uninsured Americans was growing, directed those patients toward not-for-profit and public institutions, which in turn attempted to decrease the burden of uncompensated care. In 1988, the value of uncompensated care as a percentage of gross patient revenues in for-profit and not-for-profit hospitals was little different, at 4.8% and 5.0%, respectively. By 1994, the proportion of uncompensated care in for-profit hospitals had declined by almost one-fifth to 3.9%, while at not-for-profit hospitals the decline was much more marginal, to 4.8%. But both types of hospitals were dramatically different in this regard from public hospitals, in which uncompensated care amounted to 13.3% of gross patient revenues in 1988 and 12.9% in 1993 (Greene 1995: 52). The differences were even more dramatic among hospitals associated with chains or systems: uncompensated care amounted to 1.8% of net patient revenues in for-profit systems in 1994, compared to 4.1% in not-for-profit systems and 24.1% in public systems, according to the annual survey conducted by *Modern Healthcare* magazine (Greene and Lutz 1995: 49).

As these strategies unfolded, the lines of distinction between for-profit and not-for-profit facilities began to blur. Not-for-profit entities established for-profit subsidiaries and entered into joint ventures with for-profit firms. Several Blue Cross/Blue Shield plans—in Wisconsin, Indiana, California, and Missouri—created for-profit subsidiaries in the early 1990s, and Blue Cross/Blue Shield of Ohio entered into a joint venture with Columbia/HCA as already noted. Indeed, the Blue Cross/Blue Shield Association, the mainstay of the not-for-profit sector, decided in 1994 to allow its member plans to convert to for-profit status. By 1996, Blue Cross of California had converted to for-profit status, and Blue Cross and Blue Shield plans in at least eighteen other states were either contemplating or in the process of conversion to for-profit status (Bell 1996: 60). The liquidity of not-for-profit organizations generally increased dramatically in the 1990s, triggering a number of legislative efforts at the state level to require certain levels of expenditure for uncompensated care or community service by not-for-profits in order to retain tax-exempt status, and fueling speculation about further for-profit conversions (Greene 1995; Major 1995).

The rise of for-profits, together with increased levels of vertical and horizontal integration in the health care arena, faced physicians with stark challenges. In many areas of the country, independent solo practice simply became infeasible. Individual physicians had to affiliate with managed care organizations—either directly through contracts or outright employment or indirectly through affiliation with medical groups or hospitals that in turn entered into managed care arrangements. Those who sought to establish medical groups or IPAs confronted the need for capital and for managerial expertise. Hospitals provided one possible source for meeting these needs. But the market generated others, notably a number of publicly traded for-profit physician management companies. The choice between these two major alternatives confronted physicians with difficult trade-offs:

> As facilities burdened with excess acute care beds, hospital systems are not attractive organizational partners under managed care. As tax-advantaged, bond-financed multidivisional corporations, however, hospital systems are major players and are succeeding in organizing the delivery system around themselves in some local markets. Investor-owned physician management companies also are eager to offer capital, with strings attached, to medical groups. From the perspective of the medical groups, these outside investors are attractive because of their lack of encumbrance with hospital beds, yet are disturbing because of their lack of local community commitment and their strict subordination to equity markets. Many medical groups prefer a homegrown integrated system to one made on Wall Street. (Robinson and Casalino 1996: 18–19)

More generally, the transformation of the American medical marketplace presented unprecedented challenges to the medical profession—challenges which, as described in the next section, threatened the foundations of medical influence.

## Performance Monitoring and the Role of Clinical Judgment

The rise of managed care, particularly of for-profit entities, has led many analysts and observers of the American system to remark upon the declining clinical autonomy of physicians. As previously noted, the increasing focus on cost minimization in the 1980s broke the symmetry between professional objectives to use skill and technology fully, subject only to professional norms, and the profit-maximization objectives of owners of practices, facilities, and health insurance firms. The subsequent history of organizational change can be seen in large part as a variety of attempts to realign the incentives facing these various actors. In the process, the clinical autonomy of the medical profession—the discretion to use clinical judgment in individual cases according to professional norms—came under severe pressure.

In nations in which the state plays a larger role in the financing of medical care—including (as we shall see in subsequent chapters) Canada and Britain—the entry of state agencies as the primary purchasers of medical care confronted the profession with a trade-off between the preservation of the clinical autonomy and the entrepreneurial discretion of individual physicians. The compromise that in various forms underlies most systems of publicly financed health care is one in which the profession accepts the legitimacy of the state setting budgetary parameters, while the state recognizes the legitimacy of the role of physicians, both individually and collectively, in allocating resources within those parameters through the exercise of their clinical judgment. This meant, to different degrees in different nations, that the profession ceded the entrepreneurial discretion of individual physicians over the price of their services and in some cases the location of their practices. But it also preserved the clinical autonomy of the profession, particularly at the collective level, to a marked degree.[8]

In the United States, in contrast, organized medicine strongly defended the entrepreneurial as well as the clinical autonomy of physicians through various episodes of actual or attempted change in public policy and, in so doing, allied itself with insurance and other business interests. That strategy left it vulnerable, however, when entrepreneurial and clinical interests in the provision of health care began to pull in different directions.

The preservation of entrepreneurial discretion yielded American physicians generally higher incomes than their counterparts in other nations (table 5.2). The income levels suggested in table 5.2 should be treated with great caution, given the variety of definitions of both the numerator and the denominator in calculating net professional incomes of physicians in different nations. The *trends* revealed in table 5.2, however, are less vulnerable to these cross-national differences in definition, and they are instructive. The United States is the only one of these nations in which the ratio of net professional physician income to average employee compensation increased between 1970 and 1989. In Canada, Germany, and Switzerland, in which this ratio was higher than the American ratio in 1970, the relative position of physicians declined markedly. Relative to U.S. incomes, only Japanese doctors appear to have improved their position (from a very low base); but this ratio was affected by changes in the purchasing power of national currencies as well as by definitional differences.

It should also be noted that the high average incomes of American physicians were in part a function of specialty mix. Although the different definitions of primary care or generalist and specialist physicians also vary across

TABLE 5.2  Relative Average Physician Incomes

| | Ratio of Average Physician Income to Average Employee Compensation | | | Ratio of Average Physician Income to Average U.S. Physician Income @ PPP | | |
|---|---|---|---|---|---|---|
| | 1970 | 1980 | 1989 | 1970 | 1980 | 1989 |
| Canada | 5.0 | 3.5 | 3.6 | 0.72 | 0.54 | 0.55 |
| Germany | 6.5[a] | 5.0 | 4.3[c] | 0.91 | 0.81 | 0.73[c] |
| Japan | 2.2 | 2.2 | 2.1 | 0.19 | 0.29 | 0.29 |
| Sweden | 3.7 | 2.0 | 2.0 | 0.47 | 0.27 | 0.25 |
| Switzerland | 5.0 | 4.6 | 3.9 | 0.79 | 0.90 | 0.76 |
| United Kingdom | 2.6[b] | 2.7 | 2.4[d] | 0.49 | 0.35 | 0.31 |
| United States | 4.7 | 4.8 | 5.2 | 1.0 | 1.0 | 1.0 |

*Source:* Calculated from OECD 1993, vol. 1: 156; vol. 2: 43, 45.

[a] 1971.

[b] 1975.

[c] 1986.

[d] 1987.

nations and make precise comparisons very difficult with existing data, it is nonetheless the case that the United States had a very high proportion of specialist physicians relative to most other OECD nations. The General Accounting Office of the U.S. Congress reported that the proportion of U.S. physicians engaged in general or family practice decreased from 19% to about 13% between 1970 and 1988. (If general internists and general pediatricians are included in the definition of "general practitioners" the proportion stood at 34% in 1988.) By way of contrast, the proportion of physicians who were general practitioners (not including internists or pediatricians) remained roughly stable at about 51% in Canada in the same 1970–1988 period, and declined from 50% to 42% in Britain (General Accounting Office 1991: 38; Merry 1997: 165).

There is some evidence, however, that the income gains of American physicians began to erode in the 1990s. The growth in average physician incomes in the 1980s was driven largely by greater service volumes per physician and greater profit margins per service (Pope and Schneider 1992). The increased attention to cost minimization under managed care continued to place great pressure on at least the first of these factors. Furthermore, the increasing demand for the "gatekeeping" role of primary care physicians under managed care to reduce the proportion of secondary and tertiary care suggested upward pressure on the incomes of primary care physicians and downward pressure on the incomes of specialists. A 1994 national physician survey found that a majority anticipated that physician incomes would decrease in the future, although respondents were about as likely to report recent declines in income as they were to report income increases.[9] This income experience, however, varied by specialty type: a national survey of physicians in various practice settings in 1995 indicated that specialists were significantly more likely than general practitioners, by a margin of 42% to 28%, to report declines in their incomes over the previous three years (Schoen and Collins 1996).[10]

In general, moreover, the trend toward physician employment in managed care organizations as opposed to self-employment seemed to imply lower incomes. The proportion of practicing physicians employed in hospitals, group practices, HMOs, and other organized settings rose from about 23% in 1983 to about 37% in 1994, according to AMA estimates (Burda 1994, 1995). Incomes of employed physicians were generally lower, and rates of increase slower, than for self-employed physicians, although these aggregate comparisons were greatly complicated by differences in the specialty mix and age structure of the two groups.

Data collected annually by the AMA suggested considerable income volatility, if not a declining trend, in the 1990s. Between 1985 and 1989 real average physician incomes increased at an average annual rate of 4.8%. Between 1990 and 1994 the average annual rate of increase was zero—an average that masked a range of variation from an increase of 3.5% in 1992 to a decrease of almost 4.5% in 1994 (calculated from Simon and Born 1996: exhibit 1). The income swings between the two periods were greatest in obstetrics and gynecology and in surgical and medical subspecialties. General practitioners' incomes showed slow but steady gains, but other "primary care" physicians (general internists and pediatricians) shared in the volatility of the specialist pattern (Simon and Born 1996: 127). In this context, the expressed unease of specialists about their future income streams was understandable.

If American physicians began to experience income declines in the 1990s, even earlier they began to experience constraints on their clinical autonomy. Until the mid-1980s, external constraints upon the clinical judgment of individual physicians were generally few and weak. As previously noted, the Professional Standards Review Organizations (PSROs) program of the 1970s and its successor the Peer Review Organization program, each based on the mandating of physician organizations to review services provided under Medicare, foundered amid conflicting expectations about the priority to be given to cost control and quality assurance in the face of the growing opposition of physicians. The PROs did benefit from the information revolution of the 1980s, drawing on the enormous Medicare database and taking advantage of burgeoning information technology (Salmon et al. 1994: 131). State officials also used a variety of utilization review techniques in the administration of Medicaid programs.

But it was the rise of managed care in the private sector that posed the greatest threat to the clinical autonomy of physicians. During the 1980s, a number of academic and medical commentators in the United States and abroad drew attention to this threat (e.g., Relman 1980; Starr 1982: 420–49; Fuchs 1983; Hoffenberg 1987; Lee and Etheredge 1989; Harrison and Schulz 1989; Döhler 1989; Salmon 1994). Empirical demonstration of the phenomenon is another and more difficult matter. Nonetheless, several important surveys in the 1990s provide supporting evidence.

In broad comparative terms, American physicians appeared to be more dissatisfied with the degree to which their clinical freedom was restricted than were their counterparts in some other nations. A 1991 survey of physicians in Canada, the United States, and western Germany suggested that, although a majority of physicians in each country believed that some fundamental changes in their health systems were necessary, satisfaction with the health system was higher among Canadian and German physicians than among American physicians. When respondents were asked to identify the most serious problems with their system, the sharpest differences arose between Canadian and American physicians, whose judgments of their respective systems appeared virtually as mirror images of each other. American physicians were much more likely than were Canadians to identify delays or disputes in processing insurance forms and in receiving payment, the inability of patients to afford some aspect of necessary medical care, external review of clinical decisions for the purpose of controlling health costs, and limitations on the length of hospital stays as serious problems with their system. On the other hand, Canadian physicians were much more likely to complain of limitations on the supply of well-equipped medical facilities (Blendon et al. 1993: 1015).

In the 1994 national survey of American physicians previously cited, 89% expressed the belief that they would have "less professional freedom to make treatment decisions" in the future (Blendon et al. 1994: 1547). Again, surveys suggested considerable variation in the experience of general practitioners and specialists in this regard. In 1995, 42% of specialists, according to Schoen and Collins (1996), believed that their ability to make decisions they think right for their patients had decreased in the previous three years, and only 10% respectively reported an increase. For general practitioners, the picture was slightly rosier: one-third reported that their ability to make decisions they think right for their patients decreased; 14% reported an increase.

The evolving role of the medical profession in the American health care arena was, indeed, very much bound up with the question of the specialist/ generalist balance. The spread of managed care portended an increased demand for primary care physicians and a dampened demand for specialists. Shortages of generalists of anywhere from 1,000 to 85,000 by the year 2020, and corresponding surpluses of specialists on the order of 55,000 to 196,000 were predicted—the difference depending on whether or not the proportion of new graduates choosing to practice as generalists could be raised from the 20% common in the early 1990s to 50% (Gamliel et al. 1995). In the past such scenarios would not have been threatening to either the economic or the political power of specialists. Under a regime of independent fee-for-service practice, increases in physician numbers did not reduce the economic power of physicians, given their ability to generate demand for their services. And in political terms, a large proportion of specialists appeared, in broad cross-national and historical terms, to be associated with a lower level of state intervention in the health care arena in an era in which the state was the profession's major protagonist (Hollingsworth et al. 1988: 148–52). In a future in which countervailing powers were exercised by large, mostly for-profit corporations and managed care entities, however, a surplus of specialists could well reduce their power.

Perceptions of limitations on clinical autonomy among American physicians were indeed related to the degree and form of their involvement in managed care plans, but with a most intriguing twist. Table 5.3 presents data from two major surveys of American physicians in different practice settings, as well as broad cross-national findings from the 1994 survey. Baker and Cantor (1993) analyzed data from a 1991 national telephone interview survey of 4,257 practicing physicians under the age of forty-five and in practice between two and nine years. Schoen and Collins (1996) reported findings from a 1995 national telephone interview survey of 1710 practicing physicians. Although each of these surveys tapped similar dimensions of satisfaction/dissatisfaction, the phrasing of the questions and the method of categorizing respondents varied somewhat across and within the respective surveys. Therefore, although the levels of dissatisfaction indicated are not strictly comparable across these surveys, the patterns across types of practice (and across nations) are enlightening.

What is most striking about these patterns is the general similarity between what might be considered the two extremes of the managed care continuum: fee-for-service practitioners not involved in managed care plans, and physicians employed in group/staff model HMOs. Both surveys that distinguished attitudes along this spectrum consistently indicated that physicians in each of the extreme categories were less likely than physicians involved in contractually based forms of managed care (network HMOs, IPAs, PPOs, etc.) to complain of problems with external review of clinical decisions, delays in approval of treatment, limitations on hospital admission or lengths of stay, or limitations on tests and referrals. Findings with regard to overall levels of satisfaction were less consistent. Baker and Cantor found that younger physicians practicing in group/staff HMOs experienced time pressures (they were less likely to feel in control of their work schedule or to believe that they could spend adequate time with patients); perhaps for that reason they were more likely to be dissatisfied with their practice than were their counterparts in other practice settings. But Schoen and Collins found that in overall terms, as well as in terms of problems related to clinical autonomy, group/staff HMO physicians were at least as satisfied with the conditions of their practice as were those in traditional fee-for-service practice and were considerably more satisfied than were physicians involved with other forms of managed care.

This somewhat counterintuitive result appears even more puzzling in the light of findings from a major national telephone survey of 108 managed care plans, with total enrollments of 33.5 million, in 1994 (Gold et al. 1995). Gold and her colleagues found that various monitoring practices were widespread in managed care plans (both HMOs and PPOs). Group/staff HMOs and network or IPA HMOs were fairly similar in the extent to which they monitored the practices of participating physicians, and both of these HMO forms were more likely to engage in such monitoring than were PPOs. Seventy-two percent of group/staff HMOs and 70% of network HMOs engaged in at least four types of utilization review, and virtually all engaged in at least one type.[11] Among PPOs, in contrast, 37% engaged in at least four types of utilization review, and 86% engaged in at least one. More than three-quarters of group/staff HMOs and of network HMOs made some use of practice guidelines, and about one-third of each type of HMO made extensive use of them. Among PPOs, the respective proportions were 28% and 7%. Seventy-six percent of group/staff HMOs and 86% of network HMOs made use of physician profiling, as opposed to 52% of PPOs (Gold et al. 1995: 1682).

If group/staff HMOs were as likely or more likely than contractually based forms of managed care to use utilization review and other monitoring techniques for the control of medical practice, why was it that their employee physicians were less likely to report limitations on clinical autonomy as a problem? Part of the answer to this question undoubtedly lies in self-selection: the physicians who chose to practice in group/staff HMO settings, knowing of the monitoring practices therein, might well have been less sensitive to incursions on clinical autonomy than those who chose other practice settings. Network- and IPA-style HMOs and PPOs, on the other hand, had in many cases been established solely as a defense against the market challenge of other forms of managed care and may have involved physicians who were more reluctant to cede any clinical discretion.

It is also necessary, however, to look inside each of these models to the vehicles through which monitoring and control is accomplished. Group/staff

TABLE 5.3 Percent of Physicians Reporting Dissatisfaction with Dimensions of Medical Practice, by Degree and Type of Involvement with Managed Care, or by Nation

| | Fee-for-service, No Managed Care | Some Managed Care Involvement | Group/Staff Model HMO | United States | Canada | Germany |
|---|---|---|---|---|---|---|
| *External review of clinical decisions* | | | | | | |
| Blendon 1993 | | | | 55 | 28 | 43 |
| Schoen and Collins 1996[a] | 50 | 63–65 | 38 | 61 | | |
| *Delays in approval of treatment* | | | | | | |
| Blendon 1993 | | | | 78 | 24 | 39 |
| Schoen and Collins 1996[b] | 68 | 92 | 74 | | | |
| *Limits on hospital admissions* | | | | | | |
| Schoen and Collins 1996[b] | 51 | 59 | 44 | | | |
| Baker and Cantor 1993[c] | 6 | 4–6 | 4 | | | |
| *Limits on hospital length of stay* | | | | | | |
| Blendon 1993 | | | | 60 | 30 | 29 |
| Baker and Cantor 1993 | 28 | 25–28 | 13 | | | |
| *Limits on tests* | | | | | | |
| Schoen and Collins 1996[b] | 72 | 95 | 73 | | | |
| Baker and Cantor 1993[c] | 11 | 14–33 | 8 | | | |
| *Limits on referrals* | | | | | | |
| Schoen and Collins 1996[b] | 37 | 82 | 62 | | | |
| *Inadequate time with patients* | | | | | | |
| Blendon 1993 | | | | 35 | 44 | 58 |
| Schoen and Collins 1996[a] | 54 | 64–79 | 73 | 69 | | |
| Baker and Cantor 1993[c] | 10 | 10–19 | 23 | | | |

| | | | | | |
|---|---|---|---|---|---|
| *Inadequate control of work schedule* | | | | | |
| Schoen and Collins 1996[a] (too much work or long hours) | 45 | 58–66 | 54 | 60 | |
| Baker and Cantor 1993[c] | 15 | 18–23 | 61 | | |
| *Overall dissatisfaction with practice* | | | | | |
| Blendon 1993 (would advise against entry) | | | | 37 | 26 | 33 |
| Schoen and Collins 1996[a] (less than very satisfied) | 65 | 72–83 | 64 | 37 | |
| Baker and Cantor 1993[d] (very or somewhat dissatisfied) | 11–15 | 9–18 | 19 | 76 | |
| *Level of autonomy is below expectations* | | | | | |
| Baker and Cantor 1993[e] | 47–50 | 47–48 | 48 | | |
| *Ability to practice quality medicine is below expectations* | | | | | |
| Baker and Cantor 1993[e] | 26–31 | 24–27 | 21 | | |
| *Ability to make decisions you think right for patients is less than very satisfactory* | | | | | |
| Schoen and Collins 1996[a] | 46 | 54–60 | 39 | 56 | |

*Sources:*

[a] See Table 8. Ranges for managed care reflect variation across categories defined by percentage of physician's patients in managed care arrangements. Percentages are the inverse of those reporting satisfaction.

[b] See Table 9.

[c] See Exhibit 3. Ranges for managed care reflect variation across categories defined by percentage of physician's revenue derived from managed care. Percentages are the inverse of those reporting satisfaction.

[d] See Exhibit 5. Ranges for managed care reflect variation across categories defined by types of managed care employment (self-employed vs. other employer).

[e] See Exhibit 6. Ranges for managed care reflect variation across categories defined by types of managed care employment (self-employed vs. other employer).

HMOs were based on essentially collegial models of control. The preeminent example of this approach was Kaiser Permanente, a California-based HMO established in 1945, the oldest and until 1994 the largest HMO in the country.[12] Kaiser Permanente followed a group model, replicated in each of the dozen regions in which it located around the country. Under this model physicians were employed on a salaried basis and formed a group practice that was constituted separately from the management of the plan and of the hospitals owned by the plan. Kaiser Permanente was renowned for the central role accorded to physicians in the control of medical practice—a characteristic that was seen as both a strength and a weakness of the model. Its purported strength lay in the "alignment of incentives" between plan managers and practicing physicians that it was able to achieve (Iglehart 1994), and its alleged weakness lay in its inflexibility in the face of market challenges from more entrepreneurially oriented plans (Kertesz 1995). In staff-model HMO plans, physicians were also employed on a primarily salaried basis but were not separately organized as a group practice. The decision-making models within staff-model HMOs have not been much studied and may vary considerably. Anecdotal evidence nonetheless suggested that the Kaiser Permanente model had a strong demonstration effect upon the development of staff-model HMOs, and that their medical staffs formed de facto group practices within them.

The work of Baker and Cantor (1993), and Schoen and Collins (1996) suggests that the constraints on individual clinical discretion were much more acceptable to physicians when they were generated and implemented through collegial processes than when they were imposed under the terms of arms-length contracts. In a sense, physicians practicing under a group/staff HMO model appeared to have made a trade-off analogous to that made by British and Canadian physicians under state-sponsored health care systems: they accepted limitations on their entrepreneurial discretion but preserved collegial control over medical practice.

It is also important to note that group/staff HMOs were generally older and more established than were network- and IPA-type HMOs, PPOs, and other contractually based types of managed care. By the 1990s, then, the newer models had not built up the trust networks that characterized collegial decision-making and had to rely on more explicit specification and enforcement of contracts and administrative rules. As we shall see in the British case, such trust networks can prove remarkably resilient in adjusting to changes in the environment. In the American case, group/staff HMOs appear also to have "insulated" their physicians to a considerable degree from environmental turbulence (Schoen and Collins 1996).

Whether or not this American version of the accommodation between physicians and fiscal managers would spread more widely in the system as other managed care organizations matured remained very much open to question in the late 1990s. Schoen and Collins estimated that only about 4% of American physicians practiced within a group/staff HMO in 1996. About 40% of this number, moreover, was accounted for by Kaiser Permanente with its approximately 9,300 physicians. Most of the growth in HMOs in the 1990s was in network or IPA, not group/staff models. Kaiser Permanente, the flagship of the model, was under severe competitive pressure to reduce costs, leading to speculation as to whether the alignment of medical and managerial incentives could be maintained in such circumstances.

Work by Stephen Shortell and his colleagues on integrated delivery systems gave some reason to believe that organizations which accorded physicians a significant role in governance might be well positioned to thrive in the evolving context of the 1990s. In a study of eleven developing systems, they found "physician-system integration" (defined as "the extent to which physicians identify with a system, use the system, and actively participate in its planning, management, and governance") to be associated with greater inpatient productivity, and with greater clinical integration which in turn was associated with greater total net revenue (Shortell et al. 1994: 52–53). These findings were preliminary and at best suggestive, however, and the question of which model of medical–managerial relations, if any, would come to dominate the U.S. health system—and to what effect—remained very much open in the latter part of the decade. In the turbulence of the 1990s, meanwhile, most physicians found themselves dealing with a wide variety of contractual and organizational arrangements, and substantial numbers were experiencing loss of income or clinical autonomy or both.

## Information and Information Technology

The monitoring of physicians' practice behavior against standardized patterns and protocols began in earnest, as noted, with the adoption of the DRG-based Prospective Payment System under the federal Medicare program. As private payers became more price sensitive in the 1980s and 1990s, DRG-type mechanisms of utilization review were increasingly adopted in private health plans as well, in a form of "private regulation" (Leyerle 1994: 63–64). The implementation of DRG-based reimbursement, however, would not have been possible without the rapid developments in information technology that occurred in the 1980s and 1990s. These developments made possible the assembly of huge computerized databases of patient records, the largest of which was the Medicare statistical database maintained by the Health Care Financing Administration, the federal agency that administers Medicare and Medicaid. As computing costs declined, the sophisticated manipulation of these databases became more and more feasible for a wide variety of organizations.

Most significantly, the DRG system demanded and information technology made possible the linkage of cost and clinical information at increasingly discrete levels. That is, it became possible to assess individual clinical decisions in terms of their cost implications and to compare these implications across physicians in ways never before possible. And as Salmon and his colleagues have noted, "as researchers and bureaucrats began to explore this burgeoning clinical and cost data, findings from the data set up a powerful dynamic themselves." These analyses demonstrated "huge variations . . . in resource utilization that do not appear to be directly linked to patient care outcomes"—findings that "created a crippling challenge to traditional quality assurance and legitimized experimentation with stricter modes of monitoring" (Salmon et al. 1994: 131). Large multi-institutional systems, with their large databases and geographic spread were, like the federal Medicare program, well positioned to undertake internal analyses of variations in practice patterns, with their cost implications.

In the end, however, DRG-type costing systems are only accounting techniques, and data analyses are of academic import alone until they are acted upon. The implementation of these techniques and findings requires an organizational structure in which "real people struggle for control" (Leyerle 1994: 65). As we shall see in the British case, the linkage of clinical and cost information may be forestalled in an organizational context in which professional control over the "audit" of medical practice is well established. In Britain that professional control was achieved at the cost of the surrender of entrepreneurial discretion. In the United States, no such implicit bargain was in place; when cost control imperatives arose, the organizational mechanisms for achieving them had to be created *de novo*. The linkage of cost and clinical information hence proceeded more rapidly in the United States, although most information systems continued through the 1990s to be more sophisticated in dealing with cost than with clinical (particularly clinical outcome) data. In a 1995 national survey of health care executives regarding information technology, "improved managed care capabilities" (i.e., improved linkages of cost and clinical data) emerged as the highest priority for the development of information systems, cited by two-thirds of respondents—well above the numbers citing improvements in patient care or accounting areas (Morrissey 1995).

The complex contractual and organizational arrangements of the American health care arena were indeed heavily dependent on an infrastructure of information technology. It was estimated that the typical hospital in a market with significant managed care penetration had 100 contracts, each with specific per diem or per procedure payment terms, pre-authorization requirements, and exceptions for outlier cases; sophisticated software was essential in monitoring these contracts (Morrissey 1994). Physicians on average contracted with about eight different plans (Schoen and Collins 1996).

As we have seen, many of the new and emerging organizational entities in U.S. health care in the 1990s (IPAs, PPOs, etc.) were in fact "virtual" organizations—networks held together by complex contractual and ownership relationships and increasingly dependent on information technology to maintain their linkages. They could not have existed in an earlier technological era. And they were extremely volatile. The *timing* of the emergence of cost sensitivity in the U.S. health care arena is hence of great importance in explaining the organizational forms that resulted. Had organizational mechanisms of cost control become broadly established in the United States in an earlier era, as they were in Britain and to a lesser extent in Canada, they may well have yielded structures that preserved professional control in clinical matters, and they would have been resistant to the changes made possible by the revolution in information technology in the 1980s and 1990s. As it was, however, information technology made it possible for owners and managers of facilities and health care plans to amass and analyze both clinical and cost data in ways that counteracted traditional professional power bases.

## The Changing Political Terrain

Chapter 3 described the emergence of political "hyperpluralism" in the health care arena—the movement from a dominant alliance of physicians, hospitals, insurance companies, and business interests to a situation of highly fractured competition. In this chapter, we can see how the playing out of the logic of the mixed system dominated by private finance led to that political result. The political fissioning of the dominant alliance in fact mirrors the fracturing of the symmetry of objectives of physicians, institutional providers, and insurance companies previously described. Some observers, such as Peterson (1993), read these circumstances in the early 1990s to be ripe for realignment—for the emergence of a winning coalition in support of change rather than the status quo. And if conditions in the broader political arena had been different, such a realignment might well have occurred, with various groups coalescing around the policy initiative of a Democratic president committed to health care reform. As it was, however, Clinton was not in a strong enough position as president to bring this about, and the fault lines in the health care arena deepened.

In the absence of the broad political conditions necessary to bring about major policy change, the complex and heterogeneous politics of the health care arena played themselves out in the Clinton reform episode. The political landscape in that episode, as indicated in chapter 3, was populated by a great variety of groups that fell into three broad categories as defined by their support of three types of proposals (the Clinton plan, a single-payer system, and various forms of "managed competition" without the degree of governmental involvement envisioned by Clinton), as well as a miscellany of groups whose activity was primarily focused on the defeat of various proposals.

Professional associations, including those representing the medical profession, tended on balance to give cautious support, at least at the level of principle, to the Clinton plan or even to a single-payer model. A group of ten physician organizations, including the American Academy of Family Physicians and the American Academy of Pediatrics, endorsed the basic features of the Clinton proposal when it was announced in September 1993. Other groups, such as the American College of Physicians, did not endorse the proposal in its entirety but supported several of its central features, such as employer mandates. The board of the American College of Surgeons, alone among major physician groups, announced its support for a single-payer system, largely on the grounds that such a system would better preserve patient choice and physician autonomy than would other reform alternatives (Ramsay 1995: 52). Both the American College of Physicians and the American College of Surgeons subsequently tempered their positions somewhat in response to a lack of consensus among their memberships.[13] The American Society of Internal Medicine (which had split from the American College of Physicians in 1956 to pursue an explicitly policy-oriented, rather than academic, agenda) also refrained from endorsing any specific proposals, but supported employer mandates while documenting the "hassle factor"—the administrative burden and intrusiveness of existing arrangements (Peterson 1995: 92).

The AMA itself vacillated throughout 1993 and 1994 on the issue of health care reform, also as a result of divisions within its own membership.[14] In 1990, the AMA had endorsed the concept of employer mandates. It greeted the Clinton plan in September 1993 with a mixture of approval and reservation. By December 1993 the AMA House of Delegates, in part in response to "cross-lobbying" by the National Federation of Independent Business (as discussed later), rescinded its earlier endorsement of employer mandates on the grounds that other options for achieving universal coverage should not be foreclosed (Rovner 1995: 200). In June 1994 the AMA continued to keep its options open; the House of Delegates defeated resolutions variously opposing an employer mandate and opposing the Clinton plan. The following month, however, the AMA joined the American Association of Retired Persons and the AFL-CIO in cosponsoring a newspaper advertisement that endorsed universal coverage "building on the current employer-based system . . . with a required level of employer contributions" (Rovner 1995: 242). By thus allying itself with supporters of the Clinton plan and by appearing to endorse employer mandates, the AMA leadership found itself subject not only to criticism from some quarters of its membership, but also to a barrage of "reverse lobbying" from Republican members of Congress (Rovner 1995: 242). The AMA's ambivalence throughout the Clinton reform episode is further reflected in the fact that its Political Action Committee was one of the few in the health care arena whose political contributions actually declined in the 1993–1994 election cycle from their 1991–1992 level (Weissenstein 1995a).

The vacillation and the internal divisions of the AMA stand in sharp contrast to the history of the organization since the 1930s, when the AMA consolidated its position to effectively hold a representational monopoly as the voice of American medicine—and in particular to its role in the last major policy reform episode in the United States, the enactment of Medicare and Medicaid. The AMA's fierce opposition to compulsory universal health insurance in the 1960s was a major factor in determining the ways in which policy-makers defined the boundaries of possible reform. The internal divisions within the AMA in the 1990s, as well as the positions taken by other groups such as the American Academy of Pediatrics and the American College of Surgeons, reveal the division of opinion within the medical profession regarding the trade-offs to be made between the protection of the entrepreneurial and the clinical autonomy of physicians, and between the roles of the public and private sectors in protecting physicians' interests in the changed context of the late twentieth century.

The medical profession was not alone in its internal political divisions in the 1990s. The American Hospital Association was split between its for-profit and not-for-profit members. The Federation of American Health Systems, representing investor-owned hospitals, refused to join the AHA and a number of other hospital groups in protesting Republican proposals to reduce Medicare and Medicaid funding in 1995 (Lutz 1995b). The health insurance industry was "sharply divided between the small firms who profit from the current insurance market distortions, on the one hand, and Blue Cross/Blue Shield and other large carriers, who are more accepting of increased market regulation, on the other, as well as among the large companies, according to their level of participation in the managed care business" (Peterson 1993: 411). In the early 1990s the five largest for-profit insurers split off from the Health Insurance Association of America to form the Coalition for Managed Care in support of the Jackson Hole proposal, as discussed in chapter 3.

In the face of all of this fracturing of coalitions and alliances, one group which appeared to be coalescing in representational terms comprised managed care organizations. The two major interest groups representing managed care organizations—the Group Health Association of America (GHAA) and the American Managed Care and Review Association (AMCRA)—merged in 1996 to form the American Association of Health Care Plans. The merger brought together a group (GHAA) that had represented exclusively HMOs and that had informal linkages with organized labor, with a group (AMCRA) that had a more diverse membership embracing PPOs and other forms of managed care. Much of GHAA's lobbying activity had been to promote the interests of HMOs versus PPOs, notably by pressing for a level regulatory playing field for the various types of managed care organizations. One of the major joint efforts of the merged organization was to begin to develop a Health Employer's Data Information System (HEDIS) of performance measures for participating plans. The ability of the managed care industry to counteract the fissionizing tendencies of the American health care arena was a key question for the future politics of the arena.

The political organization of interests on the demand side of the health care market was no more cohesive than it was among supply-side actors. Business coalitions mobilized at the state and local level, as noted, to consolidate purchasing power and to press various policy issues. What was most remarkable about this mobilization was the extent to which those coalitions severed business interests politically from their traditional alliances with provider interests in the health field (Peterson 1993: 412). Beyond that, however, business remained politically divided, at both local and national levels, over issues of health care reform.

These divisions were markedly apparent in the vacillating positions of business organizations in the 1992–1994 policy episode. At the outset, it appeared that the changing economic structure of the health care arena might be generating the basis for a broad political coalition embracing large- and medium-sized business interests on both the demand and the supply side of the health care market. The reform concept drawing together the diverse elements of this coalition, as discussed in chapter 3, was "managed competition." But the lurking fault was the concept of the employer mandate.

The employer mandate promised initially to be a "wedge" issue dividing large and small business interests, and drawing the former into a reform coalition. The National Leadership Coalition for Health Care Reform, representing a number of large businesses, in 1991 endorsed a "pay or play" plan in which employers would have been required to provide health care coverage for their workers or pay into a pool of federally provided coverage for the otherwise uninsured. The large business participants in the Jackson Hole Group (JHG), notably through the Washington Group on Health, were at least open to the consideration of an employer mandate. On the other hand, the National Federation of Independent Business, representing small business, remained adamantly opposed. The Chamber of Commerce, spanning both large and small business but heavily weighted toward the latter in membership, was caught on the fault line between the two sectors. It nonetheless took a position in 1993 in support of a system of universal coverage achieved in large part through an employer mandate (Judis 1995: 66–67).

The support of key business organizations for an employer mandate, so encouraging to advocates of reform leading to universal coverage, proved very soft as the policy process unfolded. The leadership of the Chamber of Commerce was subject to fierce "reverse lobbying" by House Republicans, who threatened to withhold support for Chamber of Commerce positions on other issues if the Chamber of Commerce maintained its position in support of employer mandates (Judis 1995: 68; Schick 1995: 243). In early 1994 the Chamber of Commerce abruptly changed its position to oppose both universal coverage and employer mandates as a way to achieve it.

Equally devastating to the Clinton plan's chances of success was the insistence of key members of the Jackson Hole Group that the Clinton version of managed competition was unacceptably different from the version proposed by the JHG. One of the key differences sharpened over time as it became clear that neither the JHG nor the Business Roundtable, the parent organization of the Washington Group on Health, would support employer mandates.[15] As Judis points out, the membership of the roundtable, though comprising large businesses, was divided among "four distinct kinds of businesses, each of whom had a different vantage on health care reform" (Judis 1995: 69). Only one of these sectors—the multistate employers, with largely full-time workforces, who insured their employees—supported a federal plan with an employer mandate, seeing it as a way of ending the cost-shifting across patients with various types of coverage (or none at all) that was driving up their costs, and avoiding regional and state-level variations in the terms on which they could negotiate coverage for their workers. Other types of roundtable members opposed employer mandates—the companies on the supply side of the health care market who feared that an employer mandate would lead to price controls, firms with a large proportion of part-time and low-wage workers to whom they offered little if any health coverage, and a miscellaneous group opposed on ideological grounds to governmental intervention in general. In the end, the JHG and the roundtable associated themselves with a rival plan to Clinton's, sponsored by Representative Jim Cooper, which incorporated much of the Jackson Hole framework and did not involve an employer mandate.

Shortly after the announcement by the roundtable that it would support the Cooper plan, the National Association of Manufacturers, which had been "hedging its bets," also declared that it was "unable to support the administration's health care reform plan in its present form" (Judis 1995: 71). This left Clinton with the support of individual companies and the National Leadership Coalition on Health Care Reform. But the promise of a broad-based large- and medium-sized business coalition consensus was dashed on the rocks of the internal divisions of American business.

A broad range of labor and consumer groups mobilized in support of the Clinton plan. But health care reform could not be accomplished on that base of support. If Clinton had been in a stronger position as president or possibly even if he had made different strategic judgments, as argued in part I, he might have been able to maintain the sense of the inevitability of reform that prevailed in 1992 to create a bandwagon effect; in such case, the segments of the medical and business communities that supported key features of his proposals might have carried the day. But that scenario is now a might-have-been.

In the wake of the failure of the large-scale Clinton initiative, health care policy and politics reverted to the pattern of incremental action and response that prevailed earlier. The vacillation and division among interest groups con- tinued. At the federal level, incremental changes to Medicare and Medicaid were proposed as in the past largely through the budget process—a process that was stalled in the stalemated partisan politics of the 104th Congress. In this process, the AMA aligned itself with Republican proposals to reform Medi- care by converting it from a "defined benefit" to a "defined contribution" program—proposals that would have had the effect of increasing substantially the private component of the financing of health care for elderly Americans (Martin 1997: 575–77).[16] While large business interests were alarmed by the potential of the Republican proposals to shift costs to them, they continued to be too politically divided to take effective action (Martin 1997: 583–85). Stale- mated on fiscal instruments, the Congress turned once again to an essentially regulatory change and in July 1996 passed insurance reform legislation requir- ing insurers to accept individuals who had been covered under employer-based plans and who had lost or changed jobs, regardless of preexisting conditions. No attempt was made to address the issue of the affordability of such coverage. A report by the General Accounting Office in 1998 found that prices and other restrictive practices by insurers were indeed hindering the ability of consumers to obtain coverage under the terms of the legislation (Pear 1998). Pressures ac- cordingly began to build for further regulatory action at the federal or state level. The mutually reinforcing cycle of incremental policy changes and market adjustments continued, generating a variety of interests which through their political mobilization greatly complicated attempts to accomplish anything other than incremental policy change.

The failure of large-scale health care reform at the federal level shifted at- tention to the states. But, as discussed in chapter 3, policy initiatives at the state level were constrained by the policy legacies of the American federal system, by the fact that the "hyperpluralistic" structure of interests that frustrated coalition building at the federal level was replicated to various degrees in state health care arenas, and by the conservative backlash that swept through state governments as well as Washington in the 1994 elections.

## Institutional and Structural Change in the Mixed Market

The basic policy parameters governing both the institutional mix of hierarchy, collegiality, and market, and the structural balance of influence across the state, the medical profession, and private finance, remained essentially unchanged since the last major successful episode of policy change in the 1960s. Institutionally, the policy framework continued to accord market elements a heavy weight, tempered by hierarchical controls as both federal and state regulations fluctuated over time in focus and stringency. Similarly, the policy foundation of the structural balance between the state and private finance changed little. The United States was one of the few nations in which public expenditures as a proportion of total health expenditures increased over the 1980s and 1990s (from 42.0% in 1980 to 43.9% in 1993), but the change was marginal and from a low base. The proportions of the population covered under private insurance or governmental plans, or remaining uninsured, shifted only marginally over the 1980s and early 1990s. The proportion with private insurance declined from 68.6% to 62.2% between 1980 and 1993, while the proportion covered by Medicare and Medicaid rose from 17.8% to 22.8% and the uninsured population rose from 13.7% to 15.0% (HCFA 1995a: 322).

And yet, despite this lack of change in basic policy parameters, the system of decision-making for the financing and delivery of health care was organizationally transformed, with profound implications for the institutional mix and structural balance of the system. Institutionally, the system remained essentially market-based, and the evolution of the market generated highly complex networks of contractually linked entities. But the system was also marked by an increase in reliance on hierarchical mechanisms—rules administered within organizations—as suppliers of health insurance and health care became more integrated both vertically and horizontally. Some large integrated systems, notably certain group/staff model HMOs, maintained a central role for collegial mechanisms of decision-making, but in general the increase in administrative rules and contractual requirements occurred at the expense of collegiality. On the demand side of the market, from the perspective of individual consumers of health insurance and health care, the choice of health insurance plan and health care provider was increasingly constrained by arrangements negotiated on their behalf by large private or public purchasers. Of those with employer-based health insurance (the vast majority of the privately insured population) 44% had no choice of plan, according to a 1993 survey (Davis et al. 1995b: 202).

In structural terms, the most pronounced shift has been the rise of the influence of private financial actors at the expense of the medical profession. The rise of cost-conscious purchasers led to changes in the profit-maximization strategies of suppliers of health insurance and health care, who focused increasingly on cost minimization rather than revenue maximization. This change of focus broke the "alignment of incentives" that in the past, had linked medical professionals, not-for-profit providers, and for-profit providers, as cost-minimization strategies came into potential or actual conflict with professional or community objectives. The rise of an aggressive for-profit sector leading dramatic change in organizational structure and market strategy was a major phenomenon of the 1980s and 1990s.

## The Logic of Entrepreneurialism

These changes, and the challenges that they presented to the traditional dominance of the medical profession in the American health care decision-making system, were driven by an underlying logic. That logic was created by the intersection of the logic of entrepreneurialism inherent in market-based systems with the logic of agency that characterizes health care delivery as discussed in chapter 1.

Under the traditional system of private fee-for-service medical practice that constituted a declining proportion of the American health care market, physicians were both independent entrepreneurs and professional experts. These two roles offered mutually reinforcing sets of incentives to provide an intensive level of service: the desire of the expert to fully employ skill and technology reinforced the entrepreneurial motivation to maximize revenue and vice versa. The level of expertise required to assess the need for health care as well as to provide it meant that physicians functioned as the agents of their patients in determining the demand for their own services. The incentives that they faced as entrepreneurs and experts, however, made them inherently biased agents; there were few counterbalancing incentives to take into account the consumer interest in the cost-effectiveness of care. The "second-level" agency relationship between the state and professional self-regulatory bodies, as discussed in chapter 1, focused almost entirely on ensuring the quality and appropriateness of care, not its cost. The rise of third-party payment (health insurance) made cost considerations even less salient in the context of the individual physician-payment relationship. And third-party payers (with the exception of group/staff HMOs) generally did not seek to establish "second-level" agency relationships with professional bodies to control costs—rather, they passed along cost increases in their premiums. And in a system in which the costs of paying premiums were diffused among employers, individual workers, and the state (through tax expenditures), sensitivity to cost increases was dampened.

In other national systems, the advent of the state as the major financer of health care brought about a redefinition of these traditional relationships. It changed the mechanism whereby the costs of health care were allocated to various sources: no longer primarily through health insurance premiums offered on a market, but rather through the governmental budgetary process—a process of negotiation and political accommodation among various actors both within and outside government (which will be discussed in subsequent chapters). The most central of these accommodations was between health ministries and the medical profession: the "second-level" agency relationship was redefined, in different ways in different nations, to deal with issues of cost control by charging the profession with the allocation of health care resources within a budget.

In the United States, however, the state never assumed the predominant role in health care financing—it constituted one (albeit substantial) set of payers among many. It did seek, within this narrower compass, to redefine its agency relationship with the profession: through the PSRO and PRO programs, it endowed locally based professional bodies with the mandate to review the utilization of hospital-based medical services under Medicare in order to control costs as well as to ensure quality. But the PSROs and PROs were limited in scope—applying only to Medicare services and even then excluding medical services provided in physicians' office practices. And even this limited attempt to elaborate the agency relationship between the profession and the state was ultimately disabled by conflicting expectations about the relative weights to be placed on the cost-control and quality-assurance prongs of the mandate of peer review agencies.

Much more than this limited attempt to redefine "second-level" agency relationships, the public policy change that had the greatest impact upon the dynamics of change in decision-making systems was the change in the basis of remuneration for hospital services under Medicare—the shift from cost-based reimbursement to prospective payment. This shift dramatically changed the incentives facing providers of care: under prospective payment, cost minimization became the route to maximizing profit margins in individual cases. For the first time, the logic of entrepreneurialism and the logic of professionalism began to drive in different directions.

Providers first sought to escape the constraints of the public program through the multiple safety valves offered by the multipayer system, using their economic power to price discriminate and to charge more to private than to public payers. But as charges to private payers increased disproportionately, and as tightening international competition drove employers to be more aggressive in seeking to reduce their labor costs, including the costs of health benefits, this strategy of cost-shifting became more and more difficult to pursue. Entrepreneurial providers had to reduce costs in order to maximize profits. And increasingly this entrepreneurial role was seized by actors not subject to the constraints of professional objectives or established relationships—that is, by for-profit firms accountable to private investors through volatile financial markets. The formidable competitive challenge presented by these firms drew not-for-profit organizations and physician practices in their wake.

In this changed context, rather than delegating broad discretion to individual physicians on the model of traditional agency relationships, the new entrepreneurial intermediaries more explicitly specified the nature of services to be rendered, both through contracts and through administrative directives in vertically and horizontally integrated organizations. And they were enabled to do so by the revolutionary developments in information technology that allowed them to amass and to analyze large databases of clinical and cost information. In other nations, as we shall see, established accommodations between the state and the medical profession around issues of cost control were able to temper and channel the impact of changes that information technology might have had on the balance of power in the health care arena. In the United States, outside group/staff HMOs, few such accommodations had been established.

The belated addressing of cost control in the United States, relative to other nations, meant that cost-control mechanisms were developed in a technological context in which there were alternatives to the delegation of broad discretion to physicians, and in which there were few established accommodations to constrain the development of these alternative mechanisms. This is, indeed, one of the multiple ironies of the American health care arena: in seeking to preserve a policy framework that shielded both their entrepreneurial discretion and their clinical autonomy from state incursion, the medical profession over time created the conditions in which entrepreneurs unconstrained by considerations of professional objectives or collegial modes of decision-making would come to play a more and more dominant role.

Other ironies of the American system are equally striking. A strategy of cautious incrementalism in public policy development has yielded volatile and turbulent change in decision-making structures, as public policy and market responses have generated a mutually reinforcing cycle of complexity. And in a final irony, the market-oriented American system has spawned decision-making structures increasingly dominated by large organizations on both the supply and the demand sides, leaving professionals more subject to administratively enforced rules and consumers of health care with little more choice of plan and often less choice of health care provider than is the case in systems in which the state plays a much larger role in the financing of the system. These ironies are thrown into sharp relief in comparing the American system with those of Britain and Canada, the subjects of the next two chapters.

# The Logic of Corporatism Meets
# the Internal Market

While the market-oriented U.S. system generated a relative increase in hierarchical mechanisms, ironically the British system moved in the other direction. The NHS's particular corporatist blend of hierarchy and collegiality was modified by the adoption of mechanisms based on market principles. This shift was brought about not through the playing out of the logic of the corporatist system but rather through a political intervention generated outside the health care arena and heavily influenced by ideas developed in the United States.

The implementation of these ideas, however, was very much mediated by the logic of the corporatist system. Central to the British reforms was the institution of contracting between organizationally distinct purchasers and providers. Faced with the high information and other transaction costs of writing and enforcing contracts for health care, however, British purchasers and providers, like their American counterparts, were drawn to stable forms of relationships that reduced the need for specificity in contracting. And unlike large numbers of their American counterparts, the British had readily available and familiar models of such stable relationships: the corporatist structures that had characterized the NHS since its inception.

This chapter first traces the evolution of British "hierarchical corporatism" in the decades following the establishment of the NHS, an evolution that shaped the system into which the "internal market" reforms of the 1990s were abruptly introduced. It then explores the interplay between the design of the reforms and the logic of the established system in shaping the development of more explicit bargaining relationships between providers and purchasers. Next the chapter traces out the implications of these developments for the relative influence of physicians and state and private sector actors in health care decision-making. Finally, as did the previous chapter regarding the American case, it concludes with an assessment of structural and institutional change in the British health arena and a distillation of the logic that in this case mediated the impact of major policy change.

## Corporatism in the NHS

The distinctive blend of hierarchy and collegiality that constituted NHS-style corporatism comprised two fundamental elements. First, it involved defined spheres of authority based on functional expertise, creating a set of parallel authority structures—some hierarchical, some collegial. Second, it brought these spheres together in hierarchical structures of "consensus management" which gave effective veto powers to the key functional groups at each level of the hierarchy. These essential features persisted through two major reorganizations of NHS structures, in 1974 and again in 1982. The 1974 reorganization replaced the tripartite structure established in 1948 (which involved separate geographically defined hierarchies for hospital services, community health, and general practice) with a unified model bringing all three sectors under the tiered authority of Area Health Authorities (AHAs), Regional Health Authorities (RHAs), and the central National Health Service.[1] The 1982 reorganization abolished the AHAs and created a larger number of more locally defined District Health Authorities (DHAs). Throughout these reorganizations, however, the general principles of NHS corporatism were maintained—notably the formal representation of the medical profession with effective veto rights on decision-making bodies at each level of the hierarchy.

Expectations regarding the roles of the various participants within these structures were fairly clear. Doctors, both general practitioners (GPs) and specialists, were to exercise their clinical judgment as independent professionals. GPs contracted independently with local "Executive Councils" and later with Family Practitioner Committees to provide services on a modified capitation basis. Hospital consultants were salaried employees of the NHS, but their employment contracts were held at the regional level, not the level of the operational unit (the hospital) in which they practiced. Consultants did not "report," then, to local managers, but rather formed self-governing hospital-based medical staffs. Referral patterns from the "gatekeeper" GPs to the specialist consultants were determined by professional networks, not administrative rules. Nurses performed within a hospital-based functional hierarchy dominated by the hospital matron (Strong and Robinson 1990: 14–19; Harrison 1995: 158–60). The role of the administrative manager in this context has been described by Harrison as that of the "diplomat" mediating across the various functional authority centers that comprised the NHS, someone always seen as in service to, rather than in authority over, the clinicians (Harrison 1995: 160).

NHS-style corporatism, then, responded in its own distinctive way to two major characteristics of the economics of health care—the localized base of delivery and the agency relationship between provider and patient. Resources were allocated through a more or less decentralized geographically defined hierarchy built around functional pillars. At both central and local levels, agency relationships between state and professional bodies entrusted physicians with making decisions about the provision of care within resource limits. Mechanisms of control within these structures relied heavily upon hierarchical lines of accountability in budgetary matters and upon collegial networks among professionals in matters relating to the quality and appropriateness of care.

These arrangements had a number of advantages for both state and professional actors. From the perspective of the clinician, they meant freedom to exercise clinical judgment and skill free from nonprofessional interference. From the perspective of state actors, these arrangements not only afforded overall budgetary control but also provided a legitimate rationing mechanism (Klein 1995: 75–78). As Harrison has put it, the respect for "clinical autonomy" within the NHS made "the process of rationing health care in a system which in theory provides comprehensive care politically invisible—reduced to individual, fragmented and unrecorded transactions between doctors and their patients and/or relatives" (Harrison 1995: 164).

For both state and professional actors, moreover, these corporatist arrangements, based as they were on mutual understandings, had the considerable advantage of requiring relatively low transaction costs. Comparing the administrative costs of national health care systems is notoriously difficult, because the definitional criteria for collecting such data vary across nations. The only series that attempts comparability across nations is that produced by the OECD, which focuses on the administrative costs of insurance (both public and private) and does not include provider overheads.[2] With this caveat in mind, it is nonetheless worth noting that Britain (like Canada) stood out in cross-national perspective for its relatively low costs of administration, as shown in table 6.1.

One person's administrative "cost" is another's budget, and it might be argued that it is in the interest of at least some state actors to maximize transaction costs. For the first few decades of the NHS, the relatively lean administrative structure might well be seen as a function of the dominance of providers,

TABLE 6.1 Administrative Share of Total Health Expenditure, 1990

| Britain | 2.5% |
|---|---|
| Canada | 1.3 |
| Germany | 6.6 |
| Netherlands | 7.3 |
| United States | 5.8 |

Source: OECD 1993, vol. 1: 108–9, 112–13.

British figures refer to the National Health Service only, and are for 1987.

particularly medical professionals, over managers. But even the "managerialism" that began to take hold in the British public service in the 1980s contained contradictory implications for administrative costs, and as we shall see, a system of decision-making that kept transaction costs low retained considerable attraction.

## Managerialism and the Griffiths Reforms

In the 1980s, the established relationships of NHS corporatism came under increasing pressure. From the right came the increasing emphasis on "managerialism" in the public service—an emphasis on tighter control of public spending through the establishment of performance targets to be met within budget limits. From the left came demands for higher levels of spending and for greater "democratization" within the NHS—in particular a greater role for patients as "consumers" (e.g., Toynbee 1984). Both of these strands were to come together in the "internal market" reforms of the 1990s. But for much of the 1980s it was managerialism that presented the greatest challenge to established patterns.

The high-water mark in the introduction of managerialism to the NHS was reached with the Griffiths review of the NHS management structure in 1983, as discussed in chapter 3. But the reforms that followed upon the Griffiths report, attempting to introduce a unified "general management" structure in place of the pillarized structures of "consensus management," did not fundamentally alter the relationship between doctors and managers, although their impact on the authority structures for nursing was much more profound (Harrison and Pollitt 1994: 48–49). Relations between managers and doctors continued to be those of negotiation rather than command (Harrison 1995: 161–62).

Some observers have attributed the lack of fundamental change in decision-making structures despite the post-Griffiths organizational changes to the fact that managers lacked the information resources necessary to exert their formal authority (Strong and Robinson 1990: 165–78). Indeed, attempts to develop the necessary information remained at a fairly nascent stage in the 1980s. The Resource Management Initiative (RMI), launched by the Department of Health and Social Services in 1986 at six pilot hospital sites, was intended to develop a clinical database and a casemix management system that would allow for the systematic integration of resource allocation decisions with clinical decision-making. Like other initiatives undertaken in the wake of the Griffiths report, RMI was also intended to develop structures for integrating clinicians more fully into the management process. While this latter objective recognized the central role of physicians in the resource allocation process, it also sought to change the criteria that physicians as well as managers brought to bear in decision-making, and to ensure that microlevel resource allocation was no longer driven entirely by professional judgments and norms.

The RMI experiment, however, had two effects that militated against change in the balance of hierarchical and collegial mechanisms and in the balance of influence between clinicians and managers: first, it induced substantial skepticism about the fiscal implications of such a system in the context of budgetary uncertainty, and second, it led the medical profession to seize the initiative in the monitoring of clinical behavior. As to the first of these effects, the RMI demonstrated the costliness of the technological and human resource infrastructure required for information-based resource management. An evaluation of the initiative as of 1990 found that implementation costs were two to four times higher than the top of the range initially projected (Buxton et al. 1991: 6–7). Unlike the private firms investing heavily in information technology in the U.S. context, moreover, managers in the NHS saw these costs not as an investment, on which a return could be expected in the form of increased revenue, but rather as a budgetary expenditure for which an ongoing case would have to be made.

In the context of budgetary constraint and uncertainty in the NHS in the 1980s, then, the adoption of new managerial techniques, particularly those that increased monitoring and other transaction costs, were slow to gain acceptance. Various performance measures relating to efficiency of "throughput" were adopted in the mid-1980s. But as Klein (1995) has acerbically put it, "this was achieved by the mass-baptism of all existing statistical series as performance indicators" (138). The performance of clinicians, moreover, generally lay beyond the reach of managerial review (Pollitt 1993: 70).

This brings us to the second effect of the RMI initiative. The involvement of clinicians in the process alerted medical practitioners to the potential of information systems not only to provide them with instruments in their dealings with managers, but also to inform their own clinical decisions (Packwood et al. 1991: 138–39). As a result, it had a "demonstration effect" regarding the potential of "medical audit" mechanisms: systems for monitoring clinical performance against agreed-upon criteria. The RMI also facilitated experimentation with new organizational channels of medical influence. Doctors had generally resisted integration into the structures of "general management" prescribed by Griffiths; contrary to the intentions and expectations expressed in the Griffiths report, only 6% of general manager positions were filled by medical professionals in the first round of appointments (Pollitt 1993: 70). But they were more open to participation in "clinical directorates," a matrix form of organization pioneered at Guy's hospital in London and modeled on structures at the Johns Hopkins University hospital in the United States. In this model, "the clinical director (usually, but not invariably, a member of consultant medical staff who continues to undertake part-time clinical work) is responsible to the hospital general manager, and is a budgetholder for the directorate" (Harrison and Pollitt 1994: 90). The clinical director thus played a critical role. In the colorful phrase of Packwood and his colleagues, "In addition to being able to 'hunt with the service providers,' the clinical director must also 'run with the unit managers' and along with fellow directors . . . contribute to determining unit plans and priorities as a member of the unit management board" (Packwood et al. 1992: 71–72, quoted in Harrison and Pollitt 1994: 91–92). The RMI incorporated and popularized the "clinical directorates" approach.

At any rate, the "rollout" of the RMI to the NHS as a whole was overtaken by the process of implementing the internal market reforms beginning in 1991. The rollout was accompanied by earmarked budgetary resources only temporarily; as more and more hospitals assumed the status of self-governing trusts, the acquisition of information systems became a matter for decision-making at the individual hospital level. In addition, most managerial resources were consumed in dealing with the unfamiliar mechanisms of contracting, as we shall see later.

In the meantime, however, the concept and practice of "medical audit" and "clinical directorates" continued to gain in popularity in both governmental and medical circles. In 1989, the Department of Health adopted a policy of support for medical audit that provided on average more than £40 million per annum in earmarked funding over the following five years. For provider units, this amounted to about 0.25% of their budgets/revenues (Buttery et al. 1994: 1). The recommendation that medical audit be made compulsory by April 1991 in all hospitals performing NHS work was one of the few recommendations of the White Paper *Working for Patients* welcomed by organized medicine, and the Royal Colleges proceeded to develop guidelines to assist clinicians to meet that deadline (Kemper and Macpherson 1994: 141; Smith et al. 1992: 177). Indeed, in the wake of the White Paper proposals the medical profession moved to establish control over the medical audit process. Harrison and Pollitt have described the type of medical audit established in the NHS as an internal "medical" model, in contrast to the "external, regulatory" audits conducted by professional review organizations (and, it might be added, by an increasing variety of monitoring agents) in the United States. In the assertion of this model, moreover, the profession did not encounter strong resistance from the DHSS and the NHS. As Harrison and Pollitt observe:

> 1989–90 was a period during which the Department and the organs of the medical profession were in open conflict over many elements of *Working for Patients*. Undoubtedly there was a sense in which both sides were relieved to find, in medical audit, a less controversial issue on which the usual processes of mutual adjustment and compromise could operate. (Harrison and Pollitt 1994: 102)

These "usual processes" yielded agreement between the government and organized medicine on a model in which the monitoring of clinical activities would take place on a regular retrospective basis (as opposed to the "prior approval" or "concurrent review" requirements imposed by various third party payers and managed care organizations in the United States [Gold et al. 1995]). Audit would be conducted by doctors and would be aimed at modifying clinical behavior through education. Clinical guidelines and protocols would be adopted locally, although guidance from national professional bodies would in practice weigh heavily in these local judgments. Enforcement of these guidelines would rest with medical staffs, not with line managers. And the audit process would be greatly hedged about with confidentiality requirements, although aggregate data would be passed to and through the managerial hierarchy (Harrison and Pollitt 1994: 101–3; Kemper and Macpherson 1994: 140–43).

As in the case of the Resource Management Initiative, there was consider-

able skepticism on the part of both managers and clinicians as to whether sufficient resources would be made available for the implementation of audit
processes. This skepticism was not allayed by the vague statement in the working paper on medical audit that accompanied the White Paper, that the costs of
developing medical audit would "have to be assessed and considered in future
public expenditure surveys" (Secretary of State for Social Services 1989, quoted
in Kemper and Macpherson 1994: 144–45). In the event, generous earmarked
funding for medical audit activities was continued on a "nonrecurring" basis
until 1994–1995, as discussed later.

A small part of this funding (about £6 million of a total of over £220 million over a five-year period) was allocated to the twelve Royal Colleges, the
self-governing educational and certifying bodies for medical specialties, in response to bids submitted by each college. There was very little central direction
as to how the funds were to be used, and a great variety of projects were
funded as a result. The resulting balance across types of projects hence may give
some indication as to the broader range of audit-related activities in the Royal
Colleges. About 46% of the funding went to clinical research, including the
identification of existing patterns of practice with an eye to identifying opportunities for improvement. Another 42% went to the development of clinical
guidelines and audit tools. The remaining 12% was directed to projects concerned with the actual implementation of research findings, guidelines, and
audit results—the small proportion perhaps reflecting the view that this was a
matter for locally based groups of clinicians (Amess et al. 1995: 55, 68–76).

Despite agreement between organized medicine and the government on
this medical audit model, practicing clinicians were somewhat slower to warm
to the idea. According to a survey conducted in one health district in 1990,
clinicians and managers overwhelmingly agreed that medical audit would enhance the quality of care provided to patients and would facilitate continuing
medical education. Clinicians, however, were considerably more likely than
managers to believe that medical audit incurred opportunity costs, interfering
with clinical workload, and diverting resources from patient care. Clinicians
were divided, moreover, on the implications of medical audit for clinical autonomy, with equal numbers agreeing and disagreeing that it would allow managers to manipulate medical practice (Smith et al. 1992: 178–79). A 1992 survey
of chairpersons of audit committees by the Royal College of Physicians also
reported "the need to build up clinicians' enthusiasm for and commitment to
the audit programme" (Walshe and Coles 1993: 23).

Notwithstanding these reservations, audit procedures became established in
hospitals doing NHS work (as will be discussed later). A significant effect of the
White Paper was thus to "persuade the medical profession to accept more collective responsibility for the way in which individual members exercise their
craft" (Klein 1995: 243). Clinical guidelines and protocols were established both
nationally and locally, and gained broad acceptance within the profession, at
least on principle. This represented a change in the practice of the profession
but not in its collegial processes. The production of guidelines and protocols is
a consensual process, and implementation depends upon peer pressure. In the

new accommodation that was in the process of being worked out between clinicians and managers in the 1980s and 1990s, the profession accepted increased collective responsibility while retaining its traditional zones of influence; the medical audit function was accomplished within the medical "pillar" of authority.

## The Purchaser–Provider Split: Bargaining in the Internal Market

The central feature of the reforms initiated by the White Paper *Working for Patients* was the organizational split between "purchasers" and "providers." The rationale for the split was to break the grip of provider dominance within the system, to take advantage of the near-monopsony position of the state by requiring providers to compete for the business of purchasers (Harrison and Pollitt 1994: 117–18). At the same time, the strategy continued to seek to buffer politicians from at least some types of rationing decisions—hospital mergers and closures, for example, could be presented as the shaking-out effect of market competition, not government planning.

As described in chapter 3, the reforms made District Health Authorities (DHAs) purchasing agencies and gave hospitals and other provider units the option of establishing themselves as independent "trusts" or remaining as "directly managed units" (DMUs). In either case they would receive their funding by contracting with DHAs to provide services. In the event, the distinction between trusts and DMUs became less and less salient as more units opted for trust status. By April 1995, there were 528 trusts across the United Kingdom accounting for well over 95% of NHS expenditure on hospital and community care (and not including general practice) (Smee 1995: 181; Adams 1995: 183).

The White Paper, and the set of policy ideas from which it derived, made much of the benefits of the competition that would follow upon the severing of purchasing and provision, as we saw in chapter 3. Competition among providers for contracts, however, was generally not to be the result. In part this was because in many areas, consistent with the economics of health care described in chapter 1, there were simply not enough hospitals and other provider agencies in the locality covered by a given District Health Authority to provide the possibility of meaningful competition. A study of the largest health region, the West Midlands, with eighteen DHAs in 1992, found that about one-quarter of the thirty-nine acute care hospitals in the region, treating just fewer than 40% of the patients, were in monopoly positions. The degree of competition, however, was assessed using a broad definition of the product—general surgery—and the survey authors point out that at the subspecialty level the degree of concentration would be higher (Appleby et al. 1994).

The lack of competition, however, also resulted from the persistence of relationships and patterns of activity that predated the internal market reforms. The NHS deliberately followed a strategy of phased implementation of contracting requirements, with the objective of increasing the degree of specificity of contracts and the degree of performance monitoring over time. Even so, compliance with NHS directives continued to lag. In the first year of contracting,

1991–1992, it was anticipated that simple "block" contracts would be the primary contracting vehicle, allowing purchasers and providers to make the transition to the contracting mode while preserving historical patterns of activity.[3] After 1991–1992, through a series of Executive Letters and Guidances, the NHS issued requirements that DHAs move to greater use of "cost and volume" contracts, specifying the number of treatments to be provided for a given price. As of the 1994–1995 contracting round, no more simple block contracts were to be written (NHS 1993a).

In practice, block contracts persisted to a considerable degree, although they became increasingly "sophisticated" (in the terms used by an NHS review of the 1994–1995 contracting round), by including specified floors and ceilings of activity and provisions for dealing with under- or overperformance. In 1991–1992, 41% of all contracts for acute services, accounting for 60% of the value of contracted services, were in simple block form, and an additional 42% of such contracts, accounting for 34% of the value of services, were in the form of block contracts with specified floors and ceilings (Robinson and Le Grand 1995: 32). A majority (57%) of DHAs reported that "existing patient flows" had the highest priority in influencing purchasing decisions, and another 34% assigned highest priority to the expressed preference of GPs in their districts (Appleby et al. 1994: 50). In the 1994–1995 contracting round, only 5% of major contracts for acute services[4] were in simple block form, but 69% were "sophisticated" block contracts with ceilings and floors.[5] Fifty-seven percent of DHAs incorporated or planned to incorporate financial sanctions for failure to meet specified expectations regarding matters such as data quality, timeliness of information, waiting times, activity levels, and quality standards in their contracts (NHS 1994a).

Most contracts, however, continued to be written at the "multiunit" or "whole-unit" level. Only 20% of contracts surveyed in the 1994–1995 round were negotiated at a specialty level, with a further 4% at subspecialty levels (NHS 1994a).[6] As of the 1995–1996 round, the NHS Executive required that at least one of three specialties—orthopedics, gynecology, or ophthalmology— be contracted for on a subspecialty basis using a "Healthcare Resource Group" (HRG) costing methodology (a British version of the American Diagnosis Related Group, or DRG, methodology described in chapter 5) (NHS 1994c). The level of preparedness for this shift is called into question by the observation that in the previous contracting round only forty (16%) of major acute service contracts involved subspecialty contracting, and of those only two involved HRG methodology and one involved DRG methodology (NHS 1994a).

Specialty and subspecialty contracting, while increasing the specificity of contracts, also tended to reduce the potential for competition among providers within a given district. Although the internal market reforms opened up the possibility for DHAs to contract with providers outside their own areas, and hence to stimulate some cross-area competition, past patterns tended also to prevail in this regard. From 1992–1993 to 1994–1995, contracts with purchasers outside the home district accounted for only about 15% to 16% of the total value of the average provider's contracts (Appleby 1994: 10). The NHS encouraged DHAs that contracted for certain highly specialized services, such as neonatal care, to form multidistrict purchasing consortia. As of the 1994–1995 round, just over one-half of the DHAs purchasing such services were purchasing some services jointly with other DHAs, but data on the value of services so purchased is not available (Appleby 1994: 30).

For the most part, then, at least the initial effect of the internal market reforms was not to increase levels of competition among providers for purchasers' contracts, but was rather to transform the managerial relationship between DHAs and the provider units in their areas into a relationship of explicit bargaining. Indeed, after only a short time under the implementation of the reforms the language of policy began to shift. "Commissioning" began to replace "purchasing" in describing the role of the DHAs, and "contestability" began to replace "competition" in describing the key feature of local internal markets (Klein 1995: 206). Even the degree of "contestability" of many local markets was open to question. Some of those who advanced the notion of contestability in this context described it as competition "for" rather than "in" markets. The high transaction costs associated with writing, executing, and enforcing contracts in the health care arena drives attempts to establish long-term stable relationships, as we have seen in the American case. As the hierarchical relationships which once provided this stability were transformed into contractual relationships, the contracts were likely, de facto if not de jure, to be long term. Indeed, as of 1994–1995, survey data suggest that more than 60% of DHAs had at least some contracts running for longer than a year, and almost all of the remainder intended to do so (Appleby 1994: 30). As Appleby and his colleagues have put it, "If long-term contracts exist, competition is likely to take place *for* markets at periodic stages of contract negotiation, rather than *in* markets on a day-to-day basis" (Appleby et al. 1994: 26).

Even so defined, however, the degree of contestability of local internal markets was questionable. High capital costs constituted a significant barrier to entry in most of the acute care sector. Even those private providers who had become well established in certain "niche" areas (as discussed later) did not see the margins obtainable on NHS business as sufficiently attractive to lead them to expand into other areas of care. Accordingly, some observers suggested that internal markets might be contested not by new provider organizations but by new management teams—but this was a conjecture whose practicality remained untested (Robinson and Le Grand 1995: 41).

In practice, then, the internal market did not approximate the classical market of atomized buyers and sellers but was rather what Ferlie (1994) calls a "relational" market—it was made up of local markets of near-monopsonists and near-monopolists who had well-established networks of relationship with each other. The "purchasers" and "providers" who made up the market were created, after all, by the division of established entities. Case study evidence suggested "a high degree of continuity in the personnel staffing at the upper reaches" of both purchasing authorities and trusts. The market was hence "socially embedded" in professional and managerial networks (Ferlie 1994: 221).

## Bargaining Roles: The Provider Side

If what was significant about the internal market reforms was not the development of competitive behavior but rather the emergence of new and more explicit forms of bargaining relationships, we need to consider more closely the roles of the various participants in these relationships. And one striking feature of these relationships was the key role played by medical professionals on both the purchaser and the provider sides. This is not surprising, given not only the traditional position of influence held by the medical profession within NHS structures but also the deliberate policy intention to involve doctors in the contracting process in a substantial way.

On the provider side, after an initial period of reluctance, clinicians became increasingly involved in the contracting process. With the exception of a few cases such as that of Guy's hospital in London, medical staffs were either divided about or opposed to the transformation of their NHS hospitals to trust status. One of the implications of the move to trust status was that consultants' contracts would henceforth be held (and potentially more thoroughly negotiated and enforced) at the level of the trust and no longer at the regional level. Hence one of the traditional buffers of clinical autonomy would be forfeited. Pay scales were also to be locally negotiated, calling into question the longstanding corporatist structures of central pay determination. On the other hand, trusts were required to involve clinicians in their management structures as a condition of gaining self-governing status.

As more and more hospitals made the shift to trust status, clinicians bowed to the inevitable and sought to shape the resulting arrangements. The threat of local pay determination was headed off through the central negotiation of a more flexible contract. Hospitals increasingly adopted a "clinical directorate" model for resource allocation. And clinician involvement in the contracting process, strongly prodded by the NHS Executive, continued to increase.

But the involvement of clinicians in contracting, and clinician–manager relations in general, were subject to great local variation. The NHS review of the 1994–1995 round of contracting previously cited found that in 40% of major contracts clinicians had had no involvement. Somewhat ironically, however, the involvement of clinicians appeared likely to increase as more specific contracts were negotiated at specialty and subspecialty levels. The ability of provider units to deliver specified levels of activity in discrete areas of service depended upon their ability to gain compliance from their clinicians, and the assumption was that compliance was more likely to be forthcoming if clinicians had been involved in the contracting process (Figueras et al. 1993: 225). And in fact a Ministerial Task Group convened to review clinical involvement in contracting in 1994 found that "there was a correlation between the level of contract sophistication (in particular the extent to which a contract was specialty focused) and the active involvement of clinicians in the contracting process" (NHS 1994b: paragraph 5.3).

The issues raised by the involvement of clinicians in the contracting process are thrown into sharpest relief by the attempt to introduce casemix categories, and in particular HRG methodology, for specifying and costing services for contract purposes. At least in the initial stages of this endeavor, the introduction of this methodology appeared likely to give an advantage to providers in their dealings with purchasers, and, within provider units, to clinicians in dealing with managers. Such expertise as existed in using this type of methodology tended to reside in provider units, particularly those that had been developing such techniques for use in their own internal management and resource allocation processes. The standardized HRG-type methodology provided a way of assessing trends in performance over time and of comparing the performance of a given unit against peer institutions. And it provided a common language for clinicians and managers, a way of aggregating complex data at a level that preserved sufficient information to satisfy clinicians while being manageable for accounting purposes. In the words of one hospital manager interviewed in a 1995 survey, "There's nothing magic about HRGs. They just happen to be about the right level of aggregation that gets you talking" (Orchard 1995: 6). The major impact of these technologies was not to replace the ongoing conversations between clinicians and managers, but rather to change the terms in which they were conducted.

In these conversations, focused as they were around clinical categories, the role of clinical directors was pivotal. As one clinical director put it, "[B]ecause, quite deliberately, casemix groupings are broad . . . you've actually got to know what's beneath them," and the role of clinical directorates in managing resources within more discrete categories was accordingly reinforced (Orchard 1995: 7). The task group on clinical involvement in contracting (previously cited) emphasized the key role played by clinical directors, while urging a broader involvement of clinicians in the contracting process (NHS 1994b: paragraph 5.9).

In this process of clinical management, the role of medical audit or (somewhat more broadly defined) clinical audit was of growing importance. Clinical audit remained almost exclusively the preserve of the medical profession, administered through peer review processes (Kerrison et al. 1994). A survey of provider units in late 1993 found that 64% had their own audit programs and 36% participated in multiunit programs. Audit committees, whether or not exclusively focused on medical audit, were dominated by medical staff, particularly from acute specialties; virtually all were chaired by a consultant. Nonmedical clinical professionals and managers were unlikely to be involved in audit committee meetings (Buttery et al. 1994). Furthermore, the involvement of purchasers in audit activities was very limited, largely confined to medical staff in the purchasing agencies.

Given the broad and almost exclusive medical control over audit activities, it is perhaps not surprising that the concept of clinical guidelines gained broad acceptance within the medical profession, although a minority remained opposed. Surveys of medical opinion from 1993 to 1995 found two-third to three-quarter majorities expressing broad approval for the use of clinical guidelines as improving the quality of care, with minorities expressing concerns regarding lack of flexibility and encroachment upon clinical autonomy (Mansfield 1995; Siriwardena 1995; British Medical Association 1995).[7] Reported use of guidelines was more variable and appeared to be heavily influenced by professional networks (Mansfield 1995)—a finding consistent with experience with clinical guidelines in other nations (Oxman et al. 1995).

## Bargaining Roles: The Purchaser Side

Expertise in the purchasing authorities was of a different type: it was focused on "needs assessment," not on clinical casemix. There was considerable variation across DHAs in this regard (as there was, indeed, across hospitals in expertise regarding casemix analysis). But in general as DHAs shed their responsibilities for managing provider units, they shed with them the personnel and infrastructure of clinical management. The personnel upon whom DHAs had relied as part of the hierarchical corporatist structures of the pre-1990 NHS were now lodged with the autonomous entities with which DHAs had to bargain.

In the division of responsibilities brought about by the internal market reforms, one of the traditional roles of the DHAs—assessing and planning for the health needs of their local populations—assumed central importance for DHAs as purchasing authorities. Since the adoption of the recommendations of a 1976 Resource Allocation Working Party (RAWP), the allocation of resources on a geographic basis within the NHS had been based on a formula that to some extent took account of local health needs, by weighting population figures by age and sex (the weights derived from utilization experience), standardized mortality rates, and certain other factors relevant to particular health conditions. Regional authorities and district authorities were expected, in their turn, to make their subregional and subdistrict allocations according to some form of needs assessment based on population characteristics. The capacity and willingness of these authorities to make such assessments on a systematic quantitative basis varied greatly (Whitehead 1994: 225–31). Among other problems, the abolition of the AHAs in 1982 meant that the epidemiological expertise relevant to needs assessment was dispersed among the larger number of DHAs.

What was more common across districts was a heavy reliance by DHAs on the advice of local general practitioners in performing the "needs assessment" role. As noted here, the expressed preferences of local general practitioners emerged as the most important factor reported as governing purchasing decisions in the first round of contracting. Later, partly in response to the increasing popularity of GP fundholding, the purchasing authorities developed a variety of mechanisms for involving GPs in purchasing decisions (discussed later in this chapter). In 1996, Family Health Service Authorities or FHSAs (the local bodies that provided the formal interface between general practitioners and the NHS) were merged with DHAs to become Health Authorities (HAs) or Health Commissions (the terminology varied across agencies but did not imply a difference in role)—a reorganization that tightened and complicated the relationship between purchasing authorities and local GPs.

An appreciation of the role played by general practitioners in purchasing requires an understanding both of the traditional relationship of general practitioners to the NHS and of certain key features of the 1990 reforms. Formally, general practitioners were never NHS employees but were rather "independent contractors"—a status successfully wrested in negotiations with government at the creation of the NHS and insisted upon since. Each general practitioner's contract was held by a local authority—first Executive Councils, then Family Practitioner Committees, and after 1991 by the FHSAs. Until the late 1980s, these authorities functioned essentially as paymasters, allocating funds to GPs on the basis of a nationally determined modified capitation formula, with little influence over the day-to-day practice of GPs. Each resident of a locality was to be enrolled with a general practice (and in practice about 93% of the population has been so enrolled). Although patients were in theory free to choose their general practitioner and GPs were free to decline to take a given patient, in practice there was little movement of patients from one GP's list to another for reasons other than change of residence. GPs also (until the 1990 reforms) had the freedom to refer patients to consultants of their choosing, and they developed strong and stable referral networks as a result.

In one sense, however, the establishment of the NHS in 1948 marked a significant downward shift in the status of general practitioners. As Glennerster and his colleagues describe it:

> For most of this century, and certainly since the inception of the National Health Service, general practice has lost ground to the hospital. . . . Before 1948 the voluntary hospitals and the consultants within them depended for their livelihood on GPs referring their paying patients to them. After 1948 the hospitals were directly funded by the state and the GPs became supplicants, seeking treatment for a patient on the consultant's waiting list. There was thus a latent desire among GPs for any change that would shift the balance of power back in their direction. (Glennerster et al. 1994: 74)

One of the most innovative features of the internal market reforms provided just such a change. GPs (at first only those in relatively large practices) were given the opportunity to hold budgets for prescription drugs and for various hospital and community services (largely elective surgery and outpatient procedures), from which they would purchase such services for patients enrolled in their practices, by contracting with providers. Unexpended funds could be retained by the GP to be invested in the practice. Earmarked additional funding to offset the transaction costs of contracting, including information systems, was also offered until 1996–1997, when these funds became part of the fundholding budget.

The fundholding option offered several advantages to GPs. It allowed them to retain their freedom to refer patients to whomever they wished, whereas nonfundholding GPs were restricted to those providers with whom their host purchasing authority had a contract. With their smaller scale, they had more flexibility than purchasing authorities to exit contract relationships. They would thus gain financial leverage in their dealings with the consultants before whom they had previously been "supplicants." The fundholding option also offered GPs the prospect of building up their practice infrastructure. And in a less tangible way, it presented them with the challenge of being on the leading edge of a major new development in the GP's role.

On the other hand, there were potential drawbacks to the option in the minds of significant numbers of GPs. It required them to assume a limited amount of risk[8] and to incur transaction costs in a way that they had never done. And it was controversial on ideological grounds: it raised the specter of "two-tier" medicine. Since the fundholders' budgets were withdrawn from the budget of their host purchasing authority, they were in a zero-sum relationship with nonfundholders. And while the nonfundholding GPs were funded on a modified capitation basis, fundholders' budgets were based on their historical patterns of activity—a more generous basis. To the extent that fundholders could use their more generous budgets, infrastructure support, and financial leverage with providers to gain preferential treatment (such as quicker access to services) for their patients, a two-tier system would result. Given that, at the outset, the majority of GPs were in practices too small to be eligible for fund-holding, this prospect was particularly rankling. Some GPs also objected to the introduction of a "cash nexus" into the GP–patient relationship—a nexus in which the GP would be seen to have a direct financial interest in the referral decision. Concerns were also raised that fundholding practices, like HMOs in the United States, faced incentives to "cream-skim"—to select healthy patients and so to preserve their budgets for reinvestment in their practices.

Furthermore, general practitioners were in no mood to respond favorably to any policy initiative from the Conservative government in 1990. They had just been through a highly conflictual round of negotiations with the government over the terms of a new GP contract, which ended with the government's imposition of a contract that had been overwhelming rejected in a ratification vote. Coupled with the exclusion of the profession from the process of the NHS review, this unilateral action fuelled medical opposition to the reforms (Klein 1995: 200–1).

The BMA accordingly objected vigorously to fundholding when it was first introduced. But when it became clear by 1993 that, as eligibility criteria were loosened, more and more GPs were opting for fundholding and that the BMA had an obligation to represent their interests as well as those of its nonfund-holding members, the BMA withdrew its opposition.[9]

The take-up of the fundholding option reflected a range of pragmatic and ideological motivations. A survey of fifty-six fundholding practices, including both early and late entrants, by the Audit Commission in 1994–1995 found that about one-half reported entering the scheme to gain increased leverage over providers to improve services, and about the same proportion indicated that preserving their freedom to refer had been a factor. Interestingly, however, the most common response (given by about 70% of the fundholders) was that the GPs had seen fundholding as the way of the future, and did not want their patients or their practices to suffer by not being associated with it (Audit Commission 1996a: 44). In general, fundholders also tended to be drawn from the socioeconomic and professional elite practices; they were less likely to be drawn from areas qualifying for "social deprivation" payments under the GP remuneration formula, and more likely to be accredited to perform minor surgery and to be approved by the Joint Committee on Postgraduate Training in General Practice as training practices (Audit Commission 1996a: 9–11). As for those who did not join the scheme, a survey of nineteen nonfundholding practices in one region in 1994 found that two-thirds of the medical partners in these practices had "clear, strong" objections to fundholding on grounds of principle, politics, or ideology. The method of selecting the sample of practices for interviewing, however, may well have overrepresented such views (Robinson and Hayter 1995).

In the first "wave" of fundholding—the contracting year 1991–1992—only practices with a minimum of 9,000 patients were eligible to enter. Slightly more than 300 practices joined, representing about 7.5% of GPs and covering a similar proportion of the population. Over the following years, the size threshold was gradually reduced to 5,000 by 1996, the range of services covered by the standard fundholding model was increased, and new models of fundholding were developed. One of the new models, introduced in 1996–1997, was more restrictive than the standard model and allowed small practices to hold budgets for the purchase of a range of community, but not hospital, services. Another model was much more expansive than the standard model: "total purchasing" allowed fundholders to purchase all hospital and community care for their patients. Fifty-three "total purchasing pilot projects" (TPPs) were established, after two years of preparation, in 1996–1997. Total purchasing fundholders, the British equivalent to HMOs (though much smaller than their American counterparts), were typically made up of groups of practices so as to spread the risk assumed. They ranged in size from about 13,000 to about 100,000 patients (averaging about 30,000–40,000 patients). Meanwhile, the standard fundholding model itself was evolving, as groups of fundholding practices took the initiative to pool a proportion of their management allowances to form "multifunds" to provide common services and coordination functions—some of them almost as large as the average HA in terms of the population covered (Audit Commission 1996a: 48–50).

By the time the Labour government froze fundholding as part of its proposed transition to Primary Care Groups, as will be discussed later in this chapter, more than one-half of all general practitioners were involved in some form of fundholding—primarily in the 3,500 GPFHs, but also including 80 TPPs and 100 multifunds (Department of Health 1997: figure 1). The spread of fundholding was one of the most remarkable and least anticipated effects of the NHS reforms—an example of the extent to which the rough sketch presented in 1989 was greatly elaborated in the process of implementation.

Given the degree to which fundholding was "brought . . . to centre stage in the NHS Executive's strategy for developing services" (Audit Commission 1996a: 5), it was the subject of intense interest as to its implications. The self-selected nature of the fundholding population, and the more generous funding of fundholders, confounded attempts at rigorous controlled evaluative studies. Nonetheless, certain tentative findings about the impact of fundholding began to emerge, and they suggested that neither the optimistic predictions of enthusiasts nor the fears of skeptics had been borne out (Coulter 1995[10]). The one area in which fundholding appeared to have made a difference was in holding down prescribing costs—a phenomenon that replicated German experience in assigning indicative drug budgets to physicians. Otherwise, fundholders' referral patterns showed little change (Coulter and Bradlow 1993; Audit Commission 1996a: 33), although a study limited to one district and one specialty found that fundholders' *rates* of referral increased less than did those of a control group (Kammerling and Kinnear 1996). There was no evidence of increased competition by fundholders for patients; the only study to have investigated the rate of movement of patients from one practice to another found no difference between pre- and postreform periods (Jones et al. 1994: 138). Nor was there strong evidence that a "two-tier" system was emerging: studies of waiting times for consultants' appointments for patients of fundholders and nonfundholders showed conflicting results, some suggesting no difference (Coulter 1995), others suggesting an advantage for patients of fundholders (Kammerling and Kinnear 1996), although the lack of data on severity of illness makes interpretation of these results difficult.

What does seem clear is that greater transaction costs were associated with fundholding, although the rise of "multifunds" promised to reduce these costs somewhat. As we shall see, fundholders generally entered into more specific forms of contracting with providers than did purchasing authorities. An Audit Commission review of fundholding pointed out that the increased administrative costs for fundholders (as measured by the allowances provided for management, clerical, and computing costs, and not including providers' transaction costs) outweighed the "efficiency savings" (the surpluses retained by fundholding practices) by a margin of £232 million to £206 million from 1991–1992 to 1994–1995. These were highly imperfect measures of costs and benefits, however, which the Audit Commission noted did not address the issue of gains in quality (Audit Commission 1996a: 7).

If the direct impact of fundholding remained unclear, its indirect impact in enhancing the role of general practitioners was arguably more demonstrable. Like HMOs and for-profit institutions in the United States, fundholders had an influence disproportionate to their numbers as other actors in the system responded to their rise. Faced with the threat to their own budgets of the growing popularity of fundholding, the HAs began to develop mechanisms to give GPs influence over purchasing without opting for fundholding status. These mechanisms ranged along a spectrum from advisory groups, often with a coordinator paid by the HA, concerned with needs assessment within a given locality (so-called "locality purchasing"), to groups of practices with notional or indicative budgets devolved from the HA for a range of hospital and community services (so-called "practice-sensitive commissioning" or "GP commissioning").

Indeed, the growth of these mechanisms for involving nonfundholders in HA purchasing decisions, as well as the expansion of the range of fundholding models, resulted in what Mays and Dixon (1996) have termed "purchaser plurality." Relative to the explosion of organizational models in the United States, however, these U.K. models exhibited a fairly limited range of variation. They varied essentially in the balance of influence that they implied between purchasing authorities and practicing GPs, but all—even the "total purchasing" fundholding model—implied some measure of influence for each.[11] In 1996 knowledgeable observers pointed to the outlines of an evolving model of purchasing, in which groups of general practices would be assigned either notional or real budgets for the purchase of hospital and community services and the focus of the HAs' activities would be on coordination, monitoring, and regulation (Mays and Dixon 1996: 17–18).[12] And it was such a model, indeed, that infused the Labour Government's proposals for Primary Care Groups (PCGs) in its December 1997 White Paper, to be discussed in more detail later. Building upon the fundholding model, the 1997 White Paper envisaged a staged evolution toward a system in which up to 85% of total NHS expenditure would be commissioned by PCGs.

As the new organizational structures of purchasing and providing evolved, they continued to be linked, both formally and informally, through medical networks. Over one-half of fundholding GPs met directly with provider consultants during contract negotiations (Audit Commission 1996b: 32). The clinical directorate, which was seen in some ways as parallel to GP fundholding, provided a focus for such contacts (Benady 1993). As for Health Authorities, in addition to the growing role of nonfundholding GPs in their purchasing decisions, the role of public health physicians was at least potentially central to the purchasing process. This role, however, varied widely across HAs and was in most cases a somewhat ambivalent one.

Before the unification of the three distinct sectors of the NHS in 1974, public health physicians (as Medical Officers of Health) and their staffs held positions of authority and autonomy within the public health sector, as employees of Local Authorities. Unification drew them into Area Health Authorities, and then DHAs, where their roles typically involved an ambiguous combination of managerial responsibility and professional advisory status (Levitt et al. 1995: 183–84). They were often the chief point of contact between the HA and provider clinicians, particularly insofar as issues of clinical quality were at stake. This represented a judgment on the part of managers about the importance of having medical professionals deal with each other on such issues. (As one observer put it to me more impishly, this was a "send a doc to catch a doc" strategy.) The low status of public health medicine within the British medical profession, however (Levitt et al. 1995: 183) presented a hurdle to be overcome by these public health "ambassadors" in dealing with clinicians. Some did so, but the degree of success in this regard varied widely across purchasing authorities.

## Clinical Audit and the Role of Clinical Judgment

In the United States, as we saw in chapter 5, the proliferation of contractual and organizational arrangements in response to the demands of price-conscious purchasers led to increasing intervention by managers into clinical decision-making. In Britain, the persistence of professional networks throughout the process of implementing the internal market reforms meant that such intervention was much less common. Unlike increasing numbers of their Amercian counterparts, British physicians were generally not subject to rules governing the treatment of individual cases or types of cases on the basis of their cost or revenue implications.

In the first place, contracts did not typically entail such rules. Despite the professional linkages between doctors on the purchaser and the provider sides, or perhaps because of the differences in professional expertise or status that they involved, judgments of clinical quality and appropriateness played a limited role in contracting. The predominance of block contracting by purchasing authorities meant that purchaser scrutiny of the vast bulk of medical practice was limited to the receipt of reports on overall levels of activity and costs. (The gradual move to costing based on HRGs promised to increase the incentive for managers in provider units to consider costs per case, but as we shall see such costing required a level of sophistication in information technology which most providers had not attained in the mid-1990s.) Only at the margins—in the case of "cost-per-case" contracts, which accounted for a small and diminishing proportion of the total value of contracts negotiated by HAs,[13] and in the case of "extracontractual referrals," largely for highly specialized tertiary care—did even the potential for the application of protocols by purchasers on a case by case basis arise. By and large, however, the performance standards specified in contracts were largely procedural and related to the centrally promulgated objectives regarding such matters as waiting times for appointments.

The situation was somewhat different in the case of contracts negotiated with providers by GP fundholders. Among GP fundholders, cost-per-case and cost-and-volume contracts predominated.[14] But GPFHs tended to rely on the feedback they received from consultants on individual cases to monitor performance—a mechanism built into the GP–consultant relationship and generally denied to HAs (Appleby 1994: 15). In general, the performance standards specified in GP fundholder contracts with providers also related to procedural issues: more than 90% specified "Patient's Charter" standards for waiting times for appointments and waiting times in consultants' clinics (see later in this chapter); fewer than 20% specified standards for outcome measures such as re-admission rates (Audit Commission 1996a: 57).

Central encouragement to purchasers to take issues of clinical effectiveness into account in contracting had limited impact. Requirements that purchasers use clinical guidelines and evidence of clinical and cost effectiveness in contracting were carefully couched to avoid antagonizing medical professionals (NHS 1993a). Again, the impact of such considerations was marginal, relating largely to extracontractual referrals (ECRs) and to decisions not to include certain services in purchasing contracts (NHS 1994a: paragraph 50). Reviews of purchasing plans in 1994–1995, 1995–1996, and 1996–1997 showed that the proportion of purchasing authorities choosing to remove some types of service from their purchasing contracts rose from about 10% to about 23% over that period. Most of these exclusions, however, had to do with cosmetic procedures. Potentially more significant was the identification of a number of diagnostic and therapeutic procedures (such as x-rays for back pain, or cesarean sections) which needed to be more carefully targetted to reduce instances of ineffective use (Redmayne 1996: 21–22). Klein et al. (1996: 72–74) refer to this approach as "rationing by selectivity": agreeing to pay for some services only under certain clinical conditions—for example, cholesterol testing only for high-risk patients. A related strategy was to reduce budget allocations for certain procedures whose routine use was judged to be of doubtful effectiveness and to leave to clinicians the judgment of whom to treat within those reduced envelopes—a microlevel version of the earlier macrolevel understanding between the profession and the state.

These explicit exclusions and partial exclusions from coverage, however, remained at the margins of medical treatment. For the most part, judgments of the appropriateness of patterns of medical care remained within the medical preserve of clinical audit. As we have already seen, clinical audit developed within provider units with little involvement on the part of managers, and the audit maintained a focus on the quality and effectiveness rather than the cost of specific procedures. Similarly, despite central requirements that audit provisions be included in contracts, there was little direct involvement of purchasers in audit activities.

As of 1994–1995 central earmarked funding for audit, which had been allocated through the RHAs, ceased and became part of the general allocations to DHAs, to be allocated through the contracting process. Increasingly, purchasers wrote into contracts a provision that providers must have in place clinical audit processes. By the time of the 1994–1995 contracting round, 95% of all DHAs included provisions for clinical audit in their purchasing contracts or had negotiated separate contracts with each provider dealing specifically with audit (NHS 1994a: 13). Most of the contract requirements were procedural in nature, such as requirements that all medical staff participate in audit, and that an annual report on medical audit be sent to the purchaser. Some purchasers, however, specified certain topics to be addressed by audit programs. But as of the 1993–1994 contracting rounds, virtually no sanctions related to audit provisions were specified in contracts. Monitoring mechanisms were broadly retrospective, and largely "reactive and paper-based" (Rumsey et al. 1994: 28–33). The task group on clinical involvement in contracting concluded in 1994 that "there was little evidence of purchasers using the outcomes of clinical audit to inform the contracting process" (NHS 1994b: paragraph 5.16).

Contracting, then, did not generally provide a vehicle for the monitoring of clinical performance, at least for purchasers other than GP fundholders in individual cases. In fact, most performance monitoring in the NHS occurred outside the contracting process and continued along lines of development that began well before the internal market reforms. Some occurred within more or less informal networks. Public health physicians in some of the larger and more sophisticated HAs, for example, worked with their provider hospitals and the Royal Colleges to develop protocols for certain procedures. While the use of these protocols might not have been specified in contracts, it formed part of a set of understandings within which the contracting process took place.

Somewhat more formal was the monitoring role played by RHAs and DHAs (later regional offices of the NHS and HAs, respectively), carried over from the pre-1991 period. Since the early 1980s (and in the case of mental health services since the 1970s), various statistical indicators of levels of activity—the statistical series subject to the "mass baptism" as performance indicators described by Klein—were published for each DHA (Harrison and Pollitt 1994: 54–60). Beginning in 1984, measures of "efficiency" of provision were monitored and targets for improvement were set.[15] These measures were highly controversial, and the measures of activity arguably lent themselves to manipulation (Radical Statistics Health Group 1995).

In 1991, another wave of performance measures was introduced, following the promulgation of the "Citizen's Charter" by the Conservative government. The emphasis of the Citizen's Charter was on improving the quality of public services by changing the incentives facing providers—through competitive mechanisms such as privatization and contracting out, performance-related pay, and the publication of the standards of service that recipients should expect. Each branch of government was to publish its own standards; in the case of the NHS this took the form of the "Patient's Charter." The Patient's Charter included broad guarantees at the level of principle, such as the right to "receive health care on the basis of clinical need, regardless of ability to pay." The only one of the ten "rights" set out in the Patient's Charter that enshrined a quantifiable standard related to the high-profile issue of waiting times: patients were "to be guaranteed [hospital] admission for treatment for a specific date within two years," subsequently reduced to eighteen months and then to a target of twelve months for some procedures. In addition to "rights," the Patient's Charter set out nine "standards," some qualitative (such as "respect for privacy, dignity, and religious beliefs") and some quantitative. Of the four quantitative standards, all related to waiting times, such as a guarantee of being seen within thirty minutes in an outpatient clinic. Local standards were also to be established governing matters such as waiting times for outpatient appointments (Warden 1991). All relevant hospitals were required to report annually data relating (as of 1996–1997) to waiting-time standards (regarding ambulance speed of response, assessment in emergency departments, assignment of bed upon admission through emergency, waiting in outpatient clinics, waiting for inpatient admission and outpatient appointments, and times to admission after cancelled operations) (NHS 1996). Similarly, purchasers were expected to take performance against these standards into account in the contracting process. More than 90% of GP fundholders included Patient's Charter standards for waiting times for inpatient procedures and waiting times in outpatient clinics in their contracts (Audit Commission 1996a: 57), but there are no systematic data about the use of these standards by purchasing authorities.

These essentially procedural standards did not constitute direct interventions into clinical decision-making—although it has been argued that the waiting time standard for elective surgery, for example, required arbitrarily that a patient who has spent a year on a waiting list be seen in preference to one with greater clinical need. In the case of general practice, however, the monitoring of performance began to touch directly upon areas of clinical judgement. The highly unpopular GP contract imposed in 1990 established targets for two types of procedure—cervical cytology and childhood immunization—and tied a portion of the GP's remuneration to the achievement of those targets. In addition, some FHSAs (now HAs) developed their own performance indicators for general practice, such as prescribing patterns and referral rates, although these were not tied to remuneration (Majeed and Voss 1995).

Another major initiative with implications for performance monitoring was the publication of a governmental White Paper, *The Health of the Nation,* in 1992. In contrast to the emphasis on procedural dimensions of performance in the Patient's Charter, *The Health of the Nation* focused on health outcomes. Targets for the reduction of the incidence of selected health problems were to be established and monitored on an ongoing basis, beginning with five areas— coronary heart disease and stroke, cancer, mental illness, HIV/AIDS and sexual health, and accidents. Taking a given base year (usually 1990), targets were established for the reduction of health problems in these categories within particular populations at risk by a given future date (usually the year 2000).[16] The complex etiologies of these various health problems mean that the health care delivery system is only one of a set of factors that could bring about changes in their incidence; hence measures of incidence are problematic as performance indicators for health care delivery. The prominent inclusion of these measures among those tracked by the NHS highlighted the importance of the "needs assessment" processes (and hence the role of public health physicians) within HAs. But no mechanism was developed to reward success in meeting targets for improvement. (In fact, the funding formula arguably rewarded those who were least successful in reducing mortality rates among their local populations.)

In sum, these various measures of success in meeting efficiency targets, observing patients' procedural "rights," and improving health outcomes did little to constrain clinical decision-making in individual cases. In particular, linking efficiency considerations to clinical judgement on a case by case basis would require a level of capacity in information systems that most sites within the NHS did not possess in the 1990s. The history of the development of information technology within the NHS was, indeed, one of considerable frustration, disillusionment, and skepticism, as the next section suggests.

## Information and Information Technology

As was pointed out earlier in this chapter, the large-scale introduction of information technology to the NHS was begun in the late 1980s in a context of great budgetary uncertainty and skepticism that the necessary resources would be made available on an ongoing basis. As it turned out, large sums of money were spent on information technology, but with results that fueled doubts about its utility.

Over the period 1990–1995, NHS acute care hospitals in England and Wales annually spent about £220 million on information systems. On average, this amounted to about 1.8% of total hospital revenue (Audit Commission 1995).

There was considerable variation around this average, however, with some hospitals spending less than 0.5% of revenues on information technology and others spending more than 4%. NHS Community Trusts spent on average 1.4% of their revenue on information technology (Audit Commission 1997: 18). Comparable data are not available for the purchaser side (including HAs and GPFHs). As was the case for trusts, purchasers employed a variety of systems; and NHS-wide projects to link general practices electronically with HA systems for purposes of patient registration and claims submission and to provide for the electronic transfer of contract-related activity information from providers to HAs were plagued by implementation problems.

Both the level of expenditure on information systems and the quality of the resulting systems were subject to widespread criticism. Criticisms focused upon the fragmentation of systems, the poor quality of the data, and the isolation of financially and clinically oriented systems. Each of these types of problems tended to feed the others, forming a reinforcing cycle of skepticism. Systems developed for particular purposes, such as invoicing, might serve those purposes well but not communicate with each other to inform broader management processes. Attempts to develop integrated systems, however, were vulnerable to the problems—usually data quality problems—of the "weakest link." An Audit Commission survey in 1995 found the widespread perception among clinical staff that errors in coding of clinical data constituted a problem in information management, and a substantial minority made little or no use of the data as a result (Audit Commission 1995). Disillusionment with integrated systems reinforced the tendency for financial managers and clinicians to rely on the separate systems that served their own purposes, and with whose shortcomings they were at least familiar.

The isolation of financial and clinical information systems also accorded with the structures of managerial and professional networks within the NHS—in which judgments of clinical quality remained within the medical preserve of clinical audit largely insulated from the contracting process. Linking considerations of cost and quality within an integrated decision-making system required an integrated information system—but the converse was also the case. An integrated information system cannot be effectively developed and used unless the decision-making system it supports is also integrated.

If the contracting process were to become more sophisticated, it would require such an integration of decision-making and information systems. There was widespread recognition in the 1990s that existing information systems were inadequate to support more sophisticated contracting, which required an integration of cost and clinical data using casemix techniques such as HRG-based costing (previously discussed). The task group on clinical involvement in contracting reported on the basis of a survey of sixteen DHAs and associated providers that the limited degree of sophistication in contracts was attributable in many cases to the fact that "purchaser and provider information systems still remained underdeveloped for contracting purposes" (NHS 1994b: paragraph 5.1). A survey of fifty-six NHS trusts in 1994 found that "less than a quarter said their existing systems dealt adequately with Casemix, but a number of

Trusts accepted that because of the type of services they provided and/or the type of contracts negotiated, this was not yet an issue" (Tilley 1994:10). Three-quarters of the respondents indicated an intention to replace their existing information systems within two years.

There was perhaps less explicit recognition that the reconfiguration of these information systems might themselves constitute a major arena of power struggle (Harrison and Pollitt 1994: 51–54). As Coombs and Cooper (1992: 125) observed fairly early in the process, "The NHS is about to learn a . . . rule of management; arguments about information systems are arguments about the very goals of the organization." Integrating considerations of cost explicitly and systematically into clinical decision-making on a case by case basis raised a potential threat to the "clinical autonomy" of doctors that had been a central feature of NHS mythology. The issues of the degree to which information systems integrated clinical and financial information, and of who "owned" (that is, controlled the use of) the resulting systems, went to the heart of the power relationship between managers and medical professionals.

There were, broadly, three possible types of resolutions of these issues. The first was essentially an evolution of the status quo in which information systems would remain largely the province of financial managers and would be heavily oriented to conventional accounting with little integration of clinical information, which would be treated within separate systems in support of clinical audit. Block contracting would continue to predominate, with casemix costing confined to relatively few procedures. A second possibility was that more sophisticated systems oriented to casemix would be developed essentially under the aegis of clinical directorates, which would come to play a larger role in the contracting process. The third possibility was that the more sophisticated systems would be developed and "owned" by financial managers on both the purchaser and the provider sides.

In the late 1990s it appeared likely that there would be considerable variety across different districts and units in the unfolding of these scenarios. But developments in the first five years of the internal market suggested that on balance the first two outcomes—an evolving status quo of nonintegrated systems in some cases, and a growing role for clinical directorates in controlling the use of integrated systems in others—were likely to predominate. The reasons for this projection will be discussed later in this chapter. First, however, it is necessary to consider two features of the internal market reforms that have been neglected in the discussion so far—the role of the private sector and the role of partisan politics.

## The Role of the Private Sector

Long before the emergence of the internal market, indeed from the inception of the NHS, a private market existed alongside the public system. The private health care sector in Britain was small: private expenditures accounted for roughly 17% of total health expenditures in 1991 (OECD 1993: 252), but this proportion included copayments for publicly provided services such as dentistry. An understanding of the private sector in British health care needs to begin, indeed, with a distinction between *finance* and *provision*. British health care services fell into four categories with respect to the aegis under which they were financed and provided (Laing and Buisson 1995: A94):

1. Publicly provided, publicly financed: This category accounted for the great preponderance of health care services, including virtually all general practice, accident and emergency care, maternity care, and nonelective surgery.

2. Publicly provided, privately financed: Into this category fell services provided in NHS "pay-beds." As part of the founding compromise on which the NHS was established, NHS hospitals could designate certain of their beds as "pay-beds," providing facilities in which consultants could treat patients on a private basis and for which those patients would be charged. About 2% of elective surgery was provided and financed on this basis in 1994 (Laing and Buisson 1995: A94). This category also included publicly provided services for which there were copayments, such as dentistry.[17]

3. Privately provided, publicly financed: This category related primarily to long-term care for the elderly, the mentally ill, and the mentally handicapped, about one-third to one-half of which was provided on this basis. As we shall see, it also included services such as elective surgery contracted for with private providers by NHS purchasers.

4. Privately financed, privately provided: This category included a relatively small proportion of elective surgery (about 17% of cases in 1994[18]) involving a relatively narrow range of procedures, as well as a small but growing proportion of dental services,[19] about one-third of expenditures for long-term residential care for the elderly, one-third of pharmaceutical expenditures, and more than two-thirds of expenditures on ophthalmic devices.

Private finance or provision can be seen, depending upon one's perspective, as either symbiotic with or parasitic on the publicly financed National Health Service. The great preponderance of services related either to long-term care or to certain elective surgical procedures. Virtually no primary or emergency care—and hence no "gatekeeping" or "backup" function complementary to elective surgery—was offered in the private sector. Moreover, most medical services provided in private facilities or privately financed were provided by clinicians whose primary base was in the public sector. Indeed, a clinician without an NHS base was unlikely to attract referrals and was hence unattractive to the owners and managers of private sector facilities.

The institutional reforms begun in 1990, on their face, might appear likely to have enhanced the position of private providers. By distinguishing between the roles of purchasers and providers and allowing for competition among providers for the business of purchasers, the new model in theory allowed for a greater role for private providers in the provision of publicly financed care, and hence an enhanced revenue base for the private sector. In addition, the government's "Waiting List Initiative" launched prior to the reforms—the allocation of substantial funding targeted at reducing waiting times for elective hospital service—promised a boon for the private sector. Long waits in the public sector tended to be for precisely those services that the private sector had moved in to provide—hence purchasing those services from private providers was an obvious way for public purchasers to clear their lists.

If the reforms provided greater incentives for the flowing of public funds to private providers, they also allowed for the converse—the infusion of private finance into NHS providers. As directly managed units of the NHS spun off as self-governing trusts, they were freer among other things to increase their emphasis on "pay-beds." The reforms, then, made for a blurring of the distinction between public and private sectors, and had the potential to allow for a migration of services over time from the first of the four categories just described to the other three.

The 1990s saw a slowing of the rapid expansion of the private sector for elective and acute services, in terms of both finance and provision, that had characterized the 1980s. Double-digit rates of real growth in private spending on acute inpatient and outpatient services in the 1980s dropped to levels of 4% to 7% after 1989—still somewhat above the rate of growth in NHS expenditure, but dramatically slower than in the previous decade (Laing and Buisson 1995: A99). Trends toward the growth of the market share of for-profit hospitals and hospital chains showed a similar pattern. The proportion of private hospitals operated on a for-profit basis increased from 41% in 1979 to 63% in 1995. The increase in the proportion of private beds operated on a for-profit basis increased even more dramatically over the same period, from 28.5% to 63.4%. Much of this change, however, occurred through the 1980s, and the trend slowed in the 1990s. Among not-for-profit hospitals, the proportion of institutions owned by multi-institutional groups rose from 37.5% in 1979 to 56.0% in 1995. The proportion of beds owned by multi-institutional groups rose from 24.0% to 41.7% in that period. Among for-profit hospitals, the share of institutions owned by multi-institutional groups rose much more dramatically, from 11.3% in 1979 to 79.0% in 1995; the proportion of beds so owned rose from 27.5% to 83.9%. Again, however, much of the change in the for-profit sector occurred in the 1980s (Independent Healthcare Association 1989: 5, 1995: 18).

It is difficult to judge the extent to which the internal market reforms affected these developments and to distinguish these effects from those of other major factors, particularly the economic recession of the early 1990s. But it is at least plausible that the major beneficiaries from the reforms in this regard may have been the NHS trusts, through the expansion of their pay-beds. Elective and acute care provided in private hospitals increased 37% in value terms between 1990 and 1994, while services provided on a private basis in NHS hospitals increased 90% (calculated from Monopolies and Mergers Commission 1994: 9; Laing and Buisson 1995: A93),[20] reversing the trends of the 1980s. The NHS share of the private elective and acute care market grew from 11.3% to 15.1% in the same four-year period (Laing and Buisson 1995: A112) and continued to increase thereafter.

At the same time, NHS purchases from private providers remained a small proportion of the total. Only a little more than 10% of the Waiting List Initiative funding was directed to private hospitals (Laing and Buisson 1995: A108). Later, it was estimated that NHS purchases amounted to about 3% of the total value of acute care services provided by private hospitals and clinics in 1992—a proportion that rose to 3.4% in 1993 and 3.7% in 1994. As the author of these estimates noted, "Though NHS purchasing may be growing at a significant rate from a small base . . . this has not yet become a major source of revenue for the independent sector as a whole" (Laing and Buisson 1995: A96, A102).

Indeed, private hospitals argued that the 1990 reforms left them at a disadvantage, subject to "unfair competition" from NHS trusts for the business of both private and public purchasers. The claim was that trusts undercut the prices of private hospitals by cross-subsidizing the services on which they competed with private providers from publicly funded services (e.g., Butler 1994), and also that they relied upon the political compulsion felt by NHS purchasers to support their local trusts. Alternatively, it may have been the mechanisms of cost control in the NHS that allowed them to charge lower prices. Pending the development of more sophisticated costing procedures in NHS trusts, it was not possible to know which of these explanations applied. To the extent that NHS trusts were to move to HRG-based costing, however, the competition with the private sector for some services was likely to sharpen.

Trusts were not competing on price alone, moreover. They were also improving the quality of their amenities, particularly for private patients. In the past, whether or not a given bed was considered a "pay-bed" depended on whether it was occupied by a private patient. Increasingly, however, trusts designated particular units as pay-bed units and equipped them accordingly. From 1992 to 1994, while the number of pay-beds did not increase, the number of designated private patient units in NHS hospitals approximately trebled (Monopolies and Mergers Commission 1994: 15). In 1995 there were seventy-four dedicated private units in NHS hospitals, representing 1,376 of the approximately 3,000 NHS pay-beds (Laing and Buisson 1995: A113–14). NHS pay-beds, moreover, had a significant competitive advantage over private hospitals; because they were located in full-service NHS hospitals, they could provide the backup services that were not available in the niche-oriented private facilities.

On the financing side, private insurance (which in the early 1990s financed about 85% of the value of private acute care received by British residents [Laing and Buisson 1995: A101]) showed the same pattern of dramatic increase in the 1980s, followed by a plateauing in the 1990s, as occurred in the case of private hospitals. The proportion of the U.K. population with private insurance coverage rose from 6.4% in 1980 to 11.6% in 1990, but thereafter began a slow decline (Monopolies and Mergers Commission 1994: 16). The number of subscribers increased at annual rates of about 7% or 8% in the last half of the 1980s but decreased slightly in 1991 and grew at annual rates of just over or under 1% between 1992 and 1994. Losses and gains in the employer-based market (which accounted for about 60% of all private insurance subscribers) and the individual market tended to counterbalance each other in the 1990s.

Commercial insurers increased their market share (measured in terms of numbers of subscribers) from about 11% in 1984 to 25% in 1992, at which point it began to plateau (calculated from Laing and Buisson 1995: A153). The provident associations (insurance companies), particularly the two largest associations British United Provident Association (BUPA) and Private Patients Plan (PPP) continued to dominate the market but had to respond to the competitive challenge of the commercial insurers.

Again, the reasons for the slowing of the growth of private insurance in the 1990s are complex, and it is impossible to isolate the effects of the internal market reforms and related changes. The reduction of waiting times for NHS services may have had some effect, because opinion surveys seem to suggest that the avoidance of waiting times was by far the predominant reason for seeking private treatment (Monopolies and Mergers Commission 1994: 18–19) and a significant factor determining the purchase of private insurance by individuals (Besley et al. 1996). The substantial increase in premiums by private insurers in 1992 in response to rising ratios of claims to premium income in the 1980s, which peaked in 1991, also appears to have dampened demand (Monopolies and Mergers Commission 1994: 17). While it may have been fed to some extent by an anticipation of increased claims as a result of the internal market reforms, the motivation for this increase was essentially a response to developments in the 1980s.

One area in which an increase in the role of private finance, and a further blurring of public–private sector boundaries, appeared likely for a time was that of joint ventures and other arrangements between NHS providers and private financial interests. State control of capital investment in NHS facilities was eased somewhat under the terms of the Private Finance Initiative (PFI)—a governmentwide initiative led by the Treasury in 1992. As it applied to the NHS, the PFI raised the threshold above which approval for capital projects had to be sought from £250,000 to £10 million, although projects below the £10 million threshold would be sampled and referred for approval. It also loosened the requirement that private capital be used only where it could be shown that the funds could not be provided at more economical rates by the Treasury. In 1994, the NHS required that every business case for capital investment demonstrate that the possibility of private finance had been tested. The resulting project proposals were initially for nonclinical projects such as waste incineration or office accommodation, although there were a few examples of private sector participation in the financing of joint ventures for the provision of clinical support services such as pathology laboratories and imaging services (Laing and Buisson 1995: A110). No major PFI project had been commenced by 1997, however, leading to widespread criticisms of "PFI gridlock" in the negotiations among trusts, private financial interests, and the central government. (Shortly after taking office in May 1997 the Labour government announced that it would "unlock PFI gridlock" by passing legislation to allow fourteen projects to proceed, canceling negotiations on twenty-three others, and dropping the requirement that all capital projects test private financial markets before proceeding) (Warden 1997a).

On balance, there was no significant change in the public–private balance in health care as a result of the internal market reforms. Indeed, by reaffirming the tax-based financing of the NHS and focusing instead on an *internal* market, the reforms put to rest the possibility of a major change in the financing of health care that had been considered in the first Thatcher government. The impact of the reforms, if anything, appears to have been to stabilize the private sector, which in the 1980s had seemed to be entering a phase of significant growth and reconfiguration.

Some observers suggested that private insurers and providers could have an impact disproportionate to their share of health care financing and delivery, to the extent that they lead the introduction of "managed care" techniques into the system. Given the apparent price sensitivity of demand, insurers increasingly turned to mechanisms of cost control to hold down premium increases. BUPA, which owned twenty-nine hospitals with about 1,700 beds in 1995 (Independent Healthcare Association 1995: 6), had by that time developed clinical guidelines on the nineteen procedures that accounted for the bulk of its expenditure. BUPA was careful to ensure medical "ownership" of these guidelines, having them developed by local groups of clinicians and in some cases adopting guidelines developed by the Royal Colleges. The intent was to use the guidelines not only in BUPA hospitals, but in preauthorizing care delivered by other providers as well as in contracting with "preferred providers" to establish service networks (Laing and Buisson 1995: A160; Fairfield and Williams 1996). With its large database of clinical and cost information, BUPA was well positioned to undertake this activity. Even so, it began to develop some guidelines in cooperation with other hospital chains, in order to ensure a sufficient geographical spread in the database.

Some saw this activity as constituting a "springboard for the introduction of the American concept of managed care" to the British system (Fairfield and Williams 1996: 1554), demonstrating its effect within the relatively narrow confines of the private sector. Two factors, however, worked against the likelihood that managed care in the private sector would have a widespread demonstration effect. The first was the niche orientation of the private sector itself, which facilitated the introduction of clinical guidelines but also limited the scope of activity for which guidelines are developed. Most crucially, the fact that the scope of the private sector did not include primary care meant that the forms of managed care that could be developed were severely truncated, excluding the key "gatekeeper" function of the primary care physician.

Second, and perhaps even more important, was the role and status of consultants in the public and private sectors. In a 1994 inquiry, the Monopolies and Mergers Commission concluded that consultants offering private medical services constituted a "complex monopoly" in determining the level of their fees,[21] and the commission argued that "in this situation the countervailing power of the insurers is of crucial importance" (Monopolies and Mergers Commission 1994: 4). With the increasing competitiveness of the insurance market, beginning in the 1980s, the commission speculated that private insurers were likely to be more "robust" in using their countervailing power than they had been in the past. Even so, by recommending that insurers continue to be allowed to publish fee "maxima" for given procedures even while recommending the elimination of the BMA guidelines for consultants' fees, the commission implicitly recognized that no single insurer, even the largest (BUPA), had sufficient market power to hold down consultants' remuneration arbitrarily (Laing and Buisson 1995: A120).

The same might be said for other terms and conditions of consultants' employment in the private sector. Consultants had their primary base in the public sector[22]: it was their font of professional legitimacy and the mechanism through which they became known to the GPs who were their sources of referrals. The value of consultants to private hospitals (and, for that matter, NHS pay-beds)—their ability to attract referrals—indeed depended upon building their NHS base. Hence consultants were in a strong position in negotiating contracts with private providers. They brought what the private sector could not provide—professional legitimacy and referral networks. Private hospitals hence competed for specialists as much as they did for patients. Whether or not they owned private hospitals, as in BUPA's case, private insurers had to tread carefully in dealing with the consultants who brought them their customer base.

"Managed care" in the private sector, then, appeared likely to remain confined to guidelines for a relatively small number of procedures, developed by groups of clinicians. It was quite possible that these guidelines would be picked up within the NHS as well—indeed there were some suggestions of cooperation between private insurers and the NHS in producing and disseminating guidelines (Fairfield and Williams 1996). A leading role for the private sector in managed care more generally would, however, require a transformation of the private sector itself—a transformation which was, if anything, less likely after the introduction of the internal market reforms than it was before.

## The Role of Partisan and Electoral Politics

A defining feature of the "internal market" was, of course, that it was *internal* to the public, tax-financed system. The state remained the source of finance. And that meant that a range of state actors, political as well as bureaucratic, with different roles and objectives, had a stake in the decision-making system. However much the institution of the internal market reforms might have been intended to provide an impartial buffer between political actors and decisions about rationing and restructuring of health care services, it remained the case that the ultimate accountability for the performance of the NHS rested with the secretary of state for health. "Market"-driven decisions (or more accurately decisions made in the context of local bargaining between purchasers and providers) that were politically sensitive were therefore likely to trigger political intervention. The nonexecutive members of RHAs and DHAs, particularly the regional chairpersons, provided the primary channel for ongoing political input into the decision-making system.

As part of the internal market reforms, the boards of RHAs and DHAs were reconstituted along lines more in keeping with the business-oriented ideology of the governing Conservative party. At both regional and district levels, boards were to be composed of roughly equal numbers of "executive" members (drawn from the senior management of the relevant authority) and "nonexecutive" members. Nonexecutive members of the RHA boards, including the chairpersons, were appointed by the secretary of state; nonexecutive members of the DHA boards were appointed by the responsible RHA. Prior to the internal market reforms the appointed members of the boards had been chosen to provide local input; in the post-1991 period the emphasis was on business skills and acumen (Levitt et al. 1995: 68). The other major change was the repudiation of the NHS's traditional corporatism, with the abolition of formal seats on the boards for consultants, GPs, nurses, and health care unions.

Within these structures both before and after the internal market changes, the role of board chairpersons, especially regional chairpersons, was particularly important. Those appointed to the post of regional chairperson were typically in good standing with the governing party, but also had substantial independent power bases. The role of the chairperson varied according to the personality and the power base of the incumbent. To a considerable extent, however, the regional boards, particularly the chairperson, functioned as a buffer between the central NHS and Department of Health bureaucracies and the regional and district authorities. The independent power base of the chairperson provided a degree of independence for the authorities from the central bureaucracy. But this buffering came at a cost; it opened the authorities to the political influences that bore upon the chairpersons either from their own power bases or from the governing party. Particularly in matters such as capital allocations, such influences could skew decisions in directions quite different from those preferred by local managers.

In the "internal market" era, some regional chairpersons became important vehicles for channeling the business orientation of the governing party into the NHS structures. But in general the independence of the chairpersons also constituted a real or potential threat to the ability of the center to regulate the evolving market. Following a "Functions and Manpower Review" in 1993, the decision was made to "streamline" the NHS structure by reducing the number of regions from fourteen to eight, abolishing the RHAs and replacing them with regional offices of the NHS Executive, and merging DHAs and FHSAs to become HAs, as previously discussed. In recognition of political realities, the incumbent regional chairpersons remained as advisors to the new regional directors and as members of the central NHS Policy Board. But these were effectively seen as vestigial positions that would atrophy as the terms of the incumbents ended.

The demise of the regional chairpersons and boards, however, did not mark the end of political intervention into NHS decision-making. Partisan and electoral considerations could bring about the direct intervention of the health secretary, or indeed the prime minister. The most notable case in this regard was the restructuring of London hospitals. Klein has succinctly summarized the significance of the London case:

If the logic of the internal market could be expected to work anywhere, it was in inner London. Here there was a plethora of providers and long standing evidence of considerable over-capacity in the provision of acute care. Yet over the decades successive governments had shirked the challenge of getting rid of beds and institutions: Ministers of all parties had regarded the task of taking on the prestigious teaching hospitals in central London as an invitation to political suicide. But market competition promised to do what Ministers had failed to do: by taking away custom from the inner city hospitals, it threatened their viability. If the logic of the market had been allowed to work its way through, therefore, the problem of over-supply would have been solved as hospitals went bankrupt. But, in the event, the Government intervened. Far from being left to the market, the re-structuring of London's health service was to become one of the most ambitious planning exercises in the history of the NHS. (Klein 1995: 207)

Given the persistence of hospital overcapacity in the U.S. market, Klein may have overstated the likely effect of market reforms left to run their course in London. But he is surely correct to point out the swift recourse to planning as soon as the working of the internal market *threatened* to squeeze capacity out of the system. The problem essentially lay in the fact than London had historically been "overbedded"—or at least oversupplied with acute care and particularly tertiary care beds—relative to its population, largely due to the presence of prestigious teaching hospitals with centuries-old histories. Prior to the internal market reforms, these hospitals served substantial numbers of patients referred to them from outside London, and were remunerated for doing so through a funding formula that recognized cross-boundary flows of patients from one DHA to another. When DHAs became purchasing authorities in the internal market, however, they were funded on the basis of their own populations, to purchase care from whichever provider they chose. In these circumstances, enough purchasers chose to purchase care from local providers, rather than from the generally higher-cost London hospitals, to begin to threaten the financial viability of the latter.

Faced with this threat, the government was swift to intervene. In part the intervention was motivated by the recognition that what was required was not simply a reduction in capacity but a reconfiguration of London's health care services, and that the state controlled one of the major instruments of restructuring—namely, access to capital (James 1995: 192). But it was also the case that the potential winners and losers in any restructuring mounted furious appeals through political channels that elected politicians could not ignore. Hence the resulting restructuring exercise was one that involved both careful and essentially disinterested analysis, as well as blunt partisan and electoral considerations.

The analysis came from a series of reports, the first from a highly regarded independent institute and the rest from governmentally appointed bodies. In 1992, the King's Fund published a set of reports analyzing problems of hospital overcapacity in London and proposing strategic directions for the future. Also in 1992, the government appointed a commission of inquiry headed by Sir Bernard Tomlinson, a retired professor of pathology and former regional chairman from northern England, with broad terms of reference to advise on the restructuring of inner London's health care services in the context of the internal market. Both the King's Fund and the Tomlinson inquiry came to similar conclusions and made similar recommendations, directed at a reduction of acute care beds in London by closing entire hospital sites, and improving nonacute services (particularly primary care). In response the government established the London Implementation Group (LIG) to develop and oversee the implementation of the proposals. The LIG oversaw six reviews of specialist tertiary services, which agreed on a set of principles for the consolidation of tertiary services based on clinical, epidemiological, and educational and research criteria (roughly similar to those that would guide similar exercises in Canada a few years later). Attempts to translate these principles into specific decisions about the closure, merger, and reconfiguration of particular hospitals, however, mobilized both potential winners and potential losers in response.

In implementing and attempting to implement specific changes, the governing Conservatives faced pressure not only from opposition (especially Labour) members of Parliament but also from their own backbench MPs in marginal constituencies. When the secretary of state for health brought a package of reforms for the restructuring of health services in greater London to Parliament for approval in the spring of 1995, a backbench revolt (capitalized upon by a searing Labour attack) threatened the package. The package eventually passed by a twelve-vote margin, with five Conservative members of Parliament from affected areas failing to support the government. The bitter episode contributed to the removal of Virginia Bottomley as secretary. And opposition to the package did not end there. As the Conservative majority in the Commons dwindled to a one-seat margin, two backbenchers essentially held the government to ransom, threatening to boycott all votes unless the government relented on its decision to consolidate accident and emergency (A-and-E) services in a north London suburban area by closing the A-and-E department of Edgeware hospital and transferring them to another. This threat escalated the decision about Edgeware to the highest levels, including the prime minister himself; and for a time it appeared that the government would capitulate. When the decision to close the Edgeware A-and-E department was nonetheless announced in December 1996, one of the dissident backbenchers carried through on his threat, effectively depriving the government of its assured majority and ensuring that it would be formally tipped into minority status with the loss of the next by-election, which occurred a week later.

That the standing of a national government should rest on the survival of an emergency department in a suburban London hospital is perhaps the starkest, but not the only, illustration of the continuing political salience of health care in the era of the internal market. The internal market was, after all, a creation of public policy—a policy for which the Conservatives were held accountable and against which opposition parties had to define their own positions. In Britain's adversarial parliamentary system, the Labour opposition severely criticized the development and implementation of the internal market reforms at every stage. In particular, it criticized the fundholding model as creating a two-tiered system. But it progressively softened its position in developing Labour alternatives;

these alternatives were most definitively laid out in its policy paper released in July 1995, which was modest and pragmatic in its ambitions for change (Labour Party 1996).[23]

Upon achieving its landslide victory in May 1997, the new Labour government faced a building crescendo of concern within the medical and popular media, reminiscent of a decade earlier, regarding the "underfunding" of the NHS—despite annual real increases of about 3% in the 1990s under the Conservatives (Warden 1997a). In response, it announced a "zero-base" review of NHS funding, within the context of a comprehensive review of all government spending announced by the Treasury (Warden 1997b). In its first budget, released in July 1997, the government announced an increase of £1.2 billion to the NHS budget for 1998–1999 (about a 5% nominal increase, or 2.25% in real terms), double that projected by the Conservatives.

In December 1997 the Labour government issued its own White Paper on the NHS, which began by stating the government's commitment to "increase spending on the NHS in real terms each year" (Department of Health 1997: paragraph 1:22). Beyond that, it proposed to move ahead with a number of marginal changes along the lines proposed in its 1995 policy paper. It continued the rhetoric of "abolishing" the internal market—but in effect that meant the abolition of the phrase and a continuation of the shift to language more connotative of cooperation than competition. It characterized the proposed changes, indeed, as "going with the grain" of the existing system.

In the face of fierce defensiveness of GP fundholders and much counsel of caution from the BMA itself, the paper stated that "the argument between fundholding and nonfundholding is yesterday's debate," and that "the time has come to move on, taking the best of both approaches" (Department of Health 1997: paragraph 5.6). The centerpiece of the proposals was the development of Primary Care Groups (PCGs)—groups of general practices that would "grow out of the range of commissioning models that have been developed in recent years but will give sharper focus to their work" (Department of Health 1997: paragraph 5.8). In effect, these groups would represent an evolutionary resolution of the "purchaser plurality" previously described here. They would function as consortia of general practices, granted authority and budgets by the HAs to enter into long-term "service agreements" with providers of hospital and community care, which would retain the trust status. On their part, trusts would continue to hold their own assets (contrary to earlier Labour proposals) as well as their authority as employers and their ability to retain and reinvest surpluses. They were, moreover, to be charged with a "duty of partnership," including the charge to participate with PCGs in developing a strategic plan for their localities under the leadership of their HA. The HAs themselves were ultimately to become planning and oversight bodies, allocating budgets and delegating commissioning authority to PCGs. Although various "milestones" for the implementation of the proposals were set out, it was implied throughout that the pace of change would be governed by ongoing experience.

Labour's proposals, then, promised to consolidate and stabilize the internal market reforms, as they had been shaped by the logic of established relationships. The White Paper also picked up a theme that had characterized the internal market reforms and accorded it even greater importance. This was the emphasis on accountability for the quality of clinical outcomes, as measured by specified performance indicators. The internal market reforms had relied, in theory, on the contracting process, informed by certain specified performance measures, to hold providers accountable for the quality of care they provided and to generate incentives for quality improvement. In practice, however,

> [c]ontracting proved a blunt instrument. Latterly the NHSE [National Health Service Executive] has adopted a more facilitative approach encouraging the development of local effectiveness strategies and acknowledging the professional development implied. However, accountability for clinical effectiveness has hovered between purchaser and provider—never properly defined. (Gillam 1998: 67)

The Labour proposals instead relied on "clinical governance" to achieve accountability for clinical effectiveness. This rich if ambiguous phrase had a number of potentially contradictory implications. It meant that trusts were required to establish structures of clinical governance, and chief executives were to be held accountable for clinical as well as financial matters. PCGs as well were to be accountable for the quality of service they commission and provide, and to establish processes of clinical governance. "Evidence-based" clinical guidelines would be produced by a National Institute of Clinical Excellence; and the performance of trusts would be monitored by a Commission for Health Improvement. The membership of each of these bodies was to be drawn from the health professions, the NHS, academics, and patient representatives. On their face, these proposals could be seen as "the latest of many attempts in the NHS to exercise greater managerial control over clinical activities" (Gillam 1998: 66). But the proposals also emphasized that structures of clinical governance were to accord a central role to clinical decision-makers—doctors, and also nurses and other professionals. The White Paper stressed the importance of self-regulation at all levels of the system.

The Labour proposals did on paper what earlier reforms had failed to do in practice: they integrated responsibility for clinical and financial decision-making. If the experience of the 1990s is any guide, however, these proposals will be greatly shaped and molded in the process of implementation. If the medical profession responds strategically as it has in the past (with the rule-proving exception of the action of the Royal College presidents that precipitated the 1989 NHS Review), it will maintain de facto control over the structures of clinical governance as they evolve, while dampening the government's zeal for reform by accommodating to its fiscal parameters. In this context, the greatest challenge to the profession is likely to be in the area of general practice, where collegial mechanisms are least well developed. Participants in fundholding groups, although they came to constitute a majority of general practitioners, were, after all, self-selected. Reluctant participants in the compulsory PCG scheme could prove to be less amenable to collegial control.

The Labour government did make one significant departure from Conservative policy, in reviving the issue of the linkage between socioeconomic inequality and health status—a concern that had led the previous Labour government in the late 1970s to commission a report by a former president of the Royal College of Physicians, Sir Douglas Black. The Black report, delivered to the Conservative government in 1980, clearly demonstrated that health status on a variety of measures declined steadily by declining socioeconomic quintile, and that this gradient had persisted and in some cases increased even as access to health care was being extended under the NHS (Black 1980). The Black report accordingly reached well beyond the NHS and the health care arena to recommend policy changes affecting a broad range of "social determinants of health," joining and informing an international stream of thought that was also influential in Canada, at least at the level of ideas, as we shall see in the next chapter. The recommendations accorded ill with the agenda of the governing Conservatives: the report was released by the secretary of state for social services with a foreword disclaiming any intention of proceeding with the recommendations, and it was ignored for the remainder of the Conservatives' period in office. As one of its first acts upon gaining power in 1997, the Labour government appointed a minister for public health, who among other initiatives commissioned a review of health inequalities to identify priority areas for policy action—areas that were likely to have relatively little to do with the NHS or the "internal market."

## Institutional and Structural Change in the Internal Market

We are now ready to summarize the institutional and structural impact of the internal market reforms on the British system, and the logic that mediated that impact. On the institutional dimension, the reforms introduced a market element into a system of hierarchical corporatism, by creating "purchaser" and "provider" roles and requiring purchasers and providers to bargain with each other in drawing up contracts for services. The introduction of this mechanism changed the formal mode whereby participants in the system related to each other and to some extent the sanctions that they could bring to bear in seeking to achieve their objectives. But the informal networks and modes of relationship that characterized the system prior to the reforms continued to exist within the form of the market. The prevalence of block contracts, the limited degree of competition, the preservation of the clinical arena as a zone of collegial decision-making, and the continued regulation of managerial behavior through central directives and "guidances" all represent the survival of an institutional mix in which hierarchy and collegiality had a heavy weight.

The balance of centralization and decentralization *within* the NHS hierarchy did shift over the course of the reforms. Arguably, district managers lost some discretionary authority both upward and downward—upward to the center, as the RHA "buffers" were abolished and replaced by regional offices of the NHS, and downward (or outward) to the "self-governing" trusts now accountable to the state through a separate bureaucratic line. The center continued to control the behavior of purchasers and providers through an essentially hierarchical mechanism. The hierarchical relationship between health authorities and provider units were tempered by market elements—HAs now had to seek to control providers through contracting rather than through the giving of administrative directives. But since competition among purchasers (including GP fundholders) was virtually nonexistent and competition among providers was limited, the effect of the internal market was not to transform authority relationships into relationships of voluntary exchange. Rather, its effect across the vast bulk of medical and hospital services was to make more explicit the bargaining relationships among local sets of actors who had little option but to deal with each other.

In this process, clinical decision-making continued to be carried out within collegial networks. Again, however, collegial networks were altered by market mechanisms in at least one important respect. The emergence of GP fundholding introduced explicit contracting and a "cash nexus" between consultants and GP fundholders, who, with their smaller scale and more limited range of contracting, were in practice freer to switch providers than were HAs. GP fundholding, initially conceived as a minor dimension of the internal market reforms, may in fact prove to be the reforms' most significant institutional legacy. When the Labour government proposed effectively to continue a version of fundholding on a comprehensive scale and under another name (Primary Care Groups), it appeared even more likely that the resulting relationships would continue to look more like collegial networks (albeit marked by more explicit bargaining than in the past) than like market competition.

As for the structural balance of the system, arguably little change occurred in the broad balance among state actors, the medical profession, and private finance, although significant changes have occurred within some of these categories. Despite fears raised by opponents of the reforms on the left, the reforms did not lead to significant gains for the private sector in terms either of finance or of provision. Indeed the rate of expansion and structural change in the private sector, which had accelerated in the 1980s, slowed in the era of the internal market.

Similarly, the overall balance between state actors and the medical profession was relatively unchanged. The profession protected clinical decision-making as a medical preserve, with the incursion of state managers in only a marginal range of cases. Managers, for their part, consolidated their authority over the budgetary process and financial management. Each group improved its collective capacity for control through the use of information technology, but the respective information systems supporting clinical audit and financial management remained largely separate. The linkage of financial and clinical data in HRG-type costing and planning remained limited, but such linkage promised to be an important terrain upon which the medical–managerial balance of influence would be contested. Some "alignment of incentives" between managers and clinicians appeared possible—particularly in the case of clinical directorates, in which doctors took responsibility for resource management within their particular clinical areas. But as the roles of doctors and state managers evolved under the internal market, the balance between them did not shift dramatically in one direction or the other.

Second, the observation of continuity in the overall balance of influence between the medical profession and state actors should not obscure shifts in the balance of influence *within* these categories. Most notable in the case of the medical profession was, of course, the increased influence of GPs, particularly GP fundholders, as a direct result of the reforms. This observation raises an important proposition. In arenas such as health care, in which the quality of service rendered depends on the expertise of professional practitioners, the capacity of state actors to enhance their power at the expense of the profession is limited by their reliance upon the profession in order to mount public programs. They can, however, choose to ally with different segments of the profession by using different policy instruments. Hence while the overall state–profession balance may not change, the relative position of different groups within the profession may change as a result of public policy. GP fundholders, who became key allies of the Conservative government in the implementation of the reforms, provide a case in point.

Within the category of state actors, moreover, we also observe shifts in position. Managers in provider units arguably gained increased discretion while managers in purchasing authorities lost some authority, as a result of the purchaser–provider split and the shifts in the balance of centralization and decentralization within the NHS bureaucracy. The considerable power of politicians within the system appeared to have changed little, despite the rhetoric of market and business judgment that accompanied the reforms. The establishment of the internal market was above all an act (or series of acts) of public policy, for which politicians were accountable, and in whose consequences they were continually driven to intervene.

These observations provide the basis for predicting an incremental pace of change under the set of proposals that succeeded the internal market—the Labour government's 1997 White Paper. By maintaining the purchaser–provider split, Labour continued the essential market-type institutional innovation of its Conservative predecessors, although Labour's emphasis on "clinical governance" may reinforce the resilient structures of hierarchical corporatism that absorbed that innovation. As for structural balance, the emphasis on accountability for clinical outcomes could be seen as a tipping of the balance of influence toward state actors at the expense of the medical profession. As Klein has noted, however, this balance will continue to be governed by the implicit concordat that has governed state-profession relations throughout the life of the NHS, as long as the profession is able to meet the challenge of more rigorous self-regulation (Klein 1998: 124). This brings us full circle to an understanding of the agency relationships that underlie the logic of the British system.

## The Logic of the Internal Market From Trust to Contract—and Back?

What explains the absorption of market elements into existing hierarchical and collegial networks and the relative lack of change in the overall balance of state, professional, and private financial actors in Britain, when market mechanisms in the United States generated sweeping institutional and structural change? To answer this question we need to return to the logic of agency and its particular manifestation in the British system.

The rationale underlying the internal market reforms was to attempt no less than a reconstitution of the agency relationships between state and professional bodies that characterized the NHS. Traditionally, these relationships implicitly charged doctors with considering resource constraints as well as quality and appropriateness of care in making clinical decisions, and they were enforced through the intersection of collegial networks and hierarchical structures. Agency relationships existed at the various tiers of the system: from the relationship between the department of health and the bodies of organized medicine at the center to the relationships between Family Practice Committees and local GPs and between hospital medical staffs and hospital management. Again traditionally, these agency relationships accorded individual physicians very broad discretion. Over time, however—more slowly in Britain than in a number of other nations, but inevitably as the pressures of managing the health care system increased—professional groups, especially at the local level, assumed increased collective authority over their members.

These hierarchical structures and collegial networks created continua of responsibility, along which the locus of accountability for the overall pattern of care could become blurred. The effect of splitting the purchasing and providing functions and hence creating a "market" was to make the responsibility and accountability of the various actors more clear-cut, by requiring them to bargain explicitly with each other and to monitor compliance with the specific contracts struck through this process.

Such was the theory. In practice, the older patterns of relationship, including agency roles, proved quite resilient. In part, this reflects the phased process of implementation of the reforms. As one observer of the process has put it, the difference between the process of developing the White Paper *Working for Patients* and the process of implementing it was the difference between a *blitzkrieg* and an occupation (Shock 1994). The need to secure compliance led to a phased implementation strategy whose effects varied greatly across areas and units, and which continued to unfold throughout the 1990s.

The resilience of the pre-1990 conception of the agency relationship between the profession and the state was suggested by the persistence of block (albeit "sophisticated" block) contracts and the confining of performance monitoring by purchasers to a relatively few process-oriented measures. In most areas of practice, hospital doctors continued to exercise broad discretion as the agents of their patients on an individual level, and of purchaser and provider managements on a collective level, within bluntly defined resource limits.[24] And in the case of GPs, and particularly GP fundholders, their agency roles on behalf of both patients and state payers were enhanced by making more explicit their responsibility for both budgetary and the "quality and appropriateness of care" dimensions. There were clearly tensions between the role of agent for the individual patient and agent for the payer. But the key point is that to the extent that doctors performed both roles these tensions were resolved within a medical milieu, and not in contests between managers and doctors.

The resilience of traditional patterns of relationships among the actors in the British health care arena derived from the centrality of trust-based relationships in the functioning of the system. Rudolf Klein has highlighted the importance of these relationships, while noting the challenge presented by the internal market reforms. He has summarized the intent of the internal market reforms as shifting the basis of relationships among actors in the system from one of "status" or "trust" to one of "contract" (Day and Klein 1991: 52; Klein 1993). The key feature of this shift was to increase the accountability of the providers of care for their decisions:

> [T]here is a new emphasis on holding clinicians and others accountable for their performance. A system hitherto based on trust—on the view that consultants and others, by the very nature of their professional status, can be trusted to manage the resources put at their disposal—is turning into a system where justification is required. . . . The NHS has always relied on trust; hence, of course, the inadequacy of so much information in the past. If clinicians and other health professionals can be trusted to do the best for their patients, why bother to collect information about their activities? . . . The hope must be that the new-style NHS can . . . move towards more accountability, a highly desirable aim, without introducing the kind of surveillance calculated to undermine the sense of professional dedication which has served it so well in the past. For no machinery of health care delivery can run successfully, however elegantly designed it may be, if the oil of trust is lacking. (Klein 1993: 74, 77)

The collegial networks among professionals and the agency relationships between doctors and managers that developed within the NHS are the most obvious form of trust-based relationship in the system. But the stability provided by hierarchical forms, even in the midst of periodic reorganizations, also allowed for the development of trust networks among managers over time. Theorists of the economics of institutions have generally seen hierarchy as a framework of incentives alternative to trust networks as a means of social control. But as sociologists such as Granovetter (1992) have observed, understanding the development of trust relationships within institutions must be a central concern of institutional analysis. In the case of the NHS, the persistence of hierarchical control within a highly regulated market was evidenced by the various "guidances" regarding contracting that continued to be promulgated centrally and communicated down the hierarchy, but the implementation of these guidances allowed for a range of tolerance that was well understood within established administrative networks.

The internal market, in short, remained in Ferlie's terms both "socially" and "institutionally" embedded. The market was institutionally embedded in a hierarchical regulatory system. And it was socially embedded in networks of relationships—case study evidence suggested that "there is a small health care elite (containing clinical, managerial and quasi-political components) which displays considerable stability at the apex of these [purchaser and provider] organisations. Long-term careers emerge and continue despite reorganization" (Ferlie 1994: 221).

The degree of continuity within the British health care arena, while striking in cross-national perspective, should not be exaggerated. Contracts gradually became more specific; the now-separate purchasing authorities and trusts began to proceed along different lines of evolution, with "very little staff movement between the two," processes that could lead to both groups gradually developing their own "cultures and value systems" (Ferlie 1994: 221). As these processes unfolded, a recurrent concern expressed by participants in the system was that the social capital built up in the form of trust relationships over time—the "oil of trust"—would be depleted as the adversarial logic of the market became more pervasive (Le Grand 1997). In this regard the Labour proposals announced in December 1997 promised to have a stabilizing effect.

This persistence of prereform collegial and hierarchical networks may not simply have been a function of habitual ties; it may also have been rational under the circumstances. In the context of budgetary uncertainty and deep reservations about the adequacy of data, modes of relationship that avoided the need for costly information- and technology-intensive mechanisms of control were compellingly attractive. As Robinson and Le Grand note, "the transactions costs-approach seems to suggest that the pre-reform hierarchical structure within a unitary health authority may have been the more efficient organizational structure after all" (Robinson and Le Grand 1995: 37).

As in the case of other aspects of the system, then, the *timing* of the establishment of agency relationships in the British system was essential in determining their nature and their durability. They developed from the beginning of the NHS, in a context in which the capability of information systems to generate aggregate representations of clinical activity was rudimentary in the extreme. By the time such technology became at least potentially available, attempts to redefine agency relationships in the new context had to swim against the tide of established relationships. Those relationships, with compelling advantages in terms of the ease and expense of interaction, proved resilient, and doctors both individually and collectively continued to play central roles as agents with broad discretion within the system.

In conclusion, it is worth noting that the most telling recognition of the extent to which the internal market reforms had been incorporated within the evolving logic of the British health care arena may have been the Labour government's decision to "go with the grain" in introducing its own set of policy proposals in 1997. The remarkable degree to which Labour moved from apocalyptic denunciation of the internal market reforms at the outset to acceptance of the basic features of the resulting model when it assumed power was not only a measure of ideological change in the Labour party with the rise of "New Labour." It was also a mark of the extent to which the internal market had become entrenched, as key participants in the system accommodated to and shaped the reforms in the process of their implementation.

# The Logic of the Single-Payer System

In Canada, more than perhaps in any other nation in the late twentieth century, the health care system functioned according to the logic of an accommodation between the medical profession and the state.[1] It was, in economic terms, the logic of an agency relationship in a bilateral monopoly. Under the terms of Canadian medicare, provincial governments were the "single payers" for most medical and hospital services; a single government plan in each province covered a comprehensive range of medical and hospital services; and no private insurance alternatives for coverage of those services existed.[2] Provincial governments, that is, were essentially monopsonists in the medical and hospital services sector. But they exercised their monopsony power in very gross terms. Decisions about the allocation of resources were made through negotiations with the monopoly providers of services, most particularly with the medical profession. And those negotiating relationships left great discretion in the hands of the organized profession to govern the behavior of its members.

As in Britain, the state developed a "second-level" agency relationship with the profession, which acknowledged the primacy of professional judgment in making decisions about the allocation of resources at the level of the clinical case, the professional practice, and the institution. In Canada, however, the profession enjoyed even more formal autonomy in this relationship: the state was a monopsonist, but not an employer or even a contractor. Through the 1970s and 1980s, the playing out of the logic of the single-payer system gave the Canadian system extraordinary structural and institutional stability. In the 1990s, the state sought both to reduce sharply the rates of increase in public spending and to substantially extend the terms of its accommodation with the profession. In so doing, it placed great strain on the profession–state relationship and on the ability of the profession to manage the complex internal balances upon which that relationship depended. This chapter traces out these effects.

## The Founding Bargain: Fee-for-Service and the Negotiation of Price

Upon its establishment, Canadian medicare essentially underwrote the costs of the existing system, based as it was upon private fee-for-service medical practice and public or voluntary not-for-profit hospitals. The terms of the founding bargain with the medical profession were foreshadowed by the Saskatoon agreement (which ended the medical strike against the introduction of governmental medical care insurance in Saskatchewan in 1962) and in the report of the federal Royal Commission on Health Services in 1964 that led up to the adoption of the Medical Care Act two years later. The mediator of the Saskatoon agreement described its objective as finding "a way of combining publicly supported universal coverage with the true essentials of profession freedom" (Taylor 1979: 323). The Royal Commission produced a "Health Charter for Canadians" that included among its elements a "comprehensive, universal Health Services Programme . . . based upon freedom of choice [by patient of physician and vice versa] and upon free and self-governing professions and institutions . . . [that is,] the right of members of health professions to practise within the law, to free choice of location and type of practice, and to professional self-government" (Royal Commission on Health Services 1964: 11–12).

In cross-national and historical context, private, fee-for-service practice would not appear to be one of the "true essentials of professional freedom" or a fundamental characteristic of a "free and self-governing profession." Nonetheless, it was so interpreted in the understanding between the profession and the state that underlay the establishment of Canadian medicare. According to the terms of this bargain, the profession accepted the role of the state as the "single payer" for medical and hospital services, recognizing that this would inevitably place constraints on the entrepreneurial discretion of individual practitioners. The state, for its part, accepted the entitlement of individual professionals to choose their mode of practice, recognizing that the continuation of private, fee-for-service practice as the predominant mode would be the result. The Saskatoon agreement, moreover, allowed physicians to opt to bill their patients (not the government plan) directly at rates of their own choosing. As other provinces subsequently entered the federal plan, most made some similar provision.[3]

If governments were to have any control over costs in such an open-ended system, some accommodation would have to be reached with the profession regarding the ongoing operation of the system. That accommodation took the form of an agency relationship: the government, as principal, established bud-

getary parameters; organized medicine, as agent, determined within those parameters how resources were to be allocated. For most of the two decades after
the establishment of Canadian medicare, the budgetary parameters in the
medical services sector were primarily related to rates of increase in the price
of medical services. But over time, and particularly in the 1990s, the terms of
the accommodation between the state and the profession were progressively
elaborated, to constrain increasingly the entrepreneurial discretion of physicians
while, as in Britain, seeking to maintain their clinical autonomy.

Let us consider first the negotiation of price. Rather than paying medical
fees that were "usual and customary" in particular localities as did U.S. Medicare, Canadian provincial governments followed the model of the physician-
sponsored insurance plans and paid physicians on the basis of fee schedules set
by the provincial medical associations, prorated by a given percentage (usually
15%). After the first few years, governments insisted that any increases to the fee
schedule be negotiated. It is important to note that in almost all provinces (the
notable exception being Quebec, as discussed later) what was negotiated was
the overall rate of increase to the schedule: the determination of the relative
value of particular items was accomplished entirely through the committee
structures of the provincial medical associations. One effect of medicare, then,
was to increase the centralization of control over medical fees that had been
well underway under the previous system of private insurance (and particularly
the system of physician-sponsored insurance plans).

So the entrepreneurial discretion of individual physicians over the price to
be charged for their services, already diminishing before the introduction of
medicare, was further reduced in the regime that followed. For a time,
individual physicians could escape the constraints of this regime by "extra
billing"—billing their patients a discretionary amount above that covered by
the government plan. Again, this practice continued the model that had been
established by the physician-sponsored plans—under which "participating"
physicians agreed to accept prorated payment directly from the plan, and "nonparticipating" physicians charged fees at their discretion and were responsible
for collecting fees from their patients who were reimbursed by the plan at the
prorated level.

As described in chapter 3, the extra-billing option was closed as a result of a
policy intervention by the federal government, prompted by broad partisan
considerations: the passage of the Canada Health Act in 1984. The Canada
Health Act introduced a new element into the accommodations between
provincial governments and the medical profession, which adjusted to the in-
trusion in distinctive ways. But the common effect was that, as the various
provinces came into compliance, the last of the individual physician's discretion
over the price of most medical services disappeared.

If they lost discretion over price, however, physicians retained entrepreneurial discretion over all other aspects of their practices: location, scheduling, labor
and other inputs, and volume and mix of services delivered. Although provincial governments expressed growing concern over increases in the volume and
mix of services billed to their plans, they approached the issue of utilization re-

view very cautiously. In several provinces, committees to review the practice profiles of individual physicians were established in the 1970s (Tuohy 1992: 127). With one exception (Quebec), these committees were set up under the aegis of professional bodies, not governments; without exception, they did not engage in ongoing routine reviews, but rather they dealt with extreme outlier cases.

Under this regime of negotiated prices, cross-provincial differences in fee schedules increased under medicare, reflecting the different accommodations between the profession and the government across provinces. On balance, however, negotiations constrained the rate of increase in medical fees. A contrast with the United States starkly demonstrates this point. Between 1971 and 1985, real fees declined 18% in Canada and rose 22% in the United States (General Accounting Office 1991: 35). The impact on physicians' net incomes was less dramatic, however. Changes in "utilization" factors—the volume and mix of services rendered—to some extent blunted the impact of real reductions in fees on medical incomes. Utilization tended to increase faster in provinces that experienced the greatest degree of fee level constraint, with the result that cross-provincial differences in incomes were considerably smaller than were differences in fee schedules (Barer and Evans 1986: 78–96). Lower administrative expenses in medical practices under medicare also need to be taken into account in considering the impact on medical incomes: in 1987, for example, office expenses for physicians in Canada amounted on average to about 36% of their gross billings, compared with 48% in the United States (General Accounting Office 1991: 5).

Income comparisons between Canadian and U.S. physicians are complicated by differences in specialty mix. Throughout the period after the adoption of medicare about one-half of Canadian physicians were general or family practitioners, but a much smaller and decreasing proportion of American physicians (19% in 1970 and 13.3% in 1988) fell into these categories (and another 20% were "primary care" practitioners in pediatrics and internal medicine in 1988) (General Accounting Office 1991: 38). Because of these differences, income comparisons are best made by specialty. One such comparison, by Iglehart, related U.S. physicians to their counterparts in Ontario.[4] In 1986, average net incomes in general practice and family practice were marginally (about 10%) higher for U.S. physicians than for Ontario physicians. The differences were most pronounced in orthopedic surgery and pathology, with U.S. physicians earning on average two-thirds more than their Ontario counterparts. In internal medicine and pediatrics, however, the net earnings of Ontario physicians were on average marginally (2% to 14%) higher than those in the United States (Iglehart 1990: 568).

Given the substantial and growing differences in specialty mix, the widening gap between the incomes of specialists in Canada and the United States made for very divergent trajectories of average physician incomes. As will be recalled from chapter 5 (table 5.2), Canadian physicians' average net earnings were five times those of the average employee in 1970; by 1989, this ratio had declined to 3.6. Over the same period, average net physician income in the United States rose from 4.7 times that of the average employee to 5.0. Put another way, the average Canadian physician income, which in 1970 stood at 72% of the U.S. average, had declined to 55% of the U.S. average by 1989.

## Provincial-Level Accommodations in the 1970s and 1980s

The general terms of the accommodation between the medical profession and the state—the ceding of professional discretion over price in return for the maintenance of private fee-for-service practice and professional control over clinical decision-making—were similar across provinces. But the particular terms, and the tenor of the relationship, varied considerably. The three largest provinces—Ontario, Quebec, and British Columbia—illustrate some of this variation.[5]

In Quebec, the accommodation of the 1970s and 1980s accorded a greater assertion of the role of the state than in any other province. In that respect it consistently anticipated developments in other provinces by a decade or more. Extra billing by physicians, for example, was effectively banned from the outset under the Quebec medicare plan. Quebec specialist physicians went on strike against the introduction of medicare in the province in 1971—the only province other than Saskatchewan in which such a protest occurred. One of the major issues in the strike was the option to extra bill. The government's response, enforced by back-to-work legislation, was to make extra billing economically unfeasible. It refused to reimburse patients of physicians for any portion of a physician's charge if that charge exceeded the government-sanctioned rate. The Quebec government also held rates of increase in medical fees to well below the national average from the beginning of its medicare plan (Barer and Evans 1986: 78–80) and was the first to institute global and individual caps on medical billings. Quebec was also one of the first provinces (along with Ontario) to establish a utilization review committee to review the practice profiles of physicians and to reduce payments to physicians identified as "overservicing." Unlike those in other provinces, moreover, Quebec's utilization review committee was located within the provincial agency administering the health insurance plan, not within a professional body. Quebec pioneered in establishing a system of reduced rates of payment to physicians locating in "overserviced" areas and increased rates to those locating in "underserviced" areas, in revising the structures of professional regulation to provide for lay representation on and increased Cabinet control of professional bodies, and in establishing a framework of local and regional councils with planning responsibilities and some limited management authority in the institutional and community care sectors.

The Quebec model of profession–state relations was, indeed, the most comprehensive, continuous, and intricate in the country. Lomas and his colleagues have described this "Gallic" model as follows:

> The "Gallic" model incorporated a comprehensive view of the issues at stake, reflected their inter-relatedness in complex bargaining structures and payment rules and, by the early 1980s, had evolved permanent rather than periodic negotiations.

The model relies extensively on data and experts from both legal and actuarial backgrounds, and deals in detail with both specific fee items and unique circumstance [sic] affecting specific physicians. This more technical approach is, however, tempered by a remarkable continuity of the personalities at the table. The Gallic model has also served to isolate fee negotiations from external conflicts between the parties over tangentially related medical care policies. This has been achieved by having clear understandings of what does and does not have standing at the bargaining table. In this sense Quebec's approach foresaw the much later development in other provinces of specifically designed mechanisms to absorb and deflect away from fee negotiations those issues that might disrupt or interfere with productive bargaining over remuneration. (Lomas et al. 1992: 169)

Quebec's greater "statism" in the health care arena reflected its broader political culture. Throughout the 1970s and 1980s, public opinion polls in Quebec indicated higher levels of support for state activism than in any other region of Canada (Tuohy 1992: 19–20). In the health care arena, moreover, the relative strength of the state was enhanced by the limited mobility of francophone professionals in the broader North American context, and by the divided organization of the medical profession. In contrast to other Canadian provinces, there were two professional voluntary associations: one representing specialists, the other representing general practitioners. On occasion, the two associations have diverged sharply in positions and tactics. In 1970, for example, it was the specialist association alone (galvanized by the issue of preserving an option to extra bill) that issued a strike call in response to the introduction of medicare.

In British Columbia, a more populist political culture, a more polarized partisan environment, and a system of industrial relations with a highly adversarial and conflictual history all combined to create a template of adversarialism for relationships between the profession and the state under medicare. British Columbia was one of a group of provinces (including Ontario, Alberta, and Manitoba) in which the profession–state relationship came early to be characterized both by a collective bargaining model (albeit without formal certification of the professional association as a bargaining agent under labor relations legislation) and by the use of confrontational tactics. Even more than in the other "adversarial" provinces, relationships between the medical profession and government in British Columbia were marked by tactics including appeals to public opinion, threats of withdrawal of service, professional boycotts of the policy process, and recourse to unilateral legislative action by government and litigation by the profession (Lomas et al. 1992: 167–72; Tuohy 1992: 125).

Notably, the British Columbia government was the first (in 1983) to attempt to institute controls over the distribution of physicians by refusing to issue new billing numbers (effectively denying payment under the provincial health insurance plan) to physicians seeking to establish practices in areas deemed "overserviced." Newly graduated physicians, physicians from outside the province, and those who had not practiced in the province for more than two years were required to apply for geographically limited billing numbers. This provision was vigorously resisted by the British Columbia Medical Association (BCMA), which boycotted the Medical Manpower Committees that were to determine the medical human-resource needs of given localities, and which supported an ultimately successful legal challenge to the billing number legislation as infringing the "liberty" and "mobility" rights of physicians under Canada's constitutional Charter of Rights and Freedoms. This conflict presaged attempts in other provinces to negotiate or impose physician supply and distribution arrangements.

The adversarial relationship between the profession and the state in British Columbia yielded substantial benefits for the profession. Throughout the 1970s and 1980s, the fee schedule for medical remuneration under the provincial health insurance plan was the highest or nearly the highest in the country (although medical incomes were close to the national average) (Barer and Evans 1986: 78, 93). The adversarialism of the relationship, moreover, did not negate the possibility of pragmatic collaboration between the profession and government. Extra billing, for example, was effectively prevented in British Columbia by agreement between the BCMA and the government, until this agreement was superseded by legislation in 1981. A utilization review committee to review the practice profiles of physicians with aberrant billing patterns was established as a committee of the voluntary association, the BCMA, not the governmental insurance agency as in Quebec nor the professional regulatory body as in Ontario. On the basis of limited evidence, it appeared that the BCMA committee penalized proportionately fewer physicians than its counterparts in Quebec and Ontario (Wilson et al. 1986).

In Ontario, the relationship between the provincial government and the voluntary association, the Ontario Medical Association (OMA), was also marked by adversarialism. The banning of extra billing in the wake of the Canada Health Act, for example, created a greater conflict in Ontario than in any other province. In each of the other six provinces in which extra billing had been allowed, the process of negotiating the ban was relatively amicable, and the medical profession achieved substantial gains in the form of fee schedule increases and binding arbitration mechanisms for future fee schedule disputes. In Ontario, however, the banning of extra billing occasioned unprecedented conflict between the OMA and the government, culminating in a four-week doctors' strike in 1986. This conflict was exacerbated by the disruption of the accommodation between the OMA and the provincial government resulting from the accession of the Liberals to power in 1985 after forty-three years of Conservative rule, a disruption that led to a misreading of signals and a locking-in of both parties to an escalating politics of "saving face" (Tuohy 1988). But the conflict of 1986 was neither the first nor, as we shall see, the last episode of hostility between the OMA and the provincial government.

Despite the periodic confrontations between the voluntary association and the provincial government, however, the profession–state relationship in Ontario was more fully elaborated to include issues well beyond medical remuneration and actors other than the OMA. Indeed, as I have argued elsewhere, the linchpin of the profession–state accommodation was the relationship between the state and a "strategic minority" of physicians primarily based in the medical schools and the regulatory body, the College of Physicians and Surgeons of Ontario

(CPSO). This strategic minority placed the highest value on the preservation of the clinical autonomy of the individual physician within professionally determined norms, and it was prepared to trade off considerable individual entrepreneurial discretion in order to preserve and enhance medical influence over clinical decision-making. The position of this minority within the executive ranks of the OMA varied over time, and so, accordingly, did the political stance of the voluntary association. But the strategic minority was well represented within the leadership of the CPSO and on the numerous advisory committees and task forces established by the provincial government through the 1970s and 1980s to deal with policy and planning issues of various degrees of generality and specificity (Tuohy 1992: 126–27). The process developed for the review of aberrant medical practice profiles is illustrative: as noted previously, this function in Ontario was located within the CPSO, not the OMA (as in the British Columbia model) or a government agency (as in the Quebec model).

Quebec, British Columbia, and Ontario do not exhaust the range of variation in provincial-level accommodations between the profession and the state in the 1970s and 1980s. As Lomas and his colleagues (1992) found, these relationships fell into three broad categories: the "Gallic" Quebec model previously discussed; the adversarial category comprising British Columbia, Ontario, Alberta, and Manitoba; and a category of relatively informal "mutual accommodation" comprising the Atlantic provinces and Saskatchewan. Over time, however, these three categories began to show a degree of convergence. Provincial governments sought both to assert their roles more forcefully and also to elaborate the terms of their accommodations with the profession. In this process, both the informal mechanisms of the "mutual accommodation" model and the more formalized but narrowly focused mechanisms of the adversarial collective bargaining model began to change. As we shall see shortly, they gave way increasingly to a set of relationships that, as had been the case in Quebec and to a lesser extent in Ontario, were both formalized and multifaceted.

If the style of profession–government relations began to converge across provinces through the 1970s and 1980s, patterns of convergence in outcomes are more mixed. On one important measure, real per capita health spending, we do observe some convergence. In 1975, real per capita health spending ranged from 78% of the national average in New Brunswick to 113% of the national average in British Columbia. Only six of the ten provinces were within 10% above or below the national average on this measure. By 1990 this range of variation had been reduced considerably, ranging from 90% of the national average in Newfoundland to 111% in Alberta, and all provinces but Alberta were within 10% above or below the national average (calculated from Health Canada 1997: table 10). As we shall see, the range continued to narrow over the course of the 1990s. Cross-provincial differences in the public–private balance of expenditure, never very wide, were essentially stable over this period. In 1975 the public share of total health expenditure ranged from more than 79% in Quebec to just less than 72% in British Columbia. By 1991, the range was from more than 79% percent in Newfoundland to less than 73% in Prince Edward Island (calculated from Health Canada 1996: tables 16 and 17).

Beneath these gross measures of convergence in spending levels, however, lay a persistent pattern of difference in provincial expenditure across categories of service (table 7.1). All provinces shifted expenditures from hospitals to other institutions over the 1975–1991 period. But the range of interprovincial variation in expenditures in these categories actually increased. Similarly, the pharmaceutical share increased at widely varying rates across provinces. In the sector most closely tied to the profession–state accommodation, however, there was a modest convergence: the range of variation in the share of expenditure allocated to professional services (about two-thirds of which represents the share for physicians' services) declined from 14.5 percentage points in 1975 to 12.1 percentage points in 1991.

As the health policy agenda unfolded in the 1990s, there was increasing commonality in both the mode of profession–state accommodation and the substance of policy initiatives. The legacies of conflict and accommodation in the past, however, continued to shape the translation of agendas into action.

## Expenditure Caps in the 1990s

Prior to the adoption of medicare, the Canadian system had been, in cross-national terms, a relatively costly one. In 1960 total health expenditures in Canada as a proportion of GDP were the highest among all OECD nations except for Iceland (Schieber and Poullier 1987: 108). The profession–state accommodation under medicare preserved this relatively costly system, and while rates of expenditure growth were lower in Canada than in a number of other OECD

TABLE 7.1 Share of Selected Sectors in Total Health Care Expenditure, by Province, 1975 and 1991 (Percentage of Total Health Expenditure)

| | Hospitals | | Other Institutions | | Professional Services | | Drugs | |
|---|---|---|---|---|---|---|---|---|
| | 1975 | 1991 | 1975 | 1991 | 1975 | 1991 | 1975 | 1991 |
| Newfoundland | 48.5 | 43.6 | 7.7 | 11.6 | 13.6 | 13.7 | 10.2 | 20.0 |
| Prince Edward Island | 44.3 | 38.6 | 14.7 | 14.9 | 17.3 | 15.5 | 11.8 | 19.3 |
| Nova Scotia | 48.1 | 44.3 | 6.1 | 8.6 | 19.1 | 17.5 | 11.4 | 17.0 |
| New Brunswick | 49.9 | 41.9 | 7.1 | 10.2 | 16.2 | 15.8 | 10.2 | 16.4 |
| Quebec | 48.7 | 42.5 | 8.1 | 11.7 | 19.5 | 17.8 | 9.5 | 13.3 |
| Ontario | 42.4 | 36.7 | 12.3 | 9.1 | 23.1 | 25.8 | 11.3 | 14.4 |
| Manitoba | 44.9 | 38.7 | 14.8 | 12.6 | 18.3 | 16.8 | 10.6 | 10.7 |
| Saskatchewan | 40.6 | 34.0 | 13.3 | 17.6 | 17.4 | 16.0 | 13.4 | 12.6 |
| Alberta | 43.0 | 40.4 | 11.8 | 7.2 | 22.1 | 23.1 | 10.2 | 12.6 |
| British Columbia | 39.9 | 34.3 | 8.8 | 10.4 | 28.1 | 24.7 | 11.0 | 17.5 |
| Range of Variation (percentage points)[a] | 8.8 | 10.3 | 8.7 | 10.4 | 14.5 | 12.1 | 3.9 | 9.3 |

Source: OECD 1995: table A3.

[a] Percentage point difference between province with highest proportional allocation to sector and province with lowest proportional allocation to sector.

nations, Canada consistently ranked among the top three or four nations on the measure of total health expenditures as a proportion of GDP. By the early 1990s this proportion stood at just more than 10% (10.2% in 1992), second (albeit a distant second) only to the United States at more than 14%. In this context, and in the face of broad governmental agendas at both federal and provincial levels to reduce the level of deficit spending, governments at both levels embarked upon measures to contain public health expenditures to a greater degree than had been accomplished in the past. At the federal level, these measures took the blunt form of further constraints on federal transfers to the provinces for health care, as discussed in chapter 3. At the provincial level, governments adopted a number of more or less common strategies, most requiring that they elaborate their accommodations with the medical profession in unprecedented ways.

Virtually all of the governmental control over expenditures for physicians' services throughout the 1970s and the 1980s concerned the price of physicians' services. As already noted, utilization review was marginal to the system (although it may have had a broader deterrent effect) (Tuohy 1982). Until the 1990s the medical care sector remained largely open-ended in its demands on the public treasury. Before turning to a discussion of the attempts to deal with this problem in the 1990s, however, a contrast with the hospital sector is in order.

Early in the history of medicare, governments had closed the open-endedness of payment mechanisms in the hospital sector by establishing prospective global budgets for hospitals, replacing the earlier system of per diem payments. These budgets were essentially historically based, with across-the-board percentage increases each year, based ostensibly on some consideration of economic factors but effectively on the fiscal considerations of provincial governments. This strategy proved effective in containing hospital expenditures, relative to other sectors of the health care system, in the 1970s and 1980s. The contrast with expenditures on physicians' services is enlightening. Hospital wages were not centrally negotiated, and hospital-specific wage and unit price inflation outpaced general inflation throughout the 1970s and 1980s, even as centrally negotiated medical fee schedules failed to keep place with general inflation in the 1970s and only slightly exceeded general inflation in the 1980s.[6] But hospitals functioned under a budgetary regime of global operating budgets and separate centrally-controlled capital budgets, while the physician services budget was open-ended in a regime dominated by private fee-for-service practice. Accordingly, real per capita spending on hospital operating costs and on capital (the preponderance of which was devoted to hospitals) increased at only about half the rate of increase in real per capita spending on physician services from 1975 to 1990.[7]

In the 1990s, constraints on hospital budgets increased dramatically. Global budgets were reduced in real terms; some provinces, notably Ontario and Alberta, began to experiment with case-based funding formulas in establishing hospital budgets (Bhatia et al. 1996).[8] These formulas, developed with the collaboration and support of provincial hospital associations, sought to reward hospitals for efficiency. At first this was done by comparing a hospital's actual costs with its "expected" cost per weighted case, based on comparisons with peers, and assigning budget increases or decreases based on these comparisons. These experiments, not surprisingly, generated much strategic behavior on the part of hospital actors seeking either to escape the regime by claiming membership in one of the "excluded" groups or to assert membership in a peer group that could lay claim to higher costs. These experiments were overshadowed for a time in the mid-1990s by the wave of hospital restructuring that swept through all provinces, as discussed in Chapter 3. As a result, new baseline budgets were established for restructured hospitals. In the wake of restructuring, however, the attempt to develop global budgeting formulas based on costs-per-weighted-case and negotiated volumes of activity—a model that could come to resemble British "block contracts"—was picked up again by central government agencies and regional health bodies.

One effect of the experiments with case-based hospital funding formulas was, as happened in the United States and the United Kingdom, to accelerate the development of information systems in individual hospitals and in provincial governments (Bhatia et al. 1996: 43). Information so generated was brought to bear in the hospital restructuring exercises. In contrast to the United States and in comparison with the United Kingdom, however, this information was not used by funders to intervene in the practice decisions of individual physicians. The monitoring of medical behavior in hospitals remained firmly lodged with hospital medical staffs.

The combination of hospital restructuring and global budget constraint had dramatic effects in the hospital sector in the 1990s. Real per capita spending on hospitals decreased by 7.2% from 1990 to 1996, while total real per capita health spending increased by 1.7% (calculated from Health Canada 1997: table 5). The hospital share of total health expenditures decreased from 38.2% in 1990 to 34.9% in 1996. To put this 3.3% drop over six years in perspective, the hospital share had declined by only about 7% over the previous twenty years (OECD 1995: 43).[9] Meanwhile, the share allocated to physician services remained constant throughout both periods at about 15%.

Throughout the 1970s and 1980s, however, physicians had maintained a constant share of an expanding pie. As governments sought to constrain the expansion of the pie (or at least the public portion thereof), the contrast between the hospital and physician services sectors was not lost on them. The most important development in the physician services sector in the 1990s, not only in its direct effects on expenditures but in its broader policy ramifications and implications for the profession–state accommodation, was the decision by provincial governments to cap the budget for physician services.

Quebec, not surprisingly, had led the way in this regard.[10] Beginning in 1976 and 1977, the Quebec government negotiated separate capped budgets for general practitioners and specialists, derived by multiplying an average target income for each group by the number of physicians. A number of factors, including unanticipated changes in the physician supply and distribution across specialties or particular types of utilization increases, could justify exceeding the budget cap. With these exceptions, however, aggregate physician billings in excess of the global limit in any given year were fully recovered through fee adjustments in the subsequent year. Individual billing caps were also adopted for general practitioners in 1976; for GPs, billings above a threshold were reduced through proration.

Over the course of the 1980s a number of other provincial governments began to move in this direction (Lomas et al. 1989). In Ontario, projected "utilization increases" were taken into account in negotiating fee schedule increases, but the physician services budget was not formally capped. In the mid-1980s, Manitoba and British Columbia capped their physician expenditure budgets (although the Manitoba cap was in place for only a brief period), allowing for year-to-year increases based on factors such as projected utilization and population growth, and providing for the recovery of billings in excess of the global limit through subsequent fee schedule reductions. Saskatchewan followed suit in 1989, with a different recovery mechanism.

These budgetary limits were of varying degrees of firmness—they allowed for various factors that might justify exceeding the limits, and they did not always require that excess expenditures be fully recovered. Only Quebec, moreover, had established individual billing thresholds. In the 1990s, however, all provincial governments acted to cap their physician services budgets, and in most cases to cap them more firmly than had been done in the past. A variety of mechanisms for recapturing excess expenditures were adopted, including "clawbacks" (fee adjustments in the year following the overrun to recover the excess), "holdbacks" (holding back a portion of payments to be released after a year-end reconciliation), and "paybacks" (repayment of excesses determined by a year-end reconciliation through some mechanism other than fee adjustments) (Hurley and Card 1996).

In addition, five provinces negotiated (or at times imposed) individual billing thresholds, over which payments were prorated, usually on a sliding scale. Quebec, moreover, added billing thresholds for specialists to the GP thresholds that had been in place since the 1970s. The provinces varied in the degree to which they distinguished between specialties in the establishment of individual billing thresholds; some distinguished only between general or family practitioners and all other specialists, others divided specialists into two or more subgroups—and the categories varied not only across but also within provinces over time."[11]

The adoption of global expenditure limits for physician services placed enormous strain on the structures of organized medicine. As Hurley and his colleagues have argued in their insightful analyses of the implementation of expenditure cap policies, the capping of physician services budgets created the incentive problems associated with "common-property resources" (Hurley and Card 1996; Hurley et al. 1996; Hurley et al. n.d.). Under the "clawback" or "holdback" provisions, all physicians would share equally in the imposition of penalties for exceeding the global budget, regardless of the level of their own individual billings. (The adoption of individual billing thresholds mitigated but did not solve this problem, at least at the levels at which thresholds were established.) In sheer economic terms, if physicians assumed that the global limit would be exceeded and hence penalties would be triggered, they each had an incentive to increase the level of their own billings as a hedge against future reductions—thereby greatly increasing the likelihood that the limit would indeed be exceeded. Only some collective understanding or agreement among physicians could shape expectations in a way that would discourage such behavior. The most obvious vehicle for the development and monitoring of such understandings was the voluntary medical association with whom the global limits were negotiated.

The critical role of the provincial medical associations in this process has been demonstrated by Hurley and his colleagues in their review of the implementation of global budget limits in Alberta and Nova Scotia. In Nova Scotia, even given individual billing thresholds (a feature not present in Alberta), the global budget was less successful in constraining physician billings than was the case in Alberta. In the three years following the institution of budget limits, utilization per physician actually declined in Alberta but increased in Nova Scotia.

Hurley and his colleagues examine a number of factors that might explain this difference. For example, fees and billings per physician were lower and more slowly growing in Nova Scotia than in Alberta to begin with; Alberta launched its global budget with the "sweetener" of a budget increase, while Nova Scotia began with a budget freeze. But Alberta's relative success in constraining billings persisted even in the face of subsequent budget reductions. Hurley and his colleagues attribute the difference to the respective roles of the Alberta Medical Association (AMA) and the Medical Society of Nova Scotia (MSNS). This is a somewhat surprising finding, given the history of informal "mutual accommodation" between the professional association and the provincial government in Nova Scotia in contrast to the adversarialism of Alberta (Lomas et al. 1992). But it was precisely the more formalized institutional structures associated with the collective bargaining model that stood the AMA in good stead on this issue. These structures, after all, were designed to deal with conflict, whereas the informal processes of Nova Scotia were predicated upon the congenial personal relationships of participants. Unprecedented budgetary constraint ruptured those relationships, and there were "few institutional structures . . . through which the profession and the government could conduct discussions when relations soured" (Hurley et al. n.d.: 10).

The Alberta Medical Association, moreover, followed a ratification process that was more successful in achieving the "buy-in" of its membership than was the case for the MSNS process that only required approval of its Executive Committee. Alberta physicians showed themselves remarkably responsive in constraining utilization in response to fee schedule adjustments and communications from the AMA. And finally, the AMA negotiated an agreement allowing for considerable flexibility through structures of joint decision-making to develop mechanisms for keeping expenditures within the global budget. In ironic contrast, the MSNS gave up much of its subsequent discretion by insisting on an up-front prescription of across-the-board adjustments. In Alberta, then, the agency role of the professional association was more successfully extended to embrace the constraining of physician billings in an era of global budget limits than was the case in Nova Scotia. Indeed, success in this regard varied across the provinces in accordance with different legacies of profession–state relationships.

The tensions associated with the introduction of capped physician services budgets signaled the beginning of a new era in profession–state relationships in Canada. These policies set in motion an inexorable logic of policy development, as professional associations sought ways to manage the internal conflicts that ensued. Some medical associations sought the introduction of individual billing thresholds, in the belief that this would mitigate the "common-property resource" problems they faced—this had been the case in Quebec in 1976 and was again the case in Newfoundland and Nova Scotia in the 1990s. But individual thresholds were no panacea. As medical associations and governments sought ways to ease the pressure of fee-for-service billings against the budget cap, the policy agenda expanded to include issues that had long simmered in the background of profession–state relations—issues of supply control, the scope of coverage under the public plan, alternative payment mechanisms, and clinical protocols.

## The Expanding Agenda

### Controlling physician supply

Throughout the 1970s and 1980s, such measures as were adopted to control the supply of physicians were limited to the relatively nonconflictual mechanism of severely limiting the flow of physicians immigrating to Canada, through federal–provincial agreements. But Canadian medical schools, expanded in the late 1960s and early 1970s in anticipation of a physician "shortage" under medicare, continued to supply physicians at a greater rate than physicians withdrew from practice for retirement or other reasons. The number of practicing physicians per thousand population grew from 1.5 in 1970 to 2.3 in 1988—a level of supply and rate of growth slightly below that of the United States and well below that of most Western European nations—but well above that in the United Kingdom (OECD 1993, vol. 1: 164–65). To increasingly cost-conscious governments (and to medical associations once the risk of increased billings above a global limit was transferred to the profession), however, what mattered was not cross-national comparisons but the secular trend—the increasing number of claimants on a limited budget.

Provincial governments adopted a variety of mechanisms to control the supply or at least the geographic distribution of physicians—attempting to limit the overall number of physicians or at least to ensure that additional claimants upon the physician services budget would practice where they were "needed." The first type of measure was directed at physicians trained outside a given province—not only outside Canada but in other Canadian provinces. At different times, such policies were adopted in British Columbia and Ontario.[12] A number of provinces, moreover, attempted to limit the number of physicians establishing new practices by severely prorating their billings, by as much as 50%. As Barer et al. note, these policies were intended to discourage physicians from locating in a given province, in the expectation that they would seek to locate elsewhere. But this had "the predictable effect of doing nothing more than redistributing costs among the provinces, without any national coordination, since most of these physicians will choose to practice somewhere in Canada" (Barer et al. 1996: 221). And despite some declarations of intent, there was in fact no coordination across provinces in this regard, given the problems of interprovincial and federal–provincial relations discussed in chapter 3.

Even more common than these attempts to limit the overall supply of physicians were attempts to control the distribution of new physicians by issuing geographically restricted billing numbers and by prorating payments, reducing payments to those who located in "overserviced" areas and in some cases augmenting payment to those who located in "underserviced" areas, for the first few years of practice. Quebec and British Columbia had introduced such policies in the 1970s and 1980s, respectively, as previously noted. In the 1990s, despite the successful court challenge to the British Columbia policy of the mid-1980s, various versions of such policies were introduced in the 1990s in Manitoba, Ontario, New Brunswick, Nova Scotia, Prince Edward Island, Newfoundland, and again in British Columbia. In some cases, notably British Columbia and Ontario, the initial attempts to introduce policies were met with resistance from the profession, but negotiated arrangements were eventually reached with the professional associations that provided for joint government/professional bodies to develop the physician resource plans upon which long-term supply management policies were predicated (Barer et al. 1996: 221–23).

Although these arrangements have been negotiated between medical associations and provincial governments, the negotiations have not been without conflict. As we shall see in the discussion of the Ontario case, they have been viewed as pitting the interests of established practitioners against those of new graduates. And these arrangements have been challenged, not by the provincial medical associations, but by associations of interns and residents. Legal action was launched by such associations in both British Columbia and New Brunswick. In 1997, the British Columbia Supreme Court held that the system of prorated payments violated newly graduated physicians' mobility and equality rights under the Canadian Charter of Rights and Freedoms,[13] as well as the requirement to provide "reasonable compensation" to physicians under the Canada Health Act. This surprising decision sent shock waves across provinces, given the prevalence of such policies, and signaled the likelihood of protracted litigation over these policies.

### *"Delisting" and privatization*

Another way of relieving pressure on the global budget cap under a fee-for-service system is not by limiting the number of practitioners, but by limiting the types of service that can be billed to the plan, thus allowing physicians to bill privately for "delisted" services. This way of providing physicians with some private sources of income was more consistent with Canada's "segmented" rather than "tiered" approach to the role of the public and private sectors than was the banned "extra billing" option. It was also constrained, however, by the terms of Canadian medicare. Under the letter and the spirit of both federal and provincial legislation, services could be deinsured only if they were deemed not to be medically necessary. The Canada Health Act made even more explicit the premises of its predecessor legislation: on its face, it requires provincial health insurance plans to cover fully all "medically required" physician services and a broadly defined set of "necessary" types of hospital services in order to qualify for federal financial contributions. Provincial governments, in complying with the federal legislation, either de facto or de jure accepted "medical necessity" as the standard for coverage under their respective plans. The determination of what physician services were "medically required" and which hospital services were "necessary," however, was not defined in legislation.

In the hospital sector, under the regime of historically based global budgets and separate capital budgets, considerations of "necessity" were invoked primarily with respect to capital expenditures or through additions to hospital operating budgets as "extraglobal" funding. Such decisions typically involved negotiations between the provincial ministry of health and individual hospitals. In these negotiations physicians individually or collectively typically played an important role. In the late 1980s, governments became considerably more cautious about additional claims upon the public purse. In Ontario, for example, the provincial government debated in 1986 whether to provide special funding for hospitals to introduce two new costly pharmaceuticals, non-ionic radiographic contrast media (RCM) and a thrombolitic agent, tissue plasminogen activator (tPA). The response from the medical profession presaged internal divisions to come. The regulatory body, the College of Physicians and Surgeons of Ontario, and the voluntary association, the Ontario Medical Association (OMA), jostled for legitimacy as the arbiter of such matters (Rappolt 1997: 979). The OMA Executive, wishing to establish itself as a credible agent capable of considering cost-effectiveness criteria as well as the professional interest in technology development, advised against providing extraglobal funding for either agent on grounds of cost effectiveness. In so doing the OMA Executive placed itself in opposition to the OMA's own subgroups of radiologists and cardiologists, respectively. It found its authority undercut when the government decided to provide special RCM funding, but it was vindicated in the subsequent decision not to fund the use of tPA.[14]

As for changes to the medical fee schedule itself, the question of what physicians' services were "medically required" was not a matter of negotiation between providers and governments until the 1990s. As noted earlier, fee schedule negotiations between medical associations and provincial governments were generally focused on the overall percent increase in fees, not the relative value of items nor the scope of the services covered, which had changed little since a broad base of coverage was established in each province upon the establishment of medicare. Such additions to or deletions from the schedule as were made were generally done at the initiative of the medical associations.

The first province to open up the question of delimiting the scope of coverage of the public plan was Alberta. In 1985, as part of the negotiations between the Alberta Medical Association and the provincial government around the banning of extra billing, it was decided that several services be deinsured, including family planning counseling, tubal ligations, vasectomies, and mammoplasty. This selection was driven largely by the conservative social policy ideology of the governing Conservative party of the day. From the perspective of the medical profession, however, it focused with few exceptions on fairly lucrative procedures performed by relatively high-earning specialists. Furthermore, the deinsurance of such services freed physicians to bill for them privately at rates of their own choosing. As an internal accommodation within the profession, then, it allowed for some smoothing of differentials in medicare earnings while allowing a "safety valve" for the specialties affected. This agreement did not survive the public protest that ensued, however, and funding for most of these services was restored.

In the 1990s, the imposition of global budgets for physician services triggered a renewed interest in deinsurance options, largely on the part of the medical profession. As presaged by the earlier Alberta experience—and indeed, as consistent with experience in Britain as well (Klein et al. 1996: 118)—most of the services and procedures considered for deinsuring involved cosmetic surgery and elective services related to reproduction.[15] The cross-provincial and cross-national similarity of the candidates for deinsurance suggests a considerable degree of professional consensus about the outer periphery of needed medical services, but at the margins the selection was also shaped by political considerations for governments and economic considerations for the profession, as noted in the Alberta case.

The most obvious clash of these considerations[16] occurred in Ontario, where a committee established in 1993 under the aegis of the profession–government Joint Management Committee (discussed later in this chapter) considered a range of candidates for deinsurance, including many of the cosmetic and reproductive procedures typically considered in such exercises. Again, these were lucrative services and procedures performed by relatively high-earning specialists, and their deinsurance would allow them to be offered in private markets. But the list also included, at the urging of the medical association, the routine annual health exam—a service whose efficacy was first brought into question in the Canadian context by a consensus panel reporting to the federal and provincial health ministers in 1979, although no action was ever taken to delist it. The routine annual health examination, then, was arguably not "medically necessary"; removing it from the publicly covered set of services would reduce pressure on the global budget cap and provide a significant source of discretionary private income for primary care physicians. The OMA estimated that at least one-half of the C$20 million target in savings to the public budget through delisting could be achieving with the fell swoop of delisting the routine annual health examination. Nonetheless, the panel (whose membership comprised two physicians, two government representatives, two members of the "public," and an independent chairperson, the dean of nursing at the University of Toronto) recommended against delisting the annual health examination. The panel's recommendation was that such a delisting would be premature pending the development of practice guidelines for preventive health care. It was also consistent with the government's own fears of the political ramifications of deinsuring such a commonly offered service. In the end, eight cosmetic and reproductive procedures were delisted, and the issue of further reductions in coverage remained on the agenda.

More generally, by the late 1990s some services had been identified under government–profession agreements as "medically unnecessary" and accordingly removed from coverage under the public plan in eight provinces; the issue continued to be under active negotiation between governments and professional bodies in at least five provinces (Hurley et al. 1997). But the impact on service and on government budgets was marginal. Target savings through delisting met or under consideration by 1997 amounted to 2% or less of the respective provincial governments' expenditures on physician services.

### Clinical guidelines and the role of clinical judgment

The attempt to identify medically unnecessary services was inextricably entwined with the broader question of identifying efficacious modes of practice and shaping clinical practice accordingly. The issue of the developing of clinical protocols to guide professional practice had been of periodic and specialized interest throughout the 1970s and 1980s, but, as in the United States and Britain, it rose rapidly on the agenda in Canada in the late 1980s and 1990s. As noted, professional bodies such as the College of Physicians and Surgeons and the OMA in Ontario sought to preempt governmental involvement in this area. Most provincial governments, however, chose not to defer entirely to professional bodies as their agents in the matter but rather to establish joint profession–government or specialized arm's-length bodies to develop clinical guidelines.

In the late 1980s and early 1990s, several provinces established advisory mechanisms of "technology assessment" as arm's-length bodies to be liaisons with hospital and professional bodies as well as with governments (Feeny 1994). With two important exceptions, however, these bodies did not issue clinical guidelines. The first of these exceptions was the Task Force on the Use and Provision of Medical Services established in Ontario in 1988, with bipartite representation from the provincial government (including one representative from the finance ministry) and the OMA, and chaired by a practicing lawyer and former deputy minister of health. The task force issued two sets of guidelines, one for the testing for and treatment of high blood cholesterol levels and one for thyroid testing, before it gave way to another mechanism to be discussed shortly. In the case of thyroid testing, the guidelines, although voluntary for physicians, were reinforced by the government's decision to reduce payments to commercial laboratories and subsequently to entirely delist three tests not recommended by the task force. Utilization rates for these tests had dropped to 10% of their former level two years later (Rappolt 1996: 150). The cholesterol guidelines, however, were not backed up by financial incentives, and compliance was much lower (Rappolt 1996: 145–46). The task force process, moreover, exacerbated tensions within the OMA, between specialty groups, and between academic and community-based physicians (Linton and Naylor 1990). Under a 1991 agreement between the OMA and the provincial government, the role of the task force was subsumed by a Joint Management Committee (JMC) with equal representation from the OMA and government, as will be further discussed below. Under the aegis of the JMC, an academically based Institute for Clinical Evaluative Sciences (ICES) was established to, among other things, conduct research relevant to the development of clinical guidelines that might be issued by the JMC. As we shall see, however, the JMC process was stalemated and then derailed over a period of several years by the imposition of a firm physician-services budget cap together with budget reductions in the mid-1990s.

A second attempt to establish a body mandated to develop and issue practice guidelines was more successful. In Saskatchewan a Health Services Utilization and Research Commission (HSURC) was established in 1992, funded by government but at arm's length. Of its twelve members, five (including the chairperson) were physicians—one of whom represented the College of Physicians and Surgeons. Five members had academic affiliations. Between 1992 and 1997, the HSURC issued guidelines on thyroid, prostate specific antigen (PSA), and cholesterol testing; routine testing on admission to hospitals; electrocardiograms; prenatal ultrasound; and cervical cancer screening. Although these guidelines were voluntary, they did appear to have an impact on utilization. Utilization of tests for which guidelines were issued showed declines of between 10% and more than 30% in the year following publication (Health Services Utilization and Research Commission 1995). In British Columbia, an undertaking to develop clinical guidelines backed by legislation and fiscal sanctions formed part of an agreement negotiated between the British Columbia Medical Association and the provincial government in August 1993. No such guidelines were developed, however.

A wide variety of guidelines, of course, was developed by various professional bodies. But most surveys suggest, in Canada and other nations, that compliance with such voluntary guidelines was modest. It was likely to be greatest when guidelines were championed and explained at the individual level by local opinion leaders (Oxman et al. 1995). But this process was extremely labor intensive, and government and professional associations in Canada were reluctant to bear the cost (Rappolt 1996: 173–75). Nor, with very few exceptions such as Ontario's delisting of certain thyroid tests, did governments tie compliance with clinical guidelines to remuneration—notwithstanding the information capacity of a fee-for-service remuneration system to monitor the provision of discrete services. The requirement to seek prior approval for the delivery of a service, for example, was limited to a tiny number of procedures—notably services such as neonatal circumcision that were delisted except in particular circumstances.

Clinical guidelines, in short, played a minimal role in the funding of physician services and a modest role in clinical practice itself in Canada. Attempts to develop such guidelines, however, were a periodic significant source of intra-professional and profession–government conflict. This conflict appeared to be less under mechanisms that had strong professional input but that functioned at arm's length from professional as well as governmental bodies—a point to which I shall return shortly.

### Alternative payment mechanisms and organizational forms

A final effect of the pressure of global budgets for physician services on the policy agenda was an increased interest in forms of medical remuneration other than fee-for-service. Capitation or salaried forms of remuneration promised escape from the invidious dynamics of competition among fee-for-service practitioners under a global cap. This effect was first apparent in Quebec. For several years after the adoption of global budget limits for general practitioners and specialists in 1976 and 1977, the Quebec government attempted to develop a universal salaried structure for physician remuneration. This attempt was abandoned in 1982, but during the 1980s there was a growing interest among physicians in forms of remuneration other than fee-for-service; salaried and various "hybrid" forms of remuneration were increasingly adopted through negotiation, although the fee-for-service mode remained predominant (Lomas et al. 1992: 100).

Quebec was the province in which not only alternative payment schemes but also organizational alternatives to private fee-for-service practice were most advanced. Local Community Service Centers (CLSCs) had been in existence since the 1970s as nonprofit organizations governed by community boards and providing a range of primary health care and social services with a preventive focus. They received grants from the provincial government to serve a geographically defined community and employed physicians and other personnel on a primarily salaried basis. Fewer than 10% of Quebec physicians, however, practiced in CLSCs. And alternatives to private fee-for-service practice were even less prevalent in other provinces. Grant-funded community health centers existed in Alberta, Saskatchewan, and Ontario, often targeted at less advantaged populations. Like the CLSCs they took a broad approach to preventive health measures, engaging not only in primary health care but in some cases also in community development. Again, however, they covered only tiny fractions of the population and of practicing physicians. Finally, in Ontario, capitation-based Health Service Organizations (HSOs) had existed since the 1970s as perennial pilot projects. Most were, in fact, physician group practices that had opted for capitation-based rather than fee-for-service funding. But HSOs and community clinics together covered less than 5% of the Ontario population by the end of the 1980s (Tuohy 1992: 128).

As other provinces followed Quebec in adopting global caps on physician services budgets, they also experienced a "rush of interest from within the medical profession in alternative payment mechanisms such as sessional fees in low-volume emergency rooms, salaries for academic faculty, and capitation for primary care physicians" (Barer et al. 1996: 225). "Alternative payment plans," essentially salaried systems of varying degrees of complexity, were introduced in a number of medical schools in the 1990s. In the primary care field, interest in a British-style rostering and capitation system began to ignite as well. In 1995, an advisory committee to the Federal/Provincial/Territorial Conference of Deputy Ministers of Health recommended a capitation-based model of "primary health care organizations" (PCOs). Each PCO would serve a defined population of patients on its "roster" and would employ physicians and other health care personnel. It would be funded on the basis of capitation, adjusted for the age, sex, and other risk-related characteristics of its population (Advisory Committee on Health Services 1995).

The advisory committee report fueled the growing debate between and among medical associations and governments, as well as public concerns, about the desirability and the appropriate design of alternative payment and delivery mechanisms in primary care (Lomas et al. 1995; Schurman 1997). Professional associations resisted the notion of employment of physicians by PCOs, and some responded with alternative models. Indeed, the Canadian College of Family Physicians had been pressing for alternatives to fee-for-service before the advisory committee report, and continued to advocate its own version of a "blended funding mechanism." A discussion paper jointly prepared by the ministry of health and the medical association in New Brunswick was issued in 1995. Provincial medical associations in British Columbia, Alberta, and Ontario also issued their own reports. The Ontario Medical Association, for example, developed a model of primary care practices in which physicians would be paid on a fee-for-service basis up to a "benchmark threshold," above which they would be paid only for certain services such as obstetrics and anesthesia (Primary Care Reform Advisory Group 1996). This proposed approach differed from the existing individual billing thresholds in two important respects: the threshold would be based on the size and characteristics of the rostered population, and billings above the threshold (except for excluded services) would be denied, not simply prorated.

Several barriers to the adoption of some form of capitation-based funding for primary care existed, however. Governments were wary of the public reaction to what would likely be perceived as a restriction of patient choice of physician on a per-episode basis, even though most Canadians had fairly stable relationships with primary-care physicians (Lomas et al. 1995). Medical associations, for their part, insisted that funding for experimentation with alternative payment mechanisms not be withdrawn from the capped fee-for-service pool. Provincial governments gave a tepid reaction to the advisory committee report (previously described) and requested the committee to engage in further national consultation. The committee's final report in 1996 reflected a recognition that each province would chart its own course (Schurman 1997: 6). As of 1997, it appeared that those courses would involve limited experimentation for the foreseeable future. In 1997, for example, the Ontario government appointed the family physician who had chaired the OMA Primary Care Reform Advisory Group to chair an implementation steering committee to pilot test at least two capitation and roster-based models of primary care. The Nova Scotia government issued a discussion paper proposing a capitation-based rostered model. In response to the National Health Forum's support of experimentation with population-based funding for primary care as discussed in chapter 3, moreover, a federal "transition" fund was established to support pilot projects.

If organizational change was limited in the primary care arena, it was almost nonexistent regarding the development of vertically integrated systems. Such change was, however, a gleam in the eyes of various participants in the health care arena. Toward the end of the 1990s the development of "integrated delivery systems"—linking the full spectrum of preventive, primary, secondary, tertiary, and quaternary care—was much discussed in policy circles. Such models opened up the possibility of new loci of control in the health system, and various groups competed to advance their preferred models. Organized nursing, for example, had since the 1970s been promoting health care reform based on community health centers in which nonphysician personnel would play larger roles (Tuohy 1992: 146–47). Hospitals, for their part, took a particular interest in vertically-integrated models: "Hospitals . . . see that vertical integration offers potential for increasing their revenues at a time of fiscal constraint. By controlling these new health care organizations . . . they gain access to pooled funding from primary, secondary and tertiary care budgets that were previously insulated from each other" (Lomas et al. 1995: 1318). Private financial interests began to see investment opportunities in entities that would provide management services to large-scale integrated organizations (Lomas et al. 1995: 318). Even organized medicine, which had long resisted large-scale organizational reforms to the health care system in favor of advocating increased funding, either public or private or both, for the existing system, began to seek to frame the agenda of organizational change, as will be more fully discussed later in this chapter.

Despite this growing interest, no significant policy change had occurred by the late 1990s. Governments continued to be wary of changes to the long-established system, particularly if they could achieve their fiscal targets without them. One of the unforeseen consequences of global funding for fee-for-service physicians, moreover, was that it tended to "entrench or insulate a pool of fee-for-service funds" (Barer et al. 1996: 225) and hence deprive governments of the fiscal latitude necessary for experimentation. The forum for conflict and accommodation over new delivery mechanisms, then, inevitably shifted back to the profession–government table.

## Information and Information Technology

One of the puzzles of the Canadian case, especially in comparison with the United States, is why the development of highly sophisticated databases of medical and hospital services, accessible to government payers, did not prove more destabilizing to the structural balance of the system. The Canadian single-payer, fee-for-service system generated databases regarding the delivery of medical services that were among the most comprehensive anywhere. For each provincial health insurance agency, the payment system produced a computerized set of records comprising every service billed by every doctor in the province. Given the comprehensiveness of public coverage for medical services and the absence of private alternatives to public coverage, these records cap-tured the vast bulk of medical services delivered in each province.[17]

In the hospital sector, global budgeting since the 1970s meant that data on service delivery were not routinely generated in the course of payment. Nonetheless, extensive databases were generated through voluntary coopera-tion among medical and hospital associations and provincial governments. As early as 1963, the Ontario Medical Association and the Ontario Hospital Asso-ciation entered into partnership to form the Hospital Medical Records Insti-tute (HMRI). In 1977, HMRI became a national, not-for-profit corporation governed through a structure of provincial "user group committees" including government, hospital and medical representatives, health record professionals, and academic researchers (Yungblut 1992: 195). The HMRI database was built up from "abstracts" submitted by hospitals. Abstracts were data records of indi-vidual cases, prepared at the time of discharge according to HMRI reporting criteria. By the early 1990s, the HMRI database was arguably one of the most comprehensive of its kind in the world (Suttie 1998: 13) and contained ab-stracts representing more than 75% of all acute care discharges from Canadian hospitals (Yungblut 1992: 196). The Quebec government maintained a separate database of hospital discharge summaries using somewhat different reporting criteria (Sicotte et al. 1992: 237), with the result that fewer than one-third of Quebec hospitals submitted data to the HMRI (Suttie 1988: 37).

The primary use of the HMRI database throughout the 1970s and 1980s was in support of utilization review activities at the level of the individual hos-pital. The HMRI produced both standard and customized reports that allowed a hospital to compare its utilization profile with peer institutions on dimensions such as length of stay or emergency admissions. Utilization review at the hospi-tal level was generally structured as a joint undertaking of the hospital adminis-tration and the medical staff. The particular structures varied across hospitals, as did the capacity to comprehend and utilize HMRI data. In a survey of utiliza-tion review committees in twenty large Ontario hospitals in the late 1980s, for example, three-quarters of the committee chairpersons reported that HMRI data were underused, primarily because of a lack of understanding among physicians as to how to use the data (Suttie 1988: 17).

The HMRI database, as well as the provincial databases on medical services, provided rich mines for health service researchers. University-based centers in British Columbia, Manitoba, Ontario, and Quebec in particular were major contributors to the international literature of clinical epidemiology. In some cases, moreover, these databases were augmented through linkages with others to produce comprehensive population-based data incorporating socioeconomic as well as health service data (Roos et al. 1995).

Despite international recognition of the quality of the databases, however, payers were very slow to use these resources to structure mechanisms of pay-ment. As we have seen, utilization review based on the physician services data-base was targeted at extreme outliers. As for the hospital sector, systems of global budgeting did not even begin to exploit the potential of the HMRI database until well into the 1990s. In the mid-1980s, the concept of the Diagnosis Related Group (DRG), which related resource use to clinical diagnosis, was being adopted as the foundation for the Prospective Payment System of hospital reimbursement under Medicare in the United States with far-reaching consequences; the HMRI developed an analogous measure, the Case Mix Group (CMG). But unlike DRGs in the United States, CMGs did not become foundational to hospital reimbursement in Canada. CMG data were used by individual hospitals for purposes of internal management, but as previously noted provincial governments began to experiment with introducing case-based components to global funding formulas only in the 1990s—and then only in certain provinces, in limited form, through negotiation with hospital associations and with considerable caution. There was, indeed, considerable skepticism about the potential for CMG-based mechanisms to increase transaction costs and to be susceptible to manipulation (Soderstrom 1994: 248–49).

In summary, the substantial databases generated by the Canadian system were not, by and large, used to countervail the information advantage traditionally enjoyed by the medical profession. Rather, they were absorbed as resources into the ongoing accommodations between provincial governments and providers of medical and hospital services, which relied upon global caps rather than detailed prescription as the mechanism of cost control.

## Changing Profession–Government Relations and the Impact on Organized Medicine

As noted at the beginning of this chapter, the style of profession–government relations began to converge across provinces in the 1990s (Lomas et al. 1992). In provinces with adversarial styles and narrowly focused formalized collective bargaining mechanisms, the scope of discussions was expanded and various arrangements for "co-management" were put in place. In provinces in which the style of accommodation had been more informal and collaborative, arrangements were formalized, also to embrace a broader scope of discussions and to institute co-management structures. The only province in which the arrangements remained relatively unchanged was Quebec, in which a system of permanent, formalized negotiations—whose broad scope effectively made the negotiating table a co-management forum—had already been instituted in the early 1980s.

Coincident or nearly coincident with the introduction of global budgeting for physician services, bipartite joint management committees with equal representation from government (including in most cases a representative of the finance ministry[18]) and the medical association were established in Alberta, British Columbia, New Brunswick, Newfoundland, Nova Scotia, Ontario, and Prince Edward Island. These arrangements formalized and arguably expanded the influence of the medical profession in policy-making, but they also involved the provincial medical associations in controversial decisions that led to fissurous tendencies within their memberships. Again, a closer review of experience in Quebec, British Columbia, and Ontario can illustrate some of these dynamics.

In Quebec, a permanent discussion/negotiation process was established in the early 1980s between the government and each of the two medical associations—the federation of specialist organizations, the Fédération des Médecins Spécialistes du Québec (FMSQ), and the general practitioners organization, the Fédération des Médecins Omnipraticiens du Québec (FMOQ). These negotiations were much more detailed and comprehensive than those undertaken elsewhere in Canada; they involved not just the overall level percentage increase in the fee schedule but the structure of the fee schedule itself, including the value of specific items. Indeed, in the early 1980s it was agreed to tie the rate of increase in medical target incomes (taking into account both fee schedule and utilization increases, as previously described) to the rate of increase of public sector wages generally. Thus one of the major preoccupations of negotiators in other provinces was effectively removed from the table in Quebec. Rather, negotiations involved the allocation of increases among fee schedule items, re-allocations within the fee schedule, arrangements for modes of remuneration other than fee-for-service, and a host of specific arrangements. As Lomas et al. (1992) note, "the flexible approach to what is considered a monetary issue [and hence subject to negotiation] allows parties to address policy issues such as solving under-serviced-area problems, or encouraging after-hours or home care services" (91).

As comprehensive as these negotiations were, they did not exhaust the extent of the profession–state accommodation. Issues of clinical effectiveness, including the development of practice guidelines, were dealt with by the professional regulatory body, the Corporation Professionnelle des Médecins du Québec. Physicians were, moreover, formally represented on the network of regional and local health planning and management bodies described in chapter 3, and, together with health care administrators, tended to exercise the dominant influence on those bodies (Desrosiers 1986: 214–15).

There were some points of intraprofessional and profession–state conflict in these arrangements. The specialist federation in particular was beset by internal divisions. The general surgeons' association split from the federation from 1986 to 1991; and two other groups threatened to do so—anesthesiologists in 1990 and radiologists in 1986 (Hurley et al. 1997). In 1995, the provincial government acted unilaterally by cabinet order to firm up its global caps on the GP and specialist budgets by no longer adjusting them for increases in physician supply. Cuts to the health care budget in 1996 triggered a one-day withdrawal of service, called by the FMSQ and the FMOQ as well as the associations of interns and residents and medical students. Despite these periodic conflicts, however, the structure of the profession–state accommodation in Quebec was relatively stable over the course of the 1980s and 1990s.

In British Columbia, profession–state relations evolved fairly rapidly after the introduction of a global budget for physician services in 1985. A number of special-purpose joint profession–government committees were established to deal with issues such as the monitoring of utilization, and some committees of the British Columbia Medical Association (BCMA) were designated as advisory to the Medical Services Commission which administered medicare in British Columbia (Hurley et al. 1997). In 1993, sweeping changes were made by negotiated agreement. The Medical Services Commission was restructured to become a tripartite body, with one-third of its membership from the government, one-third from the BCMA, and one-third as government-appointed "public" representatives. The 1993 agreement also made ambitious provisions for both government and the profession to be responsible for finding savings within the health care budget. These latter provisions proved impracticable and were dropped from the 1996 agreement. That agreement left the profession fully at risk for expenditures above the global budget cap, but it also gave the BCMA "significant responsibility to develop management initiatives to control utilization"—greater than that accorded to a professional association in any other province (Hurley et al. 1997).

Relationships between the BCMA and the provincial government were not without conflict. In 1992–1993 the government threatened to impose individual billing thresholds unilaterally, but the relevant legislation was allowed to die. In the mid-1990s, the BCMA faced considerable dissent from within its own ranks. These divisions led the BCMA to test another model—certification as a trade union—in 1993. The certification option was defeated by a 63% majority, but it continued to be pursued by a least one specialty group. And interspecialty rivalries, exacerbated under the global budget cap, stimulated but ultimately frustrated an attempt to implement a fee schedule revision based on a Relative Value scale.

Conflicts in British Columbia, however, paled in comparison to those in Ontario—an ironic contrast given the traditionally more congenial relations between the medical profession and the government in the latter province. Ontario had employed a relatively distributed and articulated model of profession–state accommodation. One component of these arrangements was the relationship of collective bargaining with the OMA, formalized along the lines of an adversarial model. The government also relied on the regulatory body, the CPSO, for the review of the practice profiles with aberrant billing levels. And it also established a range of standing and ad hoc advisory bodies, drawing heavily upon academically based physicians (Tuohy 1992: 126–27).

The first major rupture in this relationship occurred around the banning of extra billing in Ontario in the wake of the Canada Health Act, as discussed in chapter 3. But in the distributed, multinodal model of accommodation that prevailed, this rupture affected OMA–government relations but not the entire profession–state accommodation. Even as OMA and government representatives struggled to repair the breach, other mechanisms of accommodation were available. The premier's Council on Health Strategy established by the Liberal government in 1986, for example, was chaired by the premier and composed of thirty-one members drawn from the provincial cabinet; the medical profession; other health disciplines; and business, labor, and consumer groups. Of the eight medical members, all had academic appointments (not including the deputy minister of health, a former academic physician, who sat on the Council as secretary (Tuohy 1992: 127). This body, together with a number of issue-specific task forces, continued the accommodation with the strategic minority of academically based physicians already discussed. With the accession of several academically based physicians to the executive committee of the OMA in the late 1980s, moreover, a rapprochement with government was attempted on issues such as clinical guidelines.

The breach between the government and the OMA, however, was not healed until 1991, under the social–democratic NDP government that replaced the Liberals in 1990. In the process of reconciliation, the distributed model of accommodation was essentially abandoned. A wideranging "framework agreement" was reached between the government and the OMA, which recognized the OMA as the sole representative of fee-for-service physicians for purposes of collective bargaining and provided for an automatic checkoff of OMA dues from the billings of fee-for-service physicians, regardless of whether they were members of the association. (Similar agreements were in place or about to be put in place in six other provinces.) As previously noted, a Joint Management Committee was formed between the government and the OMA, and under its aegis an Institute for Clinical Evaluative Sciences was established, based at a Toronto teaching hospital, to conduct research to inform the decisions of the JMC about utilization management, deinsurance options, and other aspects of the health care delivery system.

The prospects for OMA–government collaboration were greatly dimmed two years later, however. As part of a broad strategy to reduce public expenditures, the NDP government introduced legislation giving it broad unilateral powers to deinsure services, and to limit payments under the government health insurance plan on the basis of the utilization profile of the patient, the practitioner, or the facility involved.[19] The OMA reacted strongly and vociferously against these provisions, accusing the government of preempting the Joint Management Committee process. The government, for its part, stated that the legislative provisions constituted a "fail-safe" measure, to take effect only if a negotiated agreement with the OMA could not be reached. In the result, the OMA and the government reached agreement on a range of cost-control measures, including a three-year freeze on medical fees and a firm cap on total physicians' billings. The JMC process for determining which services were to be deinsured was reinstated, tied to tighter deadlines, given a set dollar volume (C\$20 million) by which billings were to be reduced through deinsurance, and augmented by an advisory panel including "members of the public" as well as medical and governmental representatives.

The approach taken by the NDP to the profession–state accommodation represented a sharp departure from the past. Rather than a distributed model according an important ongoing role to academic physicians, the NDP government's approach, shaped by a fundamental respect for trade unions, was to deal primarily with the OMA as the legitimate "bargaining agent" for the profession. For the first time a body central to the profession–state relationship, the JMC, had no academically based medical members.

This new accommodation between the OMA and the provincial government in Ontario was not without controversy within the profession. A minority body of opinion within the profession held that the OMA was too concerned with the preservation and enhancement of the power of organized medicine at the expense of the autonomy of the individual physician. The automatic checkoff of membership dues to the OMA was strongly contested by this minority.

The sole focus on the medical association, using the trade union model, not only left the process at the mercy of the volatile politics of the OMA, but also bore bitter and ironic fruit when the NDP government was replaced in 1995 by a Conservative government with a decidedly right-wing agenda, including a deep suspicion of trade unions. The OMA was stunned to find itself treated, in kind if not in degree, with similar suspicion. The JMC process had been sputtering to a halt even before the election, and the new Conservative government, as part of its own expenditure control package introduced in November 1995, revoked the Framework Agreement with the OMA, withdrew recognition from the OMA as the bargaining agent, disbanded the JMC, and gave the minister and the Cabinet unprecedented discretionary powers over the medical fee schedule and the supply and distribution of physicians. (The Health Services Restructuring Commission, discussed in chapter 3, was also created pursuant to that legislation.)

What followed was a period of intense conflict between the OMA and the government, and within the OMA itself. "Coalitions" of specialists and family practitioners split off from the OMA and threatened various levels of withdrawal of service over the course of 1996. A tentative agreement reached between the OMA and government in the fall of 1996 was rejected by a vote of the membership.[20] Finally, in January 1997, an "interim" agreement was reached, followed by a final agreement in May 1997. In addition to increases to the physician services budget, the agreement reinstated the recognition of the OMA as the bargaining agent for fee-for-service physicians and for physicians under other remuneration modes at their request; the government also made provisions for a number of joint committees with mandates covering a wide range of issues related to health care delivery, scope of coverage, clinical guidelines, etc. While still under the aegis of an agreement with the OMA, these provisions promised a movement in the direction of the multinodal model of accommodation of the 1970s and 1980s.

The experiences of Quebec, British Columbia, and Ontario highlight a number of features of the evolution of the profession–state accommodation in Canada in the 1990s. First, they suggest that governments were more willing to flex their legislative muscle to take unilateral action if necessary, but more typically to establish a "shadow" within which their negotiations with the profession would proceed. Second, they illustrate the continuing variety of types of accommodation even as provinces converged toward a model of formalized arrangements with comprehensive agendas. In Quebec, the relatively stable politics of the two medical federations and the resulting longevity of the membership of negotiating teams (Lomas et al. 1992: 98), as well as the existence of a network of accommodation with several nodes, gave an overall stability to the relationship. In Ontario, the more volatile politics of the OMA made a multinodal relationship even more important for stability, and the abandonment of the distributed model in favor of a sole focus on the OMA–government relationship in the 1990s had a highly destabilizing effect. In British Columbia, however, a uninodal model of accommodation between the medical association and the government was relatively successfully maintained and extended—a result largely of the legacy of the collective bargaining approach in the 1970s and 1980s, which had yielded British Columbia physicians the highest levels of tangible benefits in Canada while providing a framework for pragmatic collaboration. None of these models, for better or worse, was likely transferable across provinces. Each had evolved in a context shaped by broader features of the political cultures and political economies of the three provinces: Quebec's indigenous corporatism, the high salience of adversarial models in British Columbia's polarized political system, and the turbulence of Ontario politics after a four-decade-long unbroken string of pragmatic and managerially oriented Conservative governments gave way after 1985 to a succession of governments of widely varying partisan complexions.

Finally, a third feature of the profession–state accommodation highlighted by this three-province review is the enormous pressure placed on medical associations to manage internal conflict as the policy agenda expanded and public spending contracted (Katz et al. 1997). In all three provinces medical associations faced challenges from subgroups within their memberships. Toward the end of the 1990s, a real question existed as to whether the profession–state accommodation at the core of Canadian medicare could be maintained. To explore this question further, we need to summarize the logic of that accommodation, and its relevance to the policy agenda of the late 1990s.

## The Logic of the Profession–State Accommodation

The logic of the profession–state accommodation under Canadian medicare begins with the policy decision in the 1960s not to change the design of the system of delivery of medical and hospital services but rather to underwrite its costs. This decision made political sense, as was evident from its embrace by all political parties at the federal level. It did not incur the political risks of disrupting the established delivery system. Nor, in the buoyant economic times of the 1960s, did such disruption appear to be necessary. As public support for the medicare program built dramatically over time, moreover, governments had continuing incentives to maintain the delivery system of private fee-for-service practice (allowing maximum freedom of choice of physician by patient and vice versa) and public and voluntary hospitals.

If the state were to undertake to manage such a decentralized system, however, it would have to build up a substantial capacity for information gathering and analysis, decision-making, and communication—a capacity that would entail not only economic but also political costs. Instead, governments chose an approach that had both the appearance and the reality of being less interventionist and costly: they came to accommodations with the medical profession that provided that the system would be "managed" through professional networks within broad budgetary parameters established by the state. One result of this approach was that Canada incurred one of the lowest levels of administrative costs among OECD nations, as noted in chapter 6. Although the OECD data need to be treated with some caution, this finding is reinforced by more focused comparisons with the United States. As Evans and his colleagues have noted, Canadian public insurers in contrast to American private insurers faced "no marketing expenses, no costs of estimating risk status in order to set differential premiums or decide whom to cover, and no allocation for shareholder profits; the process of claims payment, although not free of costs, is greatly simplified and much cheaper" (Evans et al. 1989: 573). For Canadian providers, moreover, the single-payer system meant less administrative overhead; in 1987, for example, office expenses for physicians in Canada amounted on average to about 36% of their gross billings, compared with 48% in the United States (General Accounting Office 1991: 5). The General Accounting Office of the United States Congress estimated that differences in insurers' overhead accounted for about 17% of the difference in cost between the two systems in the late 1980s (General Accounting Office 1991: 29). Others estimated that if provider overheads related to the costs of the multipayer system in the United States were included, differences in administrative costs accounted for more than one-half the difference in cost between the two systems (Evans et al. 1989: 573).

Lower administrative overheads were not all that Canadian physicians gained from their accommodation with the state. Indeed, for most groups of specialists that advantage was more than outweighed by lower gross incomes. The main advantage to the medical profession from its accommodation with the state was the preservation of clinical autonomy. Canadian physicians were aware of the different trade-offs that underlay the Canadian and American systems.[21] Even in briefs critical of government policy, medical associations typically presented the Canadian system as one of the best in the world, while expressing some concerns about its future (Tuohy 1992:144–45). The twin specters of the U.S. system (intrusive regulation, corporate dominance, inadequate coverage) and the British system (inadequate resources, excessive rationing) were frequently evoked. Attitude surveys of physicians found large majorities on balance satisfied with their conditions of practice and positively oriented toward medicare—although sizable pockets of discontent remained. A 1986 survey of Canadian physicians, for example, found less than one-quarter dissatisfied with medical practice and less than one-third dissatisfied with the functioning of medicare. Sixty percent believed that medicare had positively influenced health status, but 75% believed that it had reduced the individual's personal sense of responsibility for health (Stevenson et al. 1987). Rank-and-file members and nonmembers of medical associations were, moreover, even more favorably disposed to medicare on balance than were members of medical association executives.

Polls taken in the mid-1990s, as restraint policies began to bite, reveal a profession continuing to wrestle with these trade-offs. In 1994, a survey of Ontario physicians conducted by the OMA revealed overall levels of satisfaction with the system very comparable to those found by Blendon among Canadian physicians three years earlier.[22] There was significant support, however, for the expansion of the scope of private sources of finance for the system. Eighty-one percent of respondents were "very" or "somewhat" supportive of "allow[ing] private funds (e.g., private insurance, individual payments) to be used to pay for services currently covered under medicare" (Sullivan et al. 1995: 24). This option was more likely interpreted to refer to "delisting" than to the reinstatement of extra billing. While 84% were supportive of charging user fees for nonessential uses of hospital emergency rooms, only a bare majority supported the option of charging user fees for physician visits with the revenue retained by the physician. (This contrasts with a finding of 62% support for the reestablishment of the right to extra bill among Ontario physicians eight years earlier [Stevenson et al. 1987].) Furthermore, although only one-third of respondents supported the cap on the physician services budget, this was a higher level of support than for cost-containment strategies such as limiting certain types of surgical procedures or allowing an increased scope of practice for nurses (Sullivan et al. 1995: 25). The American and British systems continued to loom as negative reference points: only 12% of respondents were even "somewhat" supportive of the U.S. model, and only 20 percent were at least somewhat supportive of the British model.

A Canadian Medical Association survey also taken in 1994 contrasted the attitudes of physicians practicing in Canada with those of physicians who had trained or practiced in Canada but who were currently practicing in the United States. Physicians in Canada were significantly more likely than those in the United States to cite clinical autonomy as a major factor in their decision to practice in Canada or the United States, respectively. About 60% of physicians in Canada expressed satisfaction with this dimension of their practice—a level considerably higher than that expressed by U.S. physicians in polls discussed in chapter 5. But surprisingly, the U.S.-based physicians in the CMA survey were even more satisfied with the levels of clinical autonomy they experienced in their practices, with 80% reporting satisfaction. It is likely, however, that the subset of physicians who left Canada for practice in the United States constituted a very distinctive group. Highly remunerative specialties such as orthopedic surgery and cardiothoracic surgery were substantially overrepresented in this group, and they were likely to have negotiated very favorable terms of employment (McKendry et al. 1996).[23]

Such grass-roots restiveness was reflected and magnified in the positions taken by medical associations in the mid-1990s. Over the course of four annual meetings from 1994 to 1997, the General Council of the Canadian Medical Association revealed deep divisions and great uncertainty about the extent to which it should press for private alternatives to the publicly funded system. In 1994, a resolution opposing user fees, developed by a CMA working group, was defeated by the council. In 1995, however, a resolution proposing the development of a private parallel system was defeated. In 1996, a welter of contradictory resolutions was passed. The council unanimously endorsed a resolution that the CMA "should continue to strongly support a publicly funded health-care system," but also supported other resolutions calling for "study," "examination," "discussion," and "debate" of various dimensions of the public–private balance (Coutts 1996).

Events in Ontario, with 40% of Canada's physicians, may have contributed strongly to this ferment. Following the (at least temporary) resolution of that conflict in 1997, the CMA (at least temporarily) abandoned its flirtation with private options. In a 1998 brief, the CMA urged the federal government to restore cash transfers through the Canada Health and Social Transfer (CHST) to 1996–1997 levels (i.e., C$15 billion, as opposed to the government's C$12.5 billion commitment) and to index the transfers to inflation (Canadian Medical Association 1998a). At the 1998 CMA annual meeting, references to private insurance were absent from the agenda. Instead the CMA passed a variety of resolutions deploring the effects of the withdrawal of federal funding, reiterating its call for the federal government to restore funding for health care through the CHST, urging the federal government to "invest in the development of an independent clinically-based measurement system to monitor and evalute access to quality health care and other performance indicators of the health care system" and taking the position that the CMA should "continue to advocate for public access to quality medical care as an integral and essential component of health care" (Canadian Medical Association 1998b).

The logic of the Canadian accommodation hence contained its own ironies and paradoxes. Blunt mechanisms of cost control such as budget caps were chosen precisely because they were consistent with the legacy of the profession–state bargain—that governments would not become closely involved with matters of clinical judgment. But in so doing they shifted risk to the providers—and in Canada's single-payer system there was nowhere for providers to shift risk in turn. And as professional bodies were required to manage that risk, they faced internal pressures that impaired their ability to do so. Toward the end of the 1990s, in adjusting to capped budgets, provincial governments and professional associations appeared to have negotiated the worst of the rocky shoals that the unfolding of the logic of their accommodation had required them to navigate. But the future course was far from clear.

## Institutional and Structural Change in a Single-Payer System

The relative structural stability of the Canadian system is illustrated in part by tables 7.2 and 7.3. The persistence of the accommodation between the medical profession and the state is reflected in the constant share of total health expenditures going to physicians between 1975 and 1996, even as the hospital share substantially declined. Funding for physician services remained almost totally public throughout that period. As for the public–private balance, what is often referred to as the "passive privatization" of the Canadian system needs to be treated on a disaggregated basis. The public share increased in all categories of expenditure except hospitals and other institutions between 1975 and 1996. (The decline of the public share in the hospital category does not reflect the rise of private hospitals, but rather the fact that publicly funded hospitals sought other sources of revenue including ancillaries and philanthropy, as well as increased charges for amenities such as private accommodation, as public funding declined. This substitution of private for public revenue was much less

TABLE 7.2 Percentage Distribution of Total Real[a] Health Care Expenditure by Category, Canada 1975–1996

| Year | Hospitals | Other Institutions | Physicians | Other Professionals | Drugs[b] | Capital | Public Health | Other Expenditures | Total |
|------|-----------|--------------------|------------|---------------------|----------|---------|---------------|--------------------|-------|
| 1975 | 44.0 | 9.2 | 15.0 | 7.3 | 10.2 | 4.4 | 3.8 | 6.1 | 100.0 |
| 1980 | 40.6 | 11.3 | 14.4 | 8.8 | 9.9 | 4.7 | 4.0 | 6.3 | 100.0 |
| 1985 | 39.7 | 10.2 | 15.0 | 8.4 | 10.8 | 4.6 | 4.2 | 7.1 | 100.0 |
| 1990 | 38.2 | 9.3 | 15.3 | 8.3 | 12.4 | 3.7 | 4.4 | 8.5 | 100.0 |
| 1996[c] | 34.9 | 10.0 | 14.9 | 8.3 | 13.9 | 2.5 | 5.2 | 10.5 | 100.0 |

*Source:* Health Canada 1997: table 5.

[a] Deflated by CPI.

[b] Includes drugs provided inside and outside hospital.

[c] Estimate.

than one-to-one, as reflected in the overall decline in the hospital share of total expenditure.)

Nonetheless, the public share overall declined from 76% in 1975 to an estimated 70% in 1996. This shift reflected not a decreased public share by category but a growth in those categories in which, in Canada's segmented system, the private sector plays a relatively larger role: notably pharmaceuticals, non-medical professional services, and "other" expenditures such as home care and various prosthetic devices including eyeglasses and hearing aids. This is in part because of higher levels of price inflation for goods and services offered in private markets. In particular, pharmaceutical price inflation increased at a faster rate during the 1980s than did price inflation for medical and hospital services. Similarly, dental price inflation outpaced medical price inflation.[24] The relative growth of the private sector, however, also reflects the so-called "passive privatization" of services—the effect of decreasing hospital capacity and utilization in a system in which some goods and services (notably pharmaceuticals and some forms of personal care) which are covered by governmental health insurance on an inpatient basis are not covered when provided on an outpatient basis.

Two aspects of this marginal relative growth of the private sector are worth noting. One is the observation, reaffirming cross-national experience, that private markets appear to be less effective than public provision in constraining the costs of health care. The second, however, is the effect of this growth on purchasers in the private sector. Whether or not the growth of the private sector was considered "marginal" depends, after all, on the base of comparison. The private sector share of total health expenditure grew by only a little more than 6 percentage points from the mid-1970s to the mid-1990s. But this represented a 25% increase in the share of the private sector itself. And this expansion had its most concentrated effects on employment-based benefit plans. Accordingly, employers saw their benefit costs rise, and employer organizations increasingly expressed the fear that the competitive advantage they enjoyed by having the costs of health care spread across the tax base would be eroded (MacBride-

TABLE 7.3 Public Share (Percent) of Total Health Care Expenditure by Category, Canada 1975–1996

| Year | Hospitals | Other Institutions | Physicians | Other Professionals | Drugs[a] | Capital | Public Health | Other Expenditures | Total |
|------|-----------|--------------------|------------|---------------------|----------|---------|---------------|--------------------|-------|
| 1975 | 94.1 | 70.8 | 98.5 | 15.0 | 26.0 | 70.3 | 100.0 | 49.4 | 76.4 |
| 1980 | 91.9 | 71.7 | 98.4 | 18.9 | 33.6 | 66.3 | 100.0 | 55.8 | 75.6 |
| 1985 | 90.5 | 74.5 | 98.6 | 18.3 | 37.2 | 77.6 | 100.0 | 54.6 | 75.7 |
| 1990 | 91.2 | 72.4 | 99.0 | 17.3 | 39.4 | 77.0 | 100.0 | 55.8 | 74.6 |
| 1996[b] | 87.7 | 68.1 | 99.0 | 14.3 | 35.2 | 72.4 | 100.0 | 52.6 | 69.9 |

Source: Health Canada 1997: table 8.

[a] Includes drugs provided inside and outside hospital.

[b] Estimate.

King 1995; Alvi 1995).[25] Business coalitions began to form in the 1990s in response to these fears, generally expressing support for the maintenance of the five fundamental principles of Canadian medicare while urging increased use of clinical guidelines, vertically and horizontally integrated delivery systems, and, especially, information systems to support such mechanisms (Employer Committee on Health Care—Ontario 1995).[26] Despite the shift in the public–private balance, however, it remained the case that private financial interests were essentially confined to health care sectors other than medical and hospital services: dental care, pharmaceuticals, prostheses, and nursing homes. Were the federal government to follow through on its proposal to introduce a national pharmacare program, the balance would shift back in the public direction, but in the late 1990s it appeared that such a move would have to await a more propitious federal–provincial climate.

As for the institutional mix in the health care arena, little change occurred. Provincial governments did not develop the capacity for nor incur the transaction costs of closely monitoring or managing the delivery system. Cost constraints, when they came, were accordingly blunt and across the board. Governments did not, by and large, exercise their roles as "purchasers" to specify contracts with providers.[27] Several provinces decentralized governmental authority in order to bring about horizontal integration in the hospital sector. These initiatives maintained the existing balance in the hierarchical, collegial, and market-oriented elements of the system, although they did represent a reorganization of the state hierarchy and a stronger assertion of the role of state actors in the structural balance in health care decision-making systems. Providers, for their part, were concerned with maintaining their own discretion within budget limits. They did not enter into elaborate contracting arrangements with each other nor initiate the development of horizontally or vertically integrated systems.

Nonetheless, as in the United States and Britain, the health care arena in Canada in the 1990s came to be marked by more explicit and comprehensive bargaining among large and relatively sophisticated entities than had been the case in the past. In the Canadian version of this phenomenon, the key actors were provincial governments and medical associations, which both formalized the processes and expanded the focus of their negotiations. In the hospital sector as well, negotiations between provincial government or regional health authorities and restructured, more horizontally integrated hospitals became somewhat more specific. However, historically based funding (with formulaic adjustments), rather than contracts, continued to be the norm.

Whether this relative stability would prove to be resiliency and not brittleness in the face of growing pressures was a major question as Canada approached the twenty-first century. The accommodations that grew up in the medicare context resulted in a system with significant advantages, including broad clinical autonomy for providers, free choice of provider for consumers, low administrative costs, and high levels of public satisfaction. But these accommodations rested on expectations of a continuing rate of increase in public funding that could not be sustained. In the late 1990s, all the participants in the system were adjusting to these changing expectations.

# Conclusion | 8

This book is essentially a work of political science. Nonetheless, it is addressed not only to political scientists but also to others concerned with policy-making about the role of the state in the health care arena. In this concluding chapter, I first summarize the experience of Britain, the United States, and Canada in the health care arena, with particular emphasis on experience in the 1990s, to demonstrate the workings of the process of "accidental logics" that drives the dynamics of change. Forces in the broader political arena have periodically opened windows of opportunity for major policy change in the health care arena in each of these nations. The systems that resulted were largely, if not entirely, "accidents" of the timing of their birth—had windows opened at different times, they might have looked quite different. Between these policy episodes, the systems were shaped by their own internal logics. This analysis then provides the platform from which several concluding observations can be made, looking toward a future marked by accelerating technological change and ongoing policy debate.

## The Health Policy Arena in Britain, the United States, and Canada

The decision-making systems in health care arenas of Britain, the United States, and Canada have been shaped by the timing of major episodes of policy change, which established the policy parameters governing the institutional mix and the structural balance of these systems. The British NHS, as an immediate postwar creation, bears the marks of the centralization and expansion of government authority, as well as the austerity, that characterized the wartime period. It represented major structural and institutional change in the health care system—an expansion of the role of the state and a concomitant decrease in the role of private finance, as well as a comprehensive reorganization of the system into a set of geographically based hierarchies. The major episodes of policy change shaping the Canadian and American systems, in contrast, took place in the boom-times of the 1960s, when an "indemnity insurance" model of health-care financing was more fully developed, and when governments were prepared to underwrite the costs of the existing delivery system without making major organizational changes. Hence the model adopted was one of state-sponsored insurance that greatly expanded the role of the state vis-à-vis private finance and reduced reliance on market mechanisms for the financing of health care, while leaving in place a health care delivery system consisting of myriad independent units. In Canada, this model was adopted to provide universal coverage for all medical and hospital services. In the United States, the politics of the day yielded state-sponsored programs of medical and hospital insurance whose coverage was restricted to certain population groups—the elderly, the disabled, and recipients of public assistance.

In each of these cases, the medical profession continued, at least initially, to play a central role in the decision-making system. In Britain and Canada, the systems were founded upon accommodations or "implicit bargains" between the state and the profession, under which the profession retained clinical autonomy to allocate resources within budgetary parameters established by the state. Collegial mechanisms of decision-making were incorporated within the structures of "hierarchical corporatism" that characterized the British system. In Canada, collegial mechanisms played an even greater role—those that permeated the delivery system prior to the introduction of medicare were left in place, and as state controls on the price and (to a much lesser extent) the volume and mix of medical services were introduced, they were negotiated and implemented through professional organizations.

In the United States, with the persistence of private markets as the predominant mechanism of resource allocation in the financing as well as the delivery of health care, individual physicians retained broad entrepreneurial discretion in the wake of the policy changes of the 1960s. Collegial mechanisms, however, began to wane in significance. Peer review organizations established to examine the utilization of services under governmental programs were plagued by conflicting mandates and professional opposition. And with the rise of various forms of "managed care" in the 1980s and 1990s, medical practice was increasingly governed by contracts between individual physicians (and groups of physicians) and managed care organizations. "Group/staff" managed care organizations maintained a central role for collegial mechanisms, but they accounted for only a small proportion of the plethora of managed care arrangements that came to dominate the U.S. health care market.

As the 1990s approached, then, the British, Canadian, and American health care arenas evinced quite different institutional mixes of hierarchical, market, and collegial mechanisms, and quite different structural balances of influence across state actors, private finance, and the medical profession. Indeed, as argued in chapter 1, these three systems constituted rough approximations of "ideal-typical" cases: Britain marked by a predominance of state actors and hierarchical mechanisms, the United States by private finance and market mechanisms, and Canada by the medical profession and collegial mechanisms. Each system, accordingly, had its own distinctive logic that conditioned change in the system in the 1990s.

In chapter 1, it was pointed out that the experience of these three systems in the 1990s presented a corresponding set of puzzles. Why was it in Britain, a nation that provided comprehensive universal health care coverage to its population at a level of cost that was modest in international perspective, that the most ambitious change in policy parameters was enacted and implemented? Why did the United States, with the least extensive system of coverage against health care costs and the most expensive system of health care delivery, fail to adopt universal health insurance and yet experience dramatic structural and institutional change in the health care arena nonetheless? And why did Canada, one of the most expensive publicly funded health care systems in the world, experience relative stability in the face of strong fiscal pressures?

We can now summarize the contribution of the framework presented in this book, emphasizing the "accidental logics" of change in the health care arena, to the unraveling of these puzzles. Major policy change occurred in Britain in the 1990s because the relatively rare conditions for opening a "window of opportunity" for policy change were present. A majority government in its third successive term had not only the consolidated authority but also the political will to enact policy changes intended to change the institutional mix and the structural balance in the health care arena. Replacing the relationship of managerial authority between Health Authorities and provider units with a relationship of contracting between independent "purchasers" and "providers" represented a pronounced shift from hierarchical to market-type mechanisms in the design of decision-making structures. These changes were intended to change the incentives facing both purchasers and providers in order to enhance the microeconomic efficiency of the system. They were also intended to redress what was perceived to be an imbalance of power in favor of providers and to increase the influence of the state as "purchaser." Notably, although these reforms did potentially provide for greater competition between publicly and privately capitalized providers in both the "internal" and the private market, the changes were not intended to enhance the role of private finance per se—that option had been hotly debated and rejected by the Conservative government in its first term.

The internal logic of the NHS facilitated these changes in some respects, but moderated them in other respects. As a system based on a "state-hierarchical" model, the NHS allowed for the implementation of changes to be ordered and communicated from the top through a series of "guidances" and directives. Ironically, then, the implementation of market-type mechanisms depended upon the existence of a centralized authority structure, and that structure persisted even as the reforms were implemented at the local level. The use of state authority rather than voluntary exchange, moreover, continued to characterize the making of major decisions, most notably the restructuring of the hospital sector in London.

The impact of the internal market reforms was also tempered by the strength of collegial mechanisms. In the hospital sector, resource allocation within budgetary parameters continued to rest with physicians, even as collegial mechanisms became more formalized as "clinical directorates." The linkage of clinical and financial data, which was critical to the writing of specific contracts, was constrained by the persistence of separate managerial and collegial structures for cost accounting and "clinical audit," respectively. The reliance on "block" contracts between purchasers and providers meant that budgetary transfers continued to look more like annual grants (albeit with conditions of various degrees of specificity) than contracts for the purchase of particular services at particular prices. In the general practice sector, collegial relationships between "fundholding" GPs and hospital-based consultants were recast in considerably more marketlike terms by the reforms. But the rise of a variety of mechanisms for the collective involvement of GPs (both fundholding and non-fundholding) in purchasing decisions appeared to be leading to a reconstitution of collegial networks—a direction that was reinforced by the policies of the Labour government that replaced the Conservatives in 1997. In summary, although the "internal market" reforms of the NHS did bring about substantial change in decision-making systems, that change amounted largely to the introduction of explicit bargaining relationships between organized bodies of purchasers and providers—a form of voluntary exchange, but far from an approximation of a competitive market.

Understanding the logic of these developments takes us back to the discussion in chapter 1 of the merits of hierarchical and collegial mechanisms in reducing the transaction costs of decision-making, particularly those relating to information. The traditional decision-making systems in the health care arena dealt with the problem of the substantial information gap between providers and potential recipients of care by establishing agency relationships—both at the level of the individual provider–patient relationship and at the level of the relationship between the medical profession and the state. Under these relationships, potential recipients of care delegated broad decision-making authority to individual professionals, and the state relied on the professional group itself to ensure that its members did not abuse their roles as agents in decision-making about the provision of their own services. In the British system, these "second-level" agency relationships were elaborated through the system of hierarchical corporatism described in chapter 6.

The "internal market" initiative constituted an attempt to introduce a model with high information costs (as necessary for writing specific "contingent claims" contracts between independent units) into a system with fewer information requirements, and well-developed hierarchical and collegial networks for the exchange of information as deemed necessary. Within a budget-limited system, it is not surprising that actors would seek to economize on information costs by continuing to rely on established networks and modes of relationship, particularly when experiments in the 1980s had led to widespread skepticism about the costs and benefits of assembling the information necessary to write sophisticated contracts. Indeed, it is a measure of how thoroughly the reforms were absorbed by the existing system that the Labour party, having vitriolically denounced the reforms at the outset, reinforced the basic features of the reforms when it came to power itself.

The British experience stands in diametric contrast to that of the United States. The Clinton proposal of 1993, while essentially building upon the existing employer-based private insurance system, would have shifted the institutional mix in a somewhat more hierarchical direction through reliance on large-scale organizations on the supply and demand sides of the market, and would have enhanced the role of the state by mandating employer-based coverage meeting federal criteria and by increased regulation of the private insurance market. The British attempt to enact major policy change, by introducing market elements to a state-hierarchical system, was successful—but the American attempt to shift the private market system in a state-hierarchical direction through major policy change failed. Why?

There is no doubt that a number of the protagonists in the saga of American health care reform in the 1990s believed that a window of opportunity for major policy change had opened with the election of Bill Clinton to the presidency in 1992. The Democrats controlled both houses of Congress as well as the presidency, and Clinton had made health care reform a centerpiece of his presidential campaign and his inaugural agenda. And yet, in retrospect, reading these factors as implying that Clinton was in a position to accomplish major policy change appears clearly as an overassessment of the strength of his position. Having received 43% of the popular vote, he could not claim the majority mandate traditionally expected of U.S. presidents. More important, the Democrats had fewer than the sixty seats in the Senate necessary to guard against a variety of procedural maneuvers by the minority Republicans. Although a variety of factors contributed to the demise of health care reform, as discussed in chapter 3, the simple explanation is that Clinton could not command a consolidated base of authority sufficient to achieve such major change. His only hope would have been to create a "bandwagon effect" by moving quickly when the momentum for reform was strong; that possibility was derailed, however, by the need for the president to divide his limited political capital among several key priorities.

In the wake of this policy failure, a version of the shift in institutional mix sought by Clinton was generated by the system itself, as large-scale organizations continued to develop on both supply and demand sides of the health insurance and health care delivery markets. (Indeed, as consistent with the emerging paradigm sketched by Chernichovsky and described in chapter 1, these two markets merged as financing, purchasing, and providing functions melded in various permutations and combinations.) In contrast to the British experience, moreover, a blizzard of highly specific contracting arrangements came to characterize the American arena.

As for the structural balance of influence across state actors, private finance, and the medical profession, the increase in state authority sought by Clinton (and with it the increase in the proportion of the population with coverage against the costs of health care) was generally not achieved, despite some incremental gains at the federal and state levels. Instead, the most dramatic change in the structural balance in the American health care arena was the decline of the influence of the medical profession in the private market-oriented system, and the rise of for-profit private financial interests.

Again, the logic of the American system, with its predominance of private finance and market mechanisms, can explain these rapid shifts in institutional mix and structural balance in the absence of major policy change. The explication of this logic provided in chapter 5 bears some repeating here. Under the traditional system of private fee-for-service medical practice and third-party payment on an "indemnity insurance" basis, physicians exercised dominant influence, both as professional experts and as independent entrepreneurs. In both capacities, they had incentives to provide an intensive level of service, up to the point at which the marginal benefit to the patient was zero. Third-party payers passed along costs in the form of higher premiums, whose costs were in turn diffused in the employer-based and tax-subsidized system.

The persistence of this system in the United States after the 1960s stands in contrast to experience in Britain, and indeed in all other nations in which the state assumed the predominant role in the financing of health care. In those nations, the overall allocation of resources to the health sector and to its various subsectors came not to be determined primarily through health insurance and health care delivery markets, but rather through the processes of political accommodation that characterize the governmental budgetary process. In that context, governments in effect elaborated their "second-level" agency relationships with the medical profession to charge the profession with allocative decisions within governmental budgetary parameters.

In the United States, both the government's proportionate financial role and its redefinition of second-level agency relationships with professional bodies remained much more limited, and professionals continued to exercise their influence both as experts and as entrepreneurs. Meanwhile, however, the conditions for the transformation of the health care arena were taking shape. Though lacking a dominant fiscal presence, the state nonetheless sought to address the equity and efficiency problems of health care delivery and insurance markets (discussed in chapter 1) through regulatory instruments. The resulting complexity gave a competitive advantage to large-scale enterprises, often with a broad geographic span, with the resources to invest in understanding the regulatory environment and responding strategically.

In the 1980s, moreover, the federal government took fiscal action in a way that was to have dramatic consequences: it adopted a payment scheme under Medicare (the Prospective Payment System, or PPS) that limited per-case payment. In response, providers increasingly shifted costs to private payers, who in turn were jolted out of what had been their essentially passive roles. A number of factors were in fact combining to raise the price consciousness of private payers; but the adoption of PPS arguably catalyzed this development, and effectively woke the sleeping dog of private finance. Increasingly, private as well as public payers changed the terms of their reimbursement arrangements with providers to limit payment per case. As cost minimization rather than revenue maximization in individual cases became the route to profit maximization, the implications of the logic of entrepreneurialism and the logic of professionalism began to diverge. And the role of entrepreneur came increasingly to be played by a set of actors once relegated to a relatively minor role in the health care arena—for-profit firms, particularly investor-owned firms. These companies were accountable to shareholders and were relatively unconstrained by commitment to professional objectives or established collegial relationships. With their access to pools of equity capital, and their broad geographic spans as well as their sophistication in dealing with the complex regulatory environment, these for-profit firms rapidly expanded market share in a flurry of mergers and acquisitions in the 1990s.

To compete in the merged markets of health insurance and health care delivery, insurers and providers had to offer "managed care": that is, to provide a full spectrum of health care services for a defined population for a given prepaid amount. In order to do so, the new entrepreneurial intermediaries developed increasingly specific mechanisms for the control of medical practice, relying not on the traditional agency relationships that gave physicians broad discretion but rather on specific contracts or employment relationships within vertically and horizontally integrated organizations. The variety of these mechanisms, and the pace of change in their configuration, was without parallel in any other system.

Finally, how do we explain the Canadian puzzle? What accounts for the relative structural and institutional stability of the Canadian system—in particular the persistent predominance of collegial mechanisms and medical influence—in one of the most costly health care systems in the OECD? Why was no attempt made in the 1990s, in contrast to Britain, the United States, and a significant number of other nations, to change the policy parameters governing the institutional mix and the structural balance of the system? The state, at the level of provincial governments, more strongly asserted its role, particularly in bringing about some horizontal and vertical integration in the hospital sector, and (in all provinces except Ontario) in creating regional health agencies. But independent private fee-for-service medical practice remained the cornerstone of the system; the pattern of care provided was still (with the exception of a very few high-technology procedures) the aggregate of decisions made by individual physicians subject only to norms enforced by collegial bodies at the hospital and provincial level; hospital budgets were still based for the most part on historical experience and across-the-board changes (albeit with some attempt to develop formulas rewarding efficiency in performance) and not on negotiated packages of service. With the exception of the restructuring of hospital facilities, governments relied on the blunt exercise of their monopsony power through budget-capping. They did not take up the contracting mechanisms that have gained popularity in Britain, the United States, and elsewhere.

Bargaining relationships remained essentially between provincial governments and provincial medical associations, and the items on the bargaining table expanded only somewhat beyond the traditional focus on the overall level of medical fees, to include in very nascent terms the issues of the geographic distribution of physicians and, in some provinces, the organization of primary care.

The absence of major policy change affecting the institutional mix and the structural balance of the Canadian system in the 1990s can be understood with reference to the two conditions for such change: the consolidation of political authority and the will to undertake health care reform as a key component of a broader agenda. These factors did not coincide in any relevant jurisdiction in Canada. Consider first the parameters established by the Canada Health Act. That legislation, establishing the criteria for federal financial contributions to provincial medicare plans, significantly constrained the role of private finance in the medical and hospital sectors, as well as the extent to which any market mechanism based on price competition could be put in place even within an "internal market" (Stoddart and Seldon 1983). The consolidation of authority in the federal–provincial arena necessary to renegotiate the terms of the Canada Health Act was highly unlikely in an era in which federal–provincial relations were dominated by a contentious debate about the appropriate degree of centralization/decentralization within the federation, fueled by (but not confined to) the issue of Quebec independence. The federal government, under a Conservative and then (after 1993) a Liberal majority government, had the consolidated authority to act unilaterally to amend the legislation. But neither government sought to do so. The Conservatives chose to escalate a "stealthy" process whereby the legislation would be gutted over time by the erosion of federal financial contributions and accordingly the fiscal leverage of the federal government to enforce its criteria. The successor Liberal government, under a party that had been closely identified with the principles embedded in the Canada Health Act and its predecessor legislation since the 1960s, retained its leverage by establishing reduced but stable levels of funding after 1995 (phasing in a return to nominal 1995 levels after 1999), while leaving in place the Canada Health Act conditions for the transfer.

At the provincial level, governments had the authority to modify the institutional mix and structural balance of their health care arenas within the constraints of the federal legislation. While that legislation constrained the role of private finance, it gave great latitude to provincial programs with regard to the organization of health care delivery, and hence allowed for a remixing of hierarchical and collegial mechanisms, a greater use of contracting, and a rebalancing of influence between state actors and the medical profession. And yet provincial governments confined themselves primarily to blunt budget instruments to slow the growth of the health care budget and to reallocate within it. They did intervene to restructure the hospital system; and in all provinces except Ontario the governments drew the hospital sector somewhat closer to the state by establishing or increasing the authority of governmentally appointed or elected regional boards for the goverance of hospitals and other institutions.

These boards continued to function at arm's length from the provincial government, however. Meanwhile, the hospital–physician relationship, based on independently constituted medical staffs, remained unchanged; and medical practice remained outside the purview of these bodies. Even these changes were highly controversial; and no governing party at the provincial level, even among those with broad neoconservative agendas, was willing to go further to adopt an agenda of major institutional and structural change in the health care arena. The political risk of doing so, given the broad public support for the medicare program and the growing public anxiety as to its future, deterred such experimentation.

In contrast to the American experience, in the absence of major policy change the logic of the Canadian system worked to maintain its existing institutional mix and, largely, its structural balance. For the logic of the system, with its predominant weighting of collegial mechanisms and medical influence, was essentially one of traditional dual-level agency relationships, elaborated in response to the evolving health policy agenda. Maintaining a system based on agency relationships between individual patients and professionals was central to the design of Canadian medicare in the first instance. But this model, especially when financed through passive third-party payment, was extraordinarily costly, as U.S. experience demonstrated. Over time, provincial governments sought to limit their fiscal liability under this essentially open-ended scheme. They turned to professional groups in order to develop and implement these policies—negotiating overall price levels with medical associations, monitoring practice patterns (on a limited basis) through professional bodies, turning to professional bodies for the development of clinical guidelines, and establishing joint profession–government committees for system-wide planning. The "second-level" agency relationship between the state and the profession, which had traditionally focused on ensuring that services were provided according to standards of quality established by the professional group, was elaborated to include considerations of the cost and appropriateness of service.

These arrangements made sense for both state and professional actors. They retained the structures of health care delivery—private medical practices, free choice of physician for patients—to which Canadians were long accustomed and which were features of an extraordinarily popular system. The accommodation between the profession and the state allowed the profession broad clinical autonomy and influence over the system as a whole; the arrangement also allowed the state overall instruments of budgetary control without incurring the transaction costs (or developing the capacity) to manage a very diffuse system. This accommodation, however, was premised on generous levels of public funding. Leaving the fine levers of decision-making in the hands of physicians, in a system of independent fee-for-service practice, yielded levels of spending that by the end of the 1980s were second (albeit a distant second) only to the United States.

In the 1990s, as discussed in chapter 7, Canadian governments began to wield their blunt budget instruments considerably more stringently. The rate of real increase in public funding of health care declined dramatically in the 1990s; in 1994 the rate turned negative for the first time since the inception of medicare. Although health care spending was protected in most provinces relative to other areas of public spending, the health care arena nonetheless experienced what Klein described in the British case as "relative deprivation over time" (Klein 1995: 99). In Britain, this relative deprivation precipitated a breakdown of the "implicit concordat" between the medical profession and the state, which in turn triggered Margaret Thatcher's personal intervention and set in train the process that led to the "internal market" reforms of the early 1990s. Such a breakdown is neither a necessary nor a sufficient condition for major policy changes directed at the institutional mix or structural balance of the system—such changes, as noted, depend on the mobilization of political authority and will on the scale that Thatcher could accomplish in her third successive majority government. In the Canadian case, a breakdown of the accommodation could mean instead that provincial governments progressively assert their existing budgetary roles more strongly, reducing and reallocating resources within the system without mandating institutional or structural change. Institutional and structural change would then depend upon the responses of actors in the system to these budgetary changes.

In this context, the response of the medical profession promised to be critical. In the face of increasing budgetary stringency, the Canadian medical profession became increasingly divided in the 1990s, at both federal and provincial levels, over whether to continue to elaborate the accommodation with the state to address issues of the organization of health care delivery, or instead to press for the adoption of a greater role for private finance and market mechanisms to enhance the entrepreneurial freedom of the individual physicians. In this pivotal debate, as discussed in chapter 7, the British and the American experience offered twin specters for Canadian physicians, and the academic observation that the clinical autonomy of the profession appeared to be better protected through alliance with the state than with private finance spilled over into the arena of professional debate.

An elaboration of the accommodation with the state could well yield institutional change in the form of an increased reliance on hierarchical or contracting mechanisms, as indicated by the discussions of integrated delivery systems that gained prominence as the decade advanced. Alternatively, an "delisting" of a substantial range of services, well beyond the marginal changes made in the first half of the decade, would lead to significant structural change in the form of an increased role for private finance and "niche" markets for private providers. For all its stability to date, the Canadian system in the late 1990s was poised on the cusp of choice as to which of these routes to emphasize.

The British, American, and Canadian cases, then, represent somewhat imperfectly the "ideal types" of state-hierarchical, private-market, and professional-collegial systems, respectively. And their experience in the 1990s is consistent with what might be predicted on the basis of these models. Given direction from the top as a result of the opening of a window of opportunity for major policy change, the state hierarchy of the British NHS significantly transformed itself by adopting contracting mechanisms. The impact of these changes was, however, tempered by the established logic of the system of hierarchical corporatism that characterized the NHS in practice, and that offered modes of decision-making alternative to contracting, with substantially lower transaction costs. The American and Canadian systems were set on different courses from a common point in the 1960s, as a result of the major policy changes that characterized that watershed period. In the absence of major policy change in the 1990s, the two systems played out their respective logics. In Canada, the terms of an accommodation between the medical profession and the state kept the system relatively stable though under increasing pressure. In the United States, the dominant role of private finance led to the system's turbulent transformation.

This review of the experience of three nations demonstrates a phenomenon often observed in comparative studies of public policy: a common logic demonstrated in different ways in particular national contexts. Each nation has manifested in a distinctive way several common features of the health care arena of the 1990s: in particular, the prevalence of risk- and cost-shifting behavior, and the increasing centrality of bargaining relationships between relatively large and sophisticated entities as the locus of decision-making. In the United States, the open-ended multipayer system offered multiple opportunities to shift costs and cost-bearing risks. In the 1980s, however, cost-conscious payers began to insist on forms of coverage that limited their own exposure, increasingly shifting risk to insurers and providers. In this process, the menu of possibilities in the health care delivery system increasingly came to be determined through negotiations between large corporate employers (and groups of employers) and the managed care entities that sprang up to manage the interfaces between payers, providers, and recipients of care. In managing these interfaces, managed care entities became more and more involved in clinical decision-making.

Under national health insurance in Canada, risks of cost increases were shifted first from the federal government to provincial governments, as the federal government closed the open end of its cost-sharing obligation in the late 1970s. The provinces were led in turn, first in the hospital sector and later in the physician services sector, to close the open end of their financial obligations as well, by capping hospital and physician services budgets. In Canada's provincial-level single-payer system, this left providers with nowhere to shift costs and drew them into expanded and intensified negotiations with governments both at the provincial level and through the regional structures established in most provinces. By the late 1990s, however, these negotiations had yielded little change in a system of decision-making that continued to accord a central role to the clinical judgment of individual physicians in establishing health care priorities.

In Britain, a hierarchical system with fixed budgets (for other than GP services) from the 1970s onward meant that opportunities for risk- and cost-shifting were limited. Local health authorities had to bear the risk that the demand for health care would yield costs in excess of their budgets, and they managed that risk by relying on physicians to mediate demand and to make clinical judgments about priorities in the allocation of resources. The separation of purchaser and provider roles under the internal market reforms created more explicit bargaining over such priorities between Health Authorities and GP fund-holders on the one hand and newly independent provider trusts on the other. These bargaining relationships nonetheless continued to rely heavily on professional networks and on clinical judgments regarding priorities.

These observations suggest a broad irony noted at the outset of this book: in the health care arena of the 1990s, those who assumed cost-bearing risks also acquired decision-making power. As they assumed the risks of cost increases under fixed budgets, providers in Canada and Britain satisfied the gross cost-control objectives of payers, and they thereby maintained their own central role in making resource-allocation decisions within budget limits. In the United States, where managed care entities increasingly assumed cost-bearing risks, they correspondingly took on a greater role in decision-making in individual cases.

## Concluding Observations

Analysis of experience in Britain, the United States, and Canada has made evident the "accidental logics" that govern the dynamics of change in the health care arena. In the context of this analysis, several observations can be made that deserve highlighting in this concluding chapter. One set of observations concerns the role of information technology. Another relates to the debate about the implications of an increased reliance on market mechanisms and private finance in the health care arena that continues to swirl in most advanced industrial nations at the end of the twentieth century. Finally, I bring the analysis in this book to bear on two sets of questions about the future of the welfare state and the health care arena, one set directed primarily at political scientists and other students of public policy, the other set aimed primarily at participants in the health care arena. What does the experience of Britain, the United States, and Canada as analyzed in this book tell us about the likely paths of welfare-state development? And how can it inform the choices facing health care decision-makers in the years ahead?

### The impact of information technology

Throughout this book, my argument about the dynamics of change in the health care arena has been premised on the existence of disparities in access to information. It is these disparities that underlie the establishment of agency relationships and that generate the potential biases and the transaction costs to which hierarchical, collegial, and market mechanisms constitute alternative modes of response. It follows that changes in the costs of acquiring and processing information, and changes in the type of information deemed relevant, should have profound implications for these dynamics. The burgeoning of information technology in the 1980s and 1990s did indeed have an impact on the dynamics of change in each of the countries reviewed. But this impact was considerably greater in the United States than in the other two countries. This phenomenon presents yet another puzzle, which deserves some extended consideration.

The ability to use power effectively in the pursuit of given objectives or interests requires access to information about the costs and benefits of different actions. Different bases of power (skill, authority, wealth) imply access to different types of information. The ability to bring information to bear in exercising power depends upon one's comparative advantage in gaining access to relevant information. Historically, the medical profession has occupied a dominant position in the health care arena by virtue of its comparative advantage in accessing the information embedded in health care technology.

The information advantage enjoyed by the medical profession has meant that other actors in the arena have had to make accommodations or alliances with the profession in the pursuit of their own objectives. The accommodation between the profession and the state has provided the central axis of the "health care state" under systems of public finance. While the nature of this relationship has varied across nations and over time, it has generally left the fine levers of decision-making in the hands of the medical profession, to be exercised according to the clinical judgment of individual physicians, while establishing various degrees and mechanisms of fiscal constraint. Changing the fundamental balance between the profession and the state in this context has required the mobilization of sheer authority to countervail the profession's inherent comparative advantage in access to information, and a willingness on the part of political actors to incur the risks of doing so.

In most nations, the accommodation between the medical profession and the state that characterizes the structure of the welfare state in the health care arena has left relatively little room for private finance. The major exception is the United States, where the profession chose at critical junctures to ally itself with private finance against the state. The policy parameters established at these junctures proved no less resistant to change than did those governing publicly financed systems. But, ironically, these parameters also allowed the role of private finance to burgeon at the expense of the profession itself.

The dynamics that allowed the greatly expanded role of private finance in the United States have much to do with the development of information technology, particularly with the timing of technological developments in the history of the evolution of decision-making systems in the health care arena. Let us consider briefly the nature of those technological developments, and the ways in which they were taken up in the U.S. arena in comparison to experience in the United Kingdom and Canada.

In the health care arena at the end of the twentieth century, it may not be an exaggeration to say that the technological developments that are most revolutionary in their implications for the institutional and structural characteristics of decision-making systems are those in information technology. The collectivization of financing of health care, whether by the state or by large corporate bodies in the private sector, provided the vehicle for the assembling of large databases of patient records. The development of information technologies of storage, retrieval, and analysis then made feasible the tapping of these databases and related information for the assessment of health care "needs" and "outcomes," as well as the costs and prices of various service options. And medical practitioners had no comparative advantage in this regard. Rather, this advantage belonged to large corporate entities whose operations gave them the opportunity to compile such databases and whose resources were substantial enough to bear the costs of investment in information technology. Chief among these corporate entities were those who purchased, underwrote, or provided services consumed by large populations of individual patients—governments, insurance companies, large employers, and organizations of health care delivery with large enrolled populations. By the late 1990s, the level of skill in accessing such information was still highly variable across institutions and, in general, had not allowed for the tapping of the full potential of available data or technology.

Even in this nascent condition, however, the potential of information technology to alter the dynamics of structural change in the health care field could be glimpsed. As large corporate actors sought to maximize revenues or minimize costs, they increasingly availed themselves of the instruments of information technology. As governments sought to stabilize or reduce their fiscal presence in the health care arena and to spend "smarter," they sought other instruments that were information-intensive but less fiscally demanding. Both public and private actors increasingly developed the capacity to monitor the activities of health care providers.

These developments had the potential to shift fundamentally the balance of influence among state actors, health care providers, and private financial interests in the health care decision-making system, even without major institutional or structural policy interventions. This process, however, was not uniform across nations. It was facilitated or constrained by the distinctive logic of each particular system.

Those logics, as we have seen, rested in part on judgments about the relative costs of market-oriented, collegial, or hierarchical approaches to the monitoring of agency relationships. In this regard, the major implication of the development of information technology in the late twentieth century was to reduce the costs of monitoring contracts, from prohibitive to merely substantial levels, and to make possible market-style responses to the potential problems posed by agency relationships that were not feasible in the past. While thus reducing the need to replace contract-based instruments with hierarchical mechanisms, information technology also enhanced the potential capacity for information flows within hierarchies. In both respects, it reduced the relative advantage of collegial mechanisms in economizing on information costs.

These developments ought to provide the means for state actors and private financial interests to countervail the information advantage traditionally enjoyed by the medical profession. Yet in Britain and Canada this happened only to a limited extent. In Britain, the linkage of clinical and financial information essential to the specification of contracts between purchasers and providers was constrained by the persistence of medical control of clinical data under systems of "clinical audit." In Canada, notwithstanding the existence of rich databases deriving from the fee-for-service remuneration system, the monitoring of the practice profiles of individual physicians was confined to outlier cases and was implemented through collegial bodies. In the hospital sector, again despite very rich databases, hospital budgets continued to be essentially historically based until well into the 1990s, when several provinces began to experiment with casemix-based formulas for hospital budgeting. In the United States, however, the use of information technology by both state actors and private firms accelerated rapidly from the mid-1980s forward, as the federal government adopted a casemix-based Prospective Payment System for hospital services under its Medicare program, and as managed care firms developed a range of utilization review mechanisms to monitor the practices of physicians whom they employed or contracted with.

As a very rough measure of the different extent to which information technology was adopted in the three countries, expenditure on information technology amounted to about 2% of total health care spending in the United States in the mid-1990s, rising to 3–5% in major acute care hospitals. In comparison, information technology accounted for only about 1% of total health care spending in Canada (Morrissey 1995: 72; Brethour 1998). Comparable aggregate data are not available for the United Kingdom; but as noted in chapter 6, information technology accounted for about 1.8% of total expenditure in the relatively information-intensive acute care hospital sector. These differences in part reflect the generally lower administrative overheads of the Canadian and British systems; but they also reinforce the finding of a lesser reliance on information-technology-intensive management tools.

Once again, the *timing* of developments in each nation is critical to an understanding of the differences between them. Hierarchical and collegial responses involving multiple-level agency relationships were broadly elaborated in Britain and Canada before the development of sophisticated information technology made possible more market-oriented responses and closer monitoring within hierarchical organizations. In particular, these multiple-level agency relationships were defined to include mechanisms of cost control and some sharing of risk for the costs of providing health care to defined populations. Information-intensive approaches, while more feasible than in the past, still required substantial investment. In the budget-limited systems of Britain and Canada, state actors were reluctant to adopt such approaches when traditional networks were available to serve as alternatives. The logic of these relationships, then, acted as a brake on the use of information technology, as more fully discussed in chapters 6 and 7.

In the United States, on the other hand, as the discussion in chapter 5 makes clear, agency relationships remained relatively narrowly defined and generally did not embrace cost control objectives. When the development of information technology in the 1980s placed tools of control in the hands of increasingly aggressive and price-sensitive purchasers of care, both public and private, these tools were less likely to be seen as alternatives to established mechanisms of cost control than as ways of gaining control over costs in the first instance. In other words, a widespread pressure for cost control arose rather later within the fragmented and diffuse system of health care financing in the United States than it did in the state-financed systems of Britain and Canada; hence it arose in the United States in a context in which technological developments had created informational tools that had been unavailable when the cost-control mechanisms of the British and Canadian systems were shaped.

The logic of agency relationships and transaction costs, then, together with an evolutionary perspective on the development of the three systems, goes a long way toward explaining differences in the adoption and deployment of information technology. But it is not the whole story. It does not fully explain why neither public nor private payers in the United States elaborated "second-level" agency relationships with medical groups on a broad scale in an earlier period. Unraveling that aspect of the puzzle brings us to the final theme of this conclusion: the implications of public versus private finance for decision-making structures in the health care arena.

### State and market; public and private finance

The experience of Britain, Canada and the United States, as analyzed in this book, suggests that the dichotomy between "state" and "market" often invoked in policy debate masks two distinct but interrelated dimensions of decision-making systems. The state may wax or wane in influence vis-à-vis private financial interests along the *structural* dimension, and hierarchical mechanisms may become more (or less) prominent than market mechanisms along the *institutional* dimension. As noted in chapter 1, there is a "natural affinity" between state actors and hierarchical mechanisms, and between private financial actors and market mechanisms. But experience in the United Kingdom and the United States as well as other nations indicates that these affinities were increasingly being shuffled in the health care arena: state actors took up marketlike instruments in Britain, and private financial interests organized themselves in vertically and horizontally integrated firms in a U.S. health care market traditionally characterized by myriad independent units.

In this shuffling of affinities, one key phenomenon has become apparent: the way various instruments function depends on who is wielding them. In particular, the logic of decision-making systems depends fundamentally on the balance between state actors and private financial actors. More particularly, it depends on the extent to which the system is dominated by public versus private finance—or, as Boycko and his colleagues have put it, the extent to which "cash flow ownership" accrues to state or private actors (Boycko et al. 1996). Put another way, although the logic of decision-making systems is the product of the intersection of structural and institutional dimensions, it is the structural dimension—particularly the balance between state and private finance—that is most fundamental. Although extrapolation from three cases is hazardous, this conclusion is strongly suggested not only by observation of the British, Canadian, and American systems but also by an analysis of the logic underlying them—an analysis that also helps to explain why the clinical autonomy of the medical profession may be better protected under systems of public finance than in private markets.

In chapter 1, the point was made that different balances of influence among the state, private finance, and the medical profession generate different logics of change in health care decision-making systems, and that the key to understanding these differences lies in the different lines of accountability to which state actors, private entrepreneurs, and medical professionals are held. This point can now be elaborated, in the light of experience in Britain, Canada, and the United States, to explain the different implications of public and private finance for the logics of decision-making systems in the health care arena.

In publicly financed systems, state actors function within a system in which, regardless of the instruments they use, those who are making allocative decisions are politically accountable and must maintain a coalition of political support. These coalitions are likely to be complex: they involve intersecting accommodations among bureaucratic units (particularly between the treasury and line departments), among levels of government, and between these various state agencies and their myriad clientele groups and beneficiaries. In these accommodations, a variety of competing and complementary objectives are brought to bear—the level of taxation (of various forms) necessary to sustain various modes and levels of health care delivery, the incidence of cross-subsidization of benefits, the maintenance of professional discretion, the employment implications of various modes of health care delivery, the significance of health care facilities as components of local communities, etc.

The need for state actors to maintain these complex coalitions contrasts with the accountability of private entrepreneurs to investors seeking to maximize the rate of return on their investments. Economists have drawn attention to this fundamental distinction to draw invidious comparisons between systems in which control rests with actors whose accountability runs through the political system on the one hand or through channels of accountability to outside investors on the other (Boycko et al. 1996). The relatively "pure" objective of investors to maximize rates of return ensures that in private systems technical efficiency will not be sacrificed to the other objectives that characterize political coalitions in the public sector. (In practice, as discussed in chapter 5, the empirical evidence for the greater efficiency of private versus public institutions in the health care field is mixed at best and is made problematic by the difficulties of defining and measuring output.)

From this fundamental difference in lines of accountability, a number of further points of difference between decision-making systems in the health care arena under public and private finance follow. The first has to do with the level (that is, group versus individual) at which calculations are focused. In the classic case of the competitive private market, the allocation of resources is determined by the actions of multiple independent buyers and sellers making assessments of the costs and benefits of units of goods and services in individual transactions. This contrasts with the classic case of public finance, in which a public "sponsor" provides an annual grant to a monopoly supplier to produce an overall level of goods or services. In the latter case the sponsor acts on behalf of a group or population and assesses the costs and benefits of an overall level of goods and services without making marginal calculations on a per-unit basis.

It is this fundamental, if oversimplified, contrast that has led economists such as William Niskanen to hypothesize that public bureaucracies are likely to provide a greater level of output (and hence to consume a greater level of resources) than is socially optimal, the level depending on the stringency of the budget limit established by the sponsor (Niskanen 1971).

Niskanen's hypotheses carry a certain degree of irony in the health care arena of the late twentieth century, in which the private-market–dominated American system devoted a proportion of resources to health care that was about 40% greater than was the case in even the most generous systems of public finance. This empirical observation highlights the fact that Niskanen's economic models beg an important (and essentially political) set of questions—those relating to the establishment of the public budget for health care, and to the "sponsor's" lines of political accountability. The budget process involves complex coalition-building among a variety of groups, both within government and between government and societal groups. Indeed, these complex coalitions are likely to include suppliers of publicly financed goods and services themselves. These coalitions and accommodations have yielded quite different levels of public budget constraints in different nations, as our examination of the British and Canadian cases has demonstrated.

Another important distinction between systems of public and private finance concerns the relative ease of exit from relationships. Private investors wield a sanction that is less effectively available to coalition partners in the public sector: through financial markets, they can quickly withdraw their capital and exit in favor of other investments. Public funders, on the other hand, operate within political systems in which they cannot escape accountability to the populations under their jurisdiction. Furthermore, these political systems are at least in part based on local constituencies; hence decisions that impose costs (or withdraw benefits) from particular localities carry considerable political risk. These locally based accountability systems intersect with and reinforce the local networks upon which the provision of health care has traditionally been based. The result is a set of relationships from which exit is costly, in terms of the loss of good-will, for all participants (relative, at least, to the fluidity of private investment capital).

These public–private distinctions are most clearly apparent in contrasting the for-profit private sector with the public sector. The so-called "third" or not-for-profit sector was for years more similar to the public sector in this respect. Not-for-profit hospitals and insurers were governed by boards whose accountability ran, if not to local communities at large, at least to local elites (Brown 1991; Schlesinger et al. 1996: 704). Not-for-profits, then, tended to have long historical and close social and political ties to their communities. Beginning in the mid-1980s, however, as discussed in chapter 5 for the U.S. case, competition from for-profits progressively eroded the distinction between for-profit and not-for-profit entities, and ultimately led to a wave of conversion of not-for-profits to for-profit status. While perhaps most visible in the U.S. due to the dramatic rise of for-profit entities in the health care arena in the 1980s and 1990s, the growing similarities of not-for-profit organizations to for-profit enterprises was apparent in other nations as well. (For commentary on British experience in this regard, see Johnson 1995: 239–40.)

The stark contrasts between systems of public and private finance implied by models drawn from economics and political science have been put to the test as each sector, in practice, adopted the instruments of the other. In the private sector in the United States, as we have seen, the predominantly employer-based system for the financing of health care meant that the purchase of health care coverage involved transactions at the level of groups. With the rise of "managed care," moreover, the transactions came somewhat to resemble annual block grants for a given level of coverage to a given population.

These private-sector group-level negotiations, however, are actually based on aggregate calculations of the risks associated with individual cases, in contrast to the governmental budgetary process in which costs and benefits are typically assessed for groups or categories of interest per se, not for individuals. Prices per unit of coverage or per unit of service are established on the basis of marginal cost-benefit calculations made by providers and purchasers of insurance or care. Private insurance practices, particularly in the small-group market, typically involve "medical underwriting" and screening provisions for assessing the risk status of individual members of the group and offering the price and scope of coverage accordingly (Cantor et al. 1995; Glazner et al. 1995).

Marginal cost-benefit calculations for individual cases, then, persisted under group-level negotiations in the U.S. private sector. Conversely, calculations of costs and benefits remained focused at the group level in Britain even under the "internal market" mechanisms that attempted to introduce marginal calculations based on price-per-unit. The prevalence of block contracting meant that budgets continued to be determined more on the model of continual annual grants for annual gross output than on the model of marginal price-per-unit calculations. Again, experience in other nations suggests a similar persistence of grantlike arrangements. New Zealand's experiment with "internal market" mechanisms yielded an initial flurry of attempts to develop highly specific and unique contracts, followed by growing pressure for longer-term and simpler contracts (Brown 1996: 306; Krieble 1997: 8). And in New Zealand, as in Britain, competition among providers was limited; local relationships between health authorities and health care providers persisted even as the vehicle shifted from hierarchy to contract (Krieble 1997: 8). The consolidation on both the "purchaser" and the "provider" sides under the policy changes of the late 1990s, moreover, further limited the potential for competition in the New Zealand system (Ham 1997). The persistent attraction of established relationships and modes of decision-making under internal market mechanisms is due in part to the considerations of transaction costs and the availability of established networks, as already discussed. But it also derives from the fact that use of market-type mechanisms by state actors does not change their lines of accountability or the need for them to maintain coalitions of support among various groups.

In summary, systems of private finance are driven by a focus on rates of return on investment, while systems of public finance are driven by the need to maintain complex coalitions of political support. The difference in these fundamental drivers has important implications for other structural and institutional features of decision-making systems, and ultimately for the dynamics of change in those systems.

Notably, systems of public finance entail a central role for the medical profession and for collegial mechanisms. State actors under systems of public finance have struck an "implicit bargain" with the medical profession, essentially turning to professional bodies to be the agents of resource allocation within budgetary parameters established by the state. Even as state actors have experimented with the exercise of microeconomic leverage through contracting and "internal market" mechanisms, they have been constrained by the terms of this fundamental bargain. In the light of the previous discussion, the prevalence of this bargain across systems of public finance can be seen not only as an empirical phenomenon but also as a logical component of such systems; an accommodation with the medical profession has been a significant component of the political coalitions of support that characterize state-financed systems. Such bargains are possible in systems of private finance, as the development of "group/staff" HMOs in the U.S. system demonstrates. But they have constituted one modality, and a minor one at that, among the many organizational entities developed by entrepreneurs seeking microeconomic leverage in order to maximize rates of return.

A second implication of the fundamental difference between systems of public and private finance concerns the pace of structural and institutional change. The ease of exit for private investors, their quest for more profitable forms of organization in which to invest, and their attraction to entities that can demonstrate growth and expanding market share have driven rapid and volatile change in the industrial structure of health care delivery and financing in the United States, and have given rise to a range of organizational innovation that is without parallel in systems dominated by public finance. In contrast, the need to maintain coalitions of political support moderated the pace and nature of change initiated by state actors in Britain; this need also kept the Canadian system, with its broad-based political support for the medicare program, remarkably stable in international perspective.

In drawing these contrasts between systems dominated by public finance and systems dominated by private finance, it is important to recognize that the balance between the public and private sectors depends not only on their relative size but also on the way the relationships between them are defined. In Britain, for example, as described in chapter 6, the relatively small private sector had a "niche" orientation, providing alternatives to the public sector in certain specialty areas and almost entirely excluding general practice. The relationship between private sector employers or financers and consultant (specialist) physicians was defined by the fact that the consultant's primary base was in the public sector. In Canada, although the private sector in health care was larger than it was in Britain, medical and hospital services were almost entirely publicly financed; private financing related to other goods and services such as pharmaceuticals and dental care. Other predominately state-financed systems also show variety in the public-private balance. In the Netherlands, about 30% of the population (essentially all of those above a given income level) was privately insured; but private insurers were bound into networks linking hospitals, doctors' associations, and social insurance funds, and their relationships with physicians were defined within that context. In Australia, another nation with a relatively large private sector (at about 32% of total health expenditures in 1991), private insurance covered a type of "user charge"—the balance of the provider's fee not covered by governmental health insurance—and hence had a somewhat symbiotic relationship with the public sector. Even in the United States, of course, the fiscal role of the state in the health care arena was a substantial one, and it periodically had an important influence on incentives in the system as a whole (most notably, in the case of the federal government's adoption of a Prospective Payment System under Medicare in the 1980s). Nonetheless, we are left with the United States, the only system in which private finance dominated and defined the system, as the case to analyze if we wish to understand the logic of a privately financed system. And if it is a singular case, it must be remembered, as pointed out in chapter 1, that the American system in the 1990s accounted for about one-half of all health-care expenditures in the entire OECD.

### The path(s) and pace of welfare state development

The argument I have made throughout this book joins an ongoing debate in the social science literature about the survival of the welfare state at the turn of the twenty-first century. In particular, it can inform two lines of thought about late twentieth-century welfare state development. Both of these lines of thought have in common the observation that, despite the rhetoric of "crisis" that surrounded welfare-state programs and institutions in the 1980s and 1990s, those programs and institutions in fact proved remarkably resilient. Such change as occurred was incremental, not radical (Heclo 1981; Klein and O'Higgins 1988; Moran 1994; Pierson 1994).

One line of analysis that flows from such observations points nonetheless to an increasing cross-national convergence in welfare-state policies. In the health care arena, Michael Moran has observed a cross-national process of cumulative incremental change. He has argued, provocatively, that structural and institutional changes in the health care arena (to paraphrase his argument using my terminology) were incrementally but steadily drawing most advanced industrial nations closer to an American model—a model in which market mechanisms were increasingly used for resource allocation, albeit within governmentally established budgets, and in which the medical profession was losing influence to increasingly sophisticated purchasers (Moran 1994: 51).

Mary Ruggie, in her analysis of health care policy in Britain, Canada, and the United States, also found a degree of convergence in those three nations. But in her case the observed convergence was toward what she called an "integrative" policy regime. In an integrative policy regime, the role of the state is based not on the exercise of authority in the Weberian sense; rather it is a "leadership" role—the ability to guide, negotiate, broker, and facilitate the emergence of consensus. The goals of the welfare state have not fundamentally changed, she argues. What has changed (to paraphrase again) is the balance across various types of social control in achieving those objectives:

> There are many types of welfare states; each uses its own mix of agents for its own preferred social outcomes. What characterizes a welfare state is, above all, a commitment to redistribution of social resources to achieve an acceptable and ever-improving level of basic provision, whether the agents of provision are state or societal. . . . [T]he argument I have been advancing [concerns] the changing role of the state in guiding a broader base of social provision. (Ruggie 1996: 269–70)

Ruggie's argument puts her in the company of a number of scholars who argue that the withdrawal of the state from the direct provision (or even from the direct funding) of welfare-state benefits does not mean the demise or even the diminution of the welfare state. As early as 1971, Allen Schick argued that the state would increasingly assume a less "bureaucratic" and more "cybernetic" role, monitoring the provision of welfare-state benefits by those it did not directly employ. Schick, indeed, used U.S. Medicare as a primary example of this phenomenon (Schick 1971). In the 1980s Rein and Rainwater pointed to the emergence of a "welfare society" to replace the welfare state (Rein and Rainwater 1987). In the 1980s and 1990s a number of British scholars drew attention to what they termed "welfare pluralism." The term essentially refers to the provision of health care and social services by various types of suppliers—not only the state itself but also the voluntary, commercial, and "informal" sectors (Johnson 1995: 234), leaving the state to influence the pattern of provision through a variety of instruments complementary to or alternative to budgetary allocations, such as contracting, regulation, and tax expenditure.

Another line of argument, however, sees the development of welfare states as "path dependent," and emphasizes national differences. As noted in chapters 1 and 4, a number of scholars have attempted to explain incrementalism in policy change by seeking to understand how certain policies create the conditions for their own continuation, and how they become self-reinforcing. Comparative analysis has been central to this enterprise, as scholars have identified different degrees of path dependency in different national contexts and have sought to identify the relevant explanatory factors. Wilsford (1995), for example, finds these factors in the design of political institutions, which vary across nations in the relative degrees of centralization and hierarchy that they exhibit and hence in their ability to take decisions to depart from an existing path. Döhler (1991) makes a related point, arguing that the "goodness of fit" between a particular policy and the existing structure of interests in the arena greatly enhances the likelihood of successful implementation, but that centralized political institutions can enforce even a policy that departs from the prevailing pattern.

As Pierson (1997) has noted, some path dependency analysts find heuristic value in biological analogies (Krasner 1988); others (such as Wilsford 1995) are informed by work in economic history on patterns of technology development and diffusion (David 1985; Arthur 1994). Like Pierson, I find the latter approach more directly relevant to the understanding of the political as well as the economic phenomena that characterize the interactions of intelligent human beings. It is in understanding the logic of these interactions that we can see how welfare state policies, at least in the health care arena, may be both path dependent and also, in a very broad sense, convergent.

Understanding path dependency requires an understanding not just of political institutions but of the political economy of a policy arena as a whole. It means understanding the interactions of political and economic actors within the parameters established by public policy. Those interactions follow a logic as actors respond rationally to the incentives they face. And that logic is shaped not only by policy parameters but also by the microeconomic and technological characteristics of the particular arena. In the health care arena, changes in the technology of health care delivery were generating some broad cross-national similarities in the interactions of actors in the 1990s. Across nations, the health care arena was increasingly characterized by bargaining relationships among relatively large and sophisticated organizations. But this similarity holds true only from a very broad perspective. In terms of the dynamics of change in these systems, as well as the interests brought to bear in decision-making about the production and distribution of health care, it matters very much who occupies these bargaining roles, and within what institutional context the roles are defined. And these factors vary across nations. In Britain, the bargaining relationships that have increased in significance are those between state agencies—Health Authorities and independent trusts—and between organized groups of general practitioners and consultant physicians. In Canada, the bargaining relationships between provincial governments and medical associations, which have been pivotal to the system since its inception, have expanded their policy scope. And in the United States, complex networks of bargaining relationships link large employers and consortia of employers, managed care organizations, and health care providers both collectively and individually.

Notwithstanding the broad similarities that derive from the common economic and technological elements of health care delivery, then, the structural and institutional characteristics of the health care arenas of particular nations follow their own distinctive logics of development and continue to show essential differences. The persistence of distinctive trajectories does not, however, mean that change in these systems can be only incremental. In the first place, the internal logics of systems can differ greatly in their capacity to generate nonincremental change. This is nowhere more apparent than in the case of the U.S. health care arena. While it is true in broad terms that the United States has continued to follow a market-oriented path within established policy parameters, the logic of the private market has transformed the system, dramatically shifting the balance of influence away from the medical profession toward private finance, and increasing the degree of reliance on hierarchical mechanisms in the form of vertically and horizontally integrated firms. Nor does the logic of a given path always militate against major change in policy parameters themselves. Turbulent changes in the American health care market have also increased the complexity of the political landscape and have hence complicated the process of assembling a coalition of support for policy change. But that very turbulence has fractured the bulwark of medical and business interests that have traditionally opposed major policy change, and may arguably be creating the conditions under which a coalition of support for health care reform could be assembled under propitious political conditions.

This brings us, finally, to a second way in which nonincremental change can occur. The dynamics of change in the welfare state appear incremental only in the medium term. In the health care arena, periodic episodes of major policy change have yielded nonincremental shifts in the balance of influence across major categories of actors or in the mix of basic types of policy instruments, not only during the period of the formation of the modern welfare state in the health care arena in the 1940s in Britain and the 1960s in the United States and Canada, but also during the period of "reform" in the 1990s in Britain. Because of the force of these systems' internal logics, the impetus necessary to set them on a different course must typically come from the broader political arena, when the government of the day can mobilize authority on an extraordinary scale and has the will to make major changes in health policy as part of a broader policy agenda. Such occasions are rare, but they do occur. If comparable circumstances were to arise in the United States or Canada (or indeed again in Britain), we could expect nonincremental change to occur in those contexts as well.

My exploration of these national differences suggests an important qualification of the argument advanced by Ruggie and others that welfare-state objectives are likely to persist even as different means are adopted, even as the state seeks to achieve some minimum acceptable level of welfare for its citizens by engaging a number of different actors in the pursuit of collective goals. This is likely to be the case in the health care arena only so long as the state maintains a dominant *fiscal presence* and exercises its role through making budgetary allocations. The use of nonfiscal instruments such as regulation, or even other fiscal instruments such as tax expenditures, leaves a significant role for private finance. Systems requiring large investments of private capital are fundamentally driven by incentives to maximize rates of return, and the state must constantly wield its nonfiscal or indirect fiscal instruments in the face of these incentives. Systems of public finance are, as previously argued, dominated by different incentives, notably the need to maintain complex coalitions of political support—coalitions centrally including the medical profession. Cross-subsidization of benefits and the preservation of professional discretion are increasingly squeezed out of privately financed systems, but these elements are key to the maintenance of systems of public finance. Public and private finance, then, involve fundamentally different sets of incentives, and turning to one versus the other shifts not only the means but the ends of the welfare state in the health care arena.

### An epilogue on policy choices

This is a work of analysis, not prescription. It seeks to understand the processes of change in the health care arena, not to propose courses of action. But it can nonetheless inform decision-making by participants in the health care arena. This final section addresses the question often asked of political scientists by decision-makers who are faced with choosing courses of action: What can we learn from this book about what we should *do* in response to the challenges we face?

There are two caricatures of what the comparative study of public policy can offer decision-makers, each a distortion of a more nuanced truth. The first is the notion that comparative public policy can offer a menu of possibilities for domestic policy-makers, drawn from experience in other jurisdictions. Consider, for example, the wave of enthusiasm for studies of corporatist arrangements for economic policy-making in the late 1970s and early 1980s. Studies in this period seemed to suggest that corporatist structures drawing "peak associations" of business and labor together with state actors had the potential to generate a consensus around policies to improve economic performance, and that nations with such structures did better in adjusting to the shocks of the international economy, other things being equal, than did nations without such structures.[1] Similarly, as we have seen, there was a strong appetite among policy-makers in the 1990s for studies of the use of market-type mechanisms in the health care arena in a variety of jurisdictions, in the hope that they could offer guidance on how to restructure incentives to yield greater efficiency.

As such studies are pursued, however, a broad set of cautions typically appears. It soon becomes apparent that policies cannot be uprooted from their local contexts and transplanted to another (Klein 1991, 1997). In this context another caricature emerges: comparative public policy analysis appears as a "dismal science" that can only warn of the constraints bearing upon those who would learn from experience in other jurisdictions. Comparative studies can help to identify the circumstances under which a given policy innovation was more or less successfully adopted—but those circumstances are not ones over which policy-makers typically have much control. German-style corporatist "concerted action," for example, which attracted such cross-national attention from economic policy-makers in the 1970s and health policy-makers in the 1980s (Kirkman-Liff 1990), appeared on analysis to require a German-style organization of interests and set of political institutions (Katzenstein 1987; Iglehart 1991).

The reality of what comparative public policy studies can offer policy-makers is more qualified than either of these broad caricatures of the field—as cafeteria of policy options or as dismal science—suggests. In practice, such studies can provide *aids to strategic judgment*. Policy-makers must continually make judgments about what can feasibly be accomplished in their local contexts, and what instruments are best suited to accomplishing those goals. First and foremost, those judgments require a close understanding of the local context. But they also require an awareness of the range of possible courses of action and an understanding of the dynamics of change in a given policy arena that can be fully developed only in a broader comparative context.

The present study is a case in point. Its strategic lessons for policy-makers are essentially twofold. The first message is that windows of opportunity for major structural and institutional change—for shifting the balance of power across the state, the medical profession, and private finance or for changing the mix of hierarchical, market-oriented, or collegial instruments—are rare. John Kingdon's admonition to policy-makers to "strike while the iron is hot"—to move swiftly and boldly as soon as a window of opportunity opens—is hence very apt (Kingdon 1984: 178). Incrementalism in the face of such opportunities is deadly, as we have seen in the case of the United States. Kingdon argues that policy-makers need to have proposals carefully worked out beforehand in order to take advantage of open windows. This counsel appears wise in the case of the United States in the 1990s, in which the decision to seize upon the new (and ill-formed) concept of "managed competition" meant that precious time was lost while the details were fleshed out. But while this counsel may increasingly hold true in a U.S. legislative system that requires that proposals be costed in detail before passage, it does not hold consistently across nations. Both the Canadian and the British cases demonstrate that nonincremental approaches to policy-making during windows of opportunity need not be fully articulated. In Canada, the Medical Care Act of 1966 established only the broad principles within which provincial plans would develop. And in Britain, the 1989 White Paper sketched out only the framework of the internal market, which would be pragmatically developed in the course of implementation.

So, for those who would seek change in the basic policy parameters that govern the balance of influence or the mix or instruments in the health care arena, the first strategic question they should ask in their particular contexts is whether this is a moment for such major change. Can the necessary authority be mobilized within the political system? And is major change in the health care arena central to the agenda of those who can mobilize authority? (Recognizing such windows of opportunity is, of course, much easier with the benefit of hindsight than it is at the time. For example, had Democratic strategists in the United States in the 1960s known what we know today, they may well have been bolder in taking advantage of the opportunity presented by the Johnson presidency and congressional supermajorities.) Unless a strategic judgment can be made that a window of opportunity for major change in policy parameters is open, policy options that involve significant shifts in structural balance or institutional mix are not likely to succeed.

Between such windows of opportunity, the ambitions of policy-makers must be tempered by the recognition that their initiatives will be absorbed by the prevailing structural and institutional configuration of the health care arena. That is not to say that no change at all is possible. But it does imply that policy initiatives are more likely to succeed if, in the words of the British Labour government's own White Paper on the NHS in 1997, they "go with the grain" of existing arrangements (Department of Health 1997).

This is a counsel, then, of ongoing prudence and periodic boldness. In substantive terms, what does it imply for the health policy arenas of Britain, the United States, and Canada at the turn of the twenty-first century? First, this is not likely to be a period of major structural or institutional change in any of these three countries. In Britain, the potential for the massive mobilization of authority certainly exists in the wake of the landslide Labour victory in the 1997 election. But the second condition for the opening of a window for major policy change—a broad agenda of change in which health care figures prominently—does not exist. The agenda of "New Labour" does not encompass sweeping change in the structures of the British welfare state in the health care arena, even as modified by internal market reforms. As Samuel Beer has perceptively argued, the agenda of the Labour government under Tony Blair has its roots in the social liberalism of Lloyd George—a liberalism that embraces both individualism and a sense of the duties and responsibilities that individuals owe each other (Beer 1998). The Labour victory of 1997 did not constitute a mandate for a reinstatement of state power or of hierarchical instruments; rather, it changed the moral tone of policy discourse to emphasize responsibilities, duties, and partnerships instead of incentives and competition. In the field of health care Labour's agenda is essentially to confirm the effects of the internal market reforms on the structural and institutional characteristics of hierarchical corporatism, while forestalling any further movement toward a competitive model.

In the United States, the likelihood that the two conditions for major policy change—a consolidation of authority and a policy agenda that gives a central place to health care reform—are each unlikely to occur. Only under conditions in which the Democrats controlled both the White House and both houses of Congress would major changes to the status quo be likely, and then only if the pall of the failure of the Clinton reforms had lifted. Neither of these eventualities appears likely in the near term. And in Canada a change in the model established by federal legislation in the 1950s and 1960s and reconfirmed in the 1980s would require a sea change in the ideological complexion of the federal government or a federal–provincial consensus supportive of a broader range of experimentation at the provincial level. As long as such developments are held hostage to the resolution of the "national unity" issue of the place of Quebec within or outside of the Canadian federation, they are not likely to occur. Nonetheless, in all three nations incremental increases in public budgets for health care are likely as fiscal constraints lessen—targeted at extending coverage to certain segments of the population in the United States or to certain services (such as home care or pharmaceuticals) in Canada and to problem areas such as the reduction of waiting lists in the United Kingdom.

If major structural and institutional change is not likely to occur in these three countries in the foreseeable future, what then is possible? How will each of these countries confront the next major cross-national set of policy ideas? Let us consider, in that regard, one of the dominant candidates as the successor to "managed competition" and market-type reforms as the cynosure of attention—the concept of the "integrated delivery system," a system linking preventive, acute, rehabilitative, and long-term care across sites in the community, clinician's offices, hospitals, long-term care facilities, and the home. The shift in language associated with this concept is notable: the emphasis is less on the *means* (competition, or management) than on the (at least intermediate) *goal* of integration. The underlying premise is unarguable: ideally, the health care delivery system should provide for a seamless transition from one level and venue of care to another as the needs of the patient and the economies of delivery dictate. In practice, the "integration" of the delivery system is hampered, in different ways in different systems, by existing mechanisms of organizing and financing health care delivery; policy-makers in different nations will face different challenges in bringing it about.

In fact, each of these nations will address common issues related to integrated delivery systems in a distinctive way, according to its particular logic. In the terms I have been using in this book, decision-makers in each nation will have to respond to the call for "integration" in the context of a different institutional mix of instruments and a different structural balance of influence among key actors. Consider first the issue of the mix of instruments to be used—the mechanism of integration. The choice here, in simplest terms, is between "vertical" and "virtual" modes of integration. "Vertical" organizations are integrated through hierarchical mechanisms of rules and reporting relationships. "Virtual" organizations link existing formal units through a variety of negotiated agreements or contracts. Each of these models has its theoretical advantages and disadvantages in a context in which integrated systems are expected to span not only various levels of acute and long-term care, but also various forms of social service. In such contexts hospital-based vertically integrated organizations are typically resisted by nonmedical providers as representing the "medicalization" of a broad scope of service. "Virtual" organizations, then, may recommend themselves as the range of clinical decision-makers, nonmedical as well as medical, expands. As hospitals come to be linked not only with physician practices but with rehabilitation facilities, nursing homes, and so on, virtual organizations may allow for greater variety in the cultures and modes of operation at various nodes in the system depending on the mix of personnel. These virtual organizations, on the other hand, generally require more specific agreements than is the case in established hierarchies. And that specificity may increasingly constrain the exercise of clinical judgment and collegial modes of decision-making.

These trade-offs will be made differently in different systems. In the United States the search for integration of delivery systems will likely fuel an even greater expansion of explicit contracting, beyond the existing forms of managed care organizations that involve horizontal integration of hospitals in multihospital systems or the vertical linkage of physician practices with hospitals. In Britain, it will take the form of long-term service agreements and de facto accommodations among commissioning bodies and trusts. The development of GP fundholding under the internal market reforms resulted in integrated budgets for the purchase of some hospital and community services with GP budgets in some practices—a development that would continue under the Labour government's proposals to provide integrated budgets to "Primary Care Groups." The Canadian version is yet to be developed; but variations are likely to be piloted by regional health authorities in some provinces and by hospitals seeking to establish themselves as the nuclei of integrated health systems in others.

Decision-makers in these three nations will also have to pursue "integration" through systems marked by different balances of influence—in particular, by differing balances of public and private finance. In the United States, these systems may well increasingly be dominated by the interests of arm's-length and highly mobile investors. To the extent that the agenda of integration expands beyond the acute care sector to embrace long-term and home care, however, it will increasingly involve the state, since most recipients of long-term and home care are concentrated among the clientele of the publicly financed programs, Medicare and Medicaid. A few demonstration projects linking acute, long-term, and home care were established in the 1990s under Medicare, for example.[2] In Britain, public finance appears likely to remain dominant, although the public sector itself remains divided in this regard, leaving nonhospital long-term care facilities outside the NHS under the purview of local authorities. Within the Canadian system the development of integrated systems is complicated by the sectorally based division of public and private financing, which places medical and hospital services in the public sector under a universal single-payer model, while leaving home care, long-term care, and other goods and services to be funded through a more disparate public-private mix.

The integration of delivery systems, within existing institutional and structural constraints, thus presents large if different challenges in each nation. In both the United States and Canada, it requires a greater articulation of arrangements linking public and private sectors, even while the center of gravity remains public in Canada and private in the United States. In Britain, the agenda of integration adds further layers of complexity to evolving arrangements within the public sector. As a result, the kinds of "integrated delivery systems" that develop in the three nations will look quite different, despite similarities in cross-national rhetoric and discourse. The distinctiveness of each of these national systems—and indeed of other national systems, for analogous reasons—is not likely to be eroded.

The analysis of the health care arena presented in this book has implications for other arenas of public policy. The distinctions that I have made with regard to the balance of influence and the mix of instruments in the health care arena have parallels elsewhere. Certainly, it is necessary to adapt this analysis to take account of the characteristics of other policy arenas. Few arenas, for example, are as strongly marked by the influence of professional actors and by collegial instruments as is health care; but other arenas have analogs in the role, for example, of community groups and volunteerism. Nor is the organization of private finance—a key factor in determining lines of accountability—the same across arenas. In particular, the significance of the for-profit investor-owned firm varies considerably. In the health care arena, the emergence of capital-intensive technologies and the significance of "insurance" and therefore of third-party payment have created the need for large capital investments for the provision and financing of health care. Under systems of public finance, responsibility for these investments is assumed by the state. Under systems of private finance, the necessary capital is tending more and more to be assembled through arm's-length investor ownership. Other arenas may lend themselves more or less well to the investor-owned form; but experience in the health care arena suggests that the competitive challenge presented by investor-owned firms gives them an influence disproportionate to the size of their market share at any given time.

This analysis suggests that the current vogue for declaring the impotence of the state in the face of the quicksilver international mobility of capital needs to be tempered. Certainly this quicksilver mobility establishes indirect, macro-level constraints on what governments can accomplish. But at the micro-level it matters precisely that these constraints are indirect. They are not the direct constraints that bear upon private entrepreneurs: they are mediated through the political process, and through the need to maintain coalitions of political support. These coalitions require the weighing of a range of interests in decision-making (albeit varying with the partisan complexions of governments); and they also make for a steadier and less turbulent process of change. Even as the traditional affinities between state and hierarchy and between private finance and markets are being shuffled, then, the balance between public and private finance will remain a defining feature of health care systems and, indeed, of other policy arenas.

# Notes

## Chapter 1

1. Government spending on "social protection" (primarily health care and income security), which had grown dramatically as a proportion of GDP in OECD nations in the 1960s and 1970s, leveled off sharply in the 1980s. Spending on social protection as a proportion of GDP doubled from an average of about 10% in OECD nations in 1960 to an average of about 20% in 1980. By 1990, the average had increased only slightly to about 22%. A similar trend was apparent in the subcategory of public spending on health care, which rose from an average of 2.5% of GDP in 1960 to 5.4% in 1980 to 5.6% in 1990 (OECD 1994: 57–61).

2. This commonality was reflected in an OECD document issued in 1994, following discussion by the social policy ministers of member nations in 1992. The document emphasized the potential of social programs to contribute to economic growth, the need to reconcile the costs of social programs with overall limits on public budgets, the need to seek an "optimal balance . . . between public and private sector responsibility . . . in light of the comparative advantages of each sector," and the need for income transfer programs to be "structured to foster self-sufficiency through earnings, without sacrificing the goals of systems of social protection" (OECD 1994: 12–16).

3. Australia, in the period from the mid-1970s to the mid-1980s, stands out as an exception in this regard. There, the highly polarized partisan context in which universal health insurance was introduced made for a decade of instability in which the structural balance between the state and private finance vacillated with partisan changes in government.

4. My argument has something in common with the argument made more than a decade ago by John Kingdon (1984). In his now classic book, *Agendas, Alternatives, and Public Policies,* based on interviews in the late 1970s with policymakers in the health care and transportation arenas, Kingdon developed a model of policy change that also centered around the opening of windows of opportunity. In Kingdon's model, windows of opportunity may be opened by events in the "political" stream or the "problem" stream, each of which flow independent of each other and of developments in the "policy" stream. My argument differs from Kingdon's in a number of respects, however—notably, in its distinction between factors external and internal to the health care arena; in its emphasis on the choice and implementation of policy options, not just the setting of the agenda and the specification of alternatives; and in its emphasis on the logics of the resulting systems that condition future change.

5. Marian Döhler (1991) makes a similar argument, although he does not trace out the logics of systems in the way that I do in this book.

6. These figures exclude Luxembourg and Turkey, for which 1970 data were not available.

7. The program was offered as an expansion of the Medicaid program which was cost-shared by federal and state governments, and required a federal waiver to proceed, as discussed in chapter 5.

8. The contracts did not specify a volume of service, but rather "set a schedule according to which the unit price [would] fall as volume increases" (Jacobs 1998: 12).

9. Although Chernichovsky asserts that, under the emerging paradigm, the financing of health care is largely public, he must make the important exception of the United States. The essential features of the paradigm, however, and in particular the significance of bargaining relationships among relatively large organizations, remain the same even when the assumption of public financing is dropped.

10. As we shall see, switches from one general practice to another continued to be rare even after the easing of constraints on such shifts in the reforms after 1990.

11. Various provinces have plans covering drugs or dental care for certain categories within the population, such as children's dental care or drugs for those over 65. In the hospital sector, various amenities, such as private rooms, can be purchased on a private basis.

12. This selection does not allow us to explore the impact of different profession–state traditions or different traditions of private finance.

## Chapter 2

1. This power is nowhere explicitly mentioned in the Canadian constitution. It has, nonetheless, effectively been accepted by federal and provincial governments and affirmed in court decisions. It allows the federal government to make transfer payments in any area it chooses and to attach conditions to those transfers, "including conditions it could not directly legislate" (Hogg 1985: 126).

2. Antonia Maioni has provided an excellent analysis of the contrasting experience of Canada and the United States at this critical juncture. She attributes the difference to institutional as well as ideological differences between the two systems that allowed:

[American] progressive regional movements [to be absorbed] within the Democratic party while ensuring a prominent place for conservative southern politicians who dominated the institutional levers of Congress. In Canada, regional discontent was less effectively absorbed within the major parties, and this led to the rise of viable regional third parties, including the momentous election of a CCF government in Saskatchewan that spurred the expansion of universal hospital and medical insurance across Canada (Maioni 1995: 26–27).

3. It should also be noted that when Newfoundland entered Confederation in 1949, it brought with it a system of hospitals owned by the state and staffed by salaried physicians, in outlying areas (Taylor 1979: 170).

4. Estimated from Somers and Somers 1961: 252, 256, 258, correcting for mislabeling of chart 13-2 (256).

5. Prior to the enactment of governmental hospital insurance at the federal level in Canada in 1957, about 45% of the Canadian civilian population was enrolled in private hospital insurance plans (Department of National Health and Welfare 1958: 1). In 1959, in contrast, an estimated 72% of the U.S. civilian population was covered by some form of private hospital insurance (Somers and Somers 1961: 249).

6. Canadian proportion reported in Berry (1965: 11); U.S. proportion calculated from Somers and Somers (1961: 550–53).

7. The physician-sponsored plans inadvertently provided the model of remuneration for the government plans subsequently adopted. In contrast to the commercial insurers that offered "indemnity" insurance, paying a certain portion of the physician's fee, the physician-sponsored plans styled themselves as "prepayment" plans. Participating physicians agreed to accept the fee covered by the plan as payment in full. Most physicians, as we shall see, "participated" in the government plans in this way.

8. Public expenditures as a proportion of total health care expenditures increased from 52.1% in 1965 to 73.2% in 1971, the first year in which the plan was in operation in all provinces (calculated from OECD 1993, vol. 1: 108–9).

9. The coverage of these categories of benefits varied across the provincial plans. Various provinces covered drugs or dental care for certain categories within the population, such as children's dental care or drugs for those over 65.

10. The same Congress that adopted Medicare also enacted a number of other pieces of legislation affecting the health care delivery system. Notably, neighborhood health centers established by the Office of Economic Opportunity (the lead agency of the War on Poverty) were intended to serve the urban poor by overcoming various non-financial barriers to care in poor neighborhoods. The program was greatly overshadowed by Medicaid, however, and utilization of services was much more limited than had been envisaged (Marmor with Morone 1983: 147–48). Similarly, the Comprehensive Health Planning and Service Act established health planning agencies in all states (Marmor with Morone 1983: 149); but these agencies were ultimately swamped by the pace of change in the health care arena.

11. Physicians could choose to be "participating" or "nonparticipating" providers under Medicare. "Participating" physicians agreed to accept a Medicare-allowed "reasonable" fee as payment in full: 80% of this fee was paid by Medicare, 20% by the patient (after the patient had met an annual deductible amount). "Nonparticipating" physicians could charge patients directly for fees determined at their own discretion, and the patient was reimbursed at the Medicare-allowed charge, minus deductibles and coinsurance requirements (Health Care Financing Administration 1995a: 6).

12. Marmor and his colleagues, in putting the contemporary concern with the rise of for-profit facilities in the health care sector into historical perspective, point out that the proprietary form was the dominant form in the hospital sector in the late nineteenth and early twentieth centuries (Marmor et al. 1994: 54–55).

## Chapter 3

1. The number of pay-beds was reduced from 3,444 in 1976 to 2,533 in 1980, when the policy was abandoned by the Conservative government (Klein 1995: 112).

2. This episode is colorfully described by Rudolf Klein, who points out (following Blackstone and Plowden 1988) that it marked the "beginning of the end" for the Central Policy Review Staff, which was later disbanded by the Conservative government (Klein 1995: 140–41).

3. In its most oft-quoted statement, the report concluded, "If Florence Nightingale were carrying her lamp through the corridors of the NHS today, she would almost certainly be searching for the people in charge" (quoted in Klein 1995: 147).

4. The Management Board was set up in response to Griffiths's 1983 recommendation. It soon became an unstable vehicle for political influence over the NHS, and its role was refocused when a Management Executive and a Policy Board were created in 1989 (Ham 1992: 152–54).

5. The Resource Allocation Working Party (RAWP) formula is discussed in chapter 6.

6. DMU staff were employees of the DHA, and pay and other terms and conditions of employment were subject to national controls. Trusts employed their own staff, including consultants, and were free to determine pay and other terms and conditions of employment. Trusts were allowed to determine the range of services they wished to provide; DMUs were subject to the DHA in this regard, and had to consult formally with local Community Health Councils before closing or changing the use of facilities. Trusts were free to seek private capital within the specific External Financing Limit; DMUs were dependent on the NHS for capital. Both types of units were expected to set prices to cover capital depreciation and to provide for a specified return on capital assets. In the case of trusts, ownership of capital assets was transferred from the secretary of state or DHA to the trust, while the Treasury held a debt of equivalent value (Smee 1995: 179–81, 206–7).

7. The closest Enthoven came to such a suggestion was his recommendation of a testing of mechanisms for allowing GPs who prescribe economically to share in the savings.

8. Labour won a greater proportion of seats in 1997 (63.9% as compared with 61.6% in 1945), but a smaller proportion of the popular vote (43.1% in 1997 as compared with 47.8% in 1945).

9. The concept of the "focusing event" is John Kingdon's (1984). It has been applied to the Pennsylvania election by both Theda Skocpol (1996: 29) and Jacob Hacker (1997: 31).

10. See for example Hacker (1997), Skocpol (1996), Steinmo and Watts (1995) as well as two symposia, in *Health Affairs* 20, 1 (Spring 1995) and in the *Journal of Health Politics, Policy, and Law* 20, 2 (Summer 1995), individual contributions to which are cited elsewhere in this section and in chapters 4 and 5.

11. Whether employers would be *required* to contribute to the plan was initially left open.

12. Ironically, the last week of September loomed large in the history of American health care reform in the early 1990s. Clinton first presented his intentions in a campaign speech on September 24, 1992. On September 22, 1993, he presented his legislative proposals in a joint address to both houses of Congress. And on September 26, 1994, Senator George Mitchell, the Democratic majority leader, announced the "death" of health care reform.

13. Indeed, Senate Minority Leader Robert Dole was to prove his willingness to use the filibuster and other procedural tactics in April 1993 to kill Clinton's key economic stimulus package.

14. The accommodation between the medical profession and the state that underlay the establishment and much of the history of the British and Canadian systems is discussed throughout this book. This accommodation was much less developed in the United States, as will be argued at greater length in chapters 5 and 8. In the case of the development of the Medicare proposals of the 1960s, extensive consultation was undertaken by bureaucratic officials with Blue Cross and other hospital interests, and with organized labor. The decision in the late 1950s to concentrate on national hospital insurance for the elderly, and to cede the ground of medical care insurance, meant that consultation with organized medicine was much more intermittent. As noted in chapter 2, it was not until the legislative stage of the Medicare episode that a proposal for medical care insurance (Medicare Part B) was included in the package—an extraordinary development attributable largely to the changed makeup of Congress after the 1964 election (Marmor 1973: 109, 113–14).

15. Ramsay's extremely helpful compendium is not exhaustive. In compiling the list, Ramsay notes that "emphasis was placed on choosing the groups that most frequently appear before congressional committees to provide testimony on health policy issues. . . . [T]he chosen gropus were consistently the most frequently mentioned in general media and academic accounts of federal health policymaking activities" (Ramsay 1995: vii).

16. As Skocpol points out, one of the primary reasons for the Clinton plan's inclusion of the cost-control mechanisms that the Jackson Hole Group and others found unacceptable was the need to satisfy Congressional Budget Office (CBO) models about the effects of the plan on health care costs, both public and private. The CBO significantly discounted assumptions that such cost savings could be achieved through market competition alone (Skocpol 1996: 177–78).

17. Under the Consolidated Omnibus Budget Reconciliation Act of 1985 (COBRA), workers were entitled to retain their employer-based health insurance coverage (upon payment of the premium plus a 2% surcharge) for up to eighteen months after leaving a job.

18. Including a filibuster-proof 60% in the Senate.

19. This section draws heavily on an earlier paper (Tuohy 1996).

20. See also the special issue of the *Journal of Health Politics, Policy, and Law* 22, 3 (June 1997).

21. In Hawaii, the state that came closest to universal coverage, an estimated 7.2% of the population remained uninsured in 1991 (Dick 1994a). The State Health Insurance Plan (SHIP), introduced in 1991 to offer transitional coverage for "gap groups," and the Health QUEST program introduced in 1994 folding together Medicaid and SHIP, undoubtedly reduced this proportion. But coverage remained incomplete among employees of employers (roughly estimated at 10% of all employers [Dick 1994b]) that did not comply with the employer mandate, among those who qualified for but did not take up QUEST coverage, and among those whose incomes were above the QUEST threshold of 300% of the FPL but who could not afford private insurance (Gardner and Neubauer 1995).

22. The reference is to the head of authority under which the waivers were granted—section 1115 of the Social Security Act.

23. It is worth noting that in Hawaii, the state that pushed the boundaries of the American model of health care reform further than any other, the structure of interests

in the health care arena was relatively less complex. The private health insurance industry was highly concentrated, with two providers (the Hawaii Medical Service Association and Kaiser Permanente) accounting for 80% of coverage (Neubauer 1993). The industrial base was dominated by three industries—tourism, government, and agriculture; the island location and late entry into American statehood yielded a degree of isolation from mainland interest-group politics; and the Democratic party had dominated the island's partisan politics since Hawaii gained statehood. It is also worth noting that the foundations of Hawaii's health policies were laid in 1974, before the full flowering of complexity in the structure of the American health care arena. Yet even the Hawaiian reformers, looking as they did toward what they saw as impending developments at the national level, remained well within the American model.

24. It should also be noted, however, that some states did not have the administrative capacity to move rapidly—as was demonstrated by the severe implementation difficulties encountered by Tennessee, which chose a rapid implementation schedule precisely to avoid risking the unraveling of support and the mobilization of opposition (Gold et al. 1996).

25. The actual number of tax points transferred was calculated as the number that would indeed have yielded an amount equivalent to half of the federal transfer in the base year to the two richest provinces, then Ontario and British Columbia.

26. It was assumed that the growth in the yield from the tax points would outpace the growth of the cash transfer, and that eventually all provinces would be as well off as or better off than they would have been if the federal government had simply converted the entire transfer to a block grant and escalated it according to nominal GNP and population.

27. In 1991, the federal Parliament passed legislation enabling the government to withhold *other* transfers to the provinces in the event that the "penalty" for noncompliance with the Canada Health Act exceeded the cash transfer thereunder. This legislation was never invoked, or tested in the courts, and may have been effectively superseded by the successor Liberal government's pledge to establish a floor on federal contributions.

28. Indeed, these payments were analogous to provincial payments to hospitals in which such services were routinely performed. Ontario had licensed "independent health facilities" and had provided similar public financial support since 1988.

29. See chapter 6.

30. The forum's second and third terms of reference were to:

- promote a dialogue with Canadians about their health system in order that renewal processes will maintain and improve the health system and lead to better health while respecting the principles on which the system was built
- identify priorities for the future and develop greater consensus for change (National Forum on Health 1994).

31. The report of one of the forum's working groups went into somewhat more detail, recommending pilot projects with "population-based funding for a broad array of preventive, diagnostic and treatment services at the level of primary care" with the "populations" potentially defined in a variety of ways: "residence, consumer choice, social or other affiliation." The projects were also to include "multidisciplinary teams" of providers (National Forum on Health 1997, vol. 2: 33).

32. Turnout in regional board elections in Saskatchewan averaged 35%—comparable to that of most municipal elections in Canada (Lomas 1996: 18).

33. Under the legislation, the HSRC was established for a four-year period with a mandate to make decisions about hospital restructuring. The HSRC was accountable to

the Cabinet, in that the Cabinet could revise the HSRC's mandate or dissolve it altogether if in the minister's view its processes or decisions were severely flawed. But the HSRC was given repeated public assurances that the Cabinet would not intervene in individual decisions.

34. For a telling critique of the omnibus legislation under which the HSRC was appointed, see Weinrib (1996: 62), who argues: "Bill 26 undeniably sets aside a costlier, less efficient, slower and messier process, forwarding its stated purpose of achieving 'fiscal savings' and promoting 'economic prosperity through public sector restructuring, streamlining and efficiency.' But it does so by implementing a revolutionary, retrograde transition to an autocratic, centralized back-room, top-down government."

35. These figures compare with 12% and 15% of American respondents, respectively, and 6% and 6% of German respondents, respectively.

36. As previously discussed, these penalties amounted to less than 1% of provincial health care budgets in the case of extra billing in the mid-1980s. Alberta's penalty for allowing facility fees was about one-tenth of 1% of the provincial health care budget.

37. There was one exception. As part of the price of the agreement of the western premiers, the provinces gained increased authority over natural resources.

## Chapter 4

1. That is, no federal law could override a provincial law relating to pensions.

2. In 1986, modest changes were made to the CPP by federal–provincial agreement, to provide for greater flexibility in the retirement age, improve the rights of surviving spouses, and enhance disability benefits to bring them in line with the Quebec Pension Plan. The most significant change was an increase in the contribution rate—a change that was in the interest of provincial governments that had otherwise faced the prospect of paying back loans from the CCP (Prince 1991: 326–27).

3. As Joe White has put it in a related context, "[W]hen I hear that both 'A' and 'not A' cause 'B,' I have to suspect that some other independent variable is more significant" (White 1995: 337).

4. Arguably one other vulnerable segment of the population—children (other than those eligible for Medicaid)—was left unprotected by the policy changes of the 1960s. It is not surprising, then, that proposals to extend childrens' health insurance coverage flowed in the wake of the defeat of proposals for universal health insurance in the 1990s.

5. Arguably, however, the Federal Employee Health Benefits Program might have been employed as a model in this regard.

## Chapter 5

1. Public spending on health care in the United States amounted to about 6% of GDP in 1991, a greater proportion than was the case in Britain. Given the much higher levels of total expenditure on health in the United States than in Britain, however, U.S. public expenditure as a share of total health expenditure is only about one-half the British share.

2. Amendments in 1976, 1978, and 1988 liberalized the regulatory requirements for organizations seeking federal qualification as HMOs but also progressively removed preferential treatment for such entities. The requirement for employers to offer an HMO option where available was eliminated, no new start-up funds were distributed after 1981, and existing funding was phased out over the 1980s.

3. Other factors include the proportion of uncompensated care provided by the hospital, a local wage index, and teaching hospital status.

4. Some economists maintain that this differential between public and private payers represents "static" cost-shifting, or price discrimination. That is, it means that hospitals exercised their local market power to charge different prices depending on the price-sensitivity of the payer. Studies of "dynamic" cost-shifting—that is, raising prices to less price-sensitive private payers as prices paid by public payers decline—suggest that the ability of hospitals to pursue this strategy is limited: not all revenue lost from public payers can be recovered from private payers (Morrisey 1994: 46–59).

5. Enrollment in self-funded plans increased from about 38 million in 1988 to about 44 million in 1993 (Lipson and De Sa 1996: 64).

6. By 1981, government and philanthropy together accounted for less than 8% of funds for capital construction in health care (Institute of Medicine 1986: 185).

7. The evidence is mixed (Gilbert and Tang 1995: 211–14). Sloan and Vraciu (1983), for example, found no evidence of systematic cost differentials between investor owned and nonprofit hospitals. Pattison and Katz (1983) and Lewin et al. (1981), however, found evidence of various revenue-maximization strategies including higher margins on and utilization of ancillary services in for-profit facilities. The Institute of Medicine reviewed studies of the pre-PPS period and concluded that for-profit chain hospitals generally charged higher prices, had higher markups, and were more profitable than hospitals with other types of ownership (including independent for-profit hospitals). It noted, however, that these comparisons were complicated by the need to adjust for the various forms of subsidy afforded to not-for-profit hospitals (Institute of Medicine 1986: 76–86).

8. There is an extensive literature on this point, which will be cited more fully later in this chapter. Two useful compendia of cross-national observations are Freddi and Björkman (1989) (particularly the chapter by Döhler) and Johnson et al. 1995.

9. Twenty-eight percent reported income decreases; 24% reported income increases (Blendon et al. 1994: 1547).

10. Thirty-two percent of general practitioners and 23% of specialists reported that their incomes had increased.

11. The types were as follows: pre-admission review for all nonemergency admissions, concurrent review, retrospective review, discharge planning that does not rely on hospital staff, and ambulatory review for resource-intensive services.

12. In 1994 Blue Cross/Blue Shield surpassed Kaiser Permanente in HMO enrollment. In 1995, Blue Cross/Blue Shield HMO enrollment stood at 8.5 million and Kaiser Permanente's was at 6.7 million (Thorpe 1997: 344).

13. A March 1994 national survey, for example, found that 50% of surgeons viewed the single-player approach as "totally unacceptable" (Blendon et al. 1994: 1546).

14. A national survey of physicians found that support for making major changes to the system declined from 76% in March 1993 to 46% in March 1994. Furthermore, physicians split almost equally in their support of four possible models of reform—an individual mandate, an employer mandate, a voluntary plan, and a single-payer plan (Blendon et al. 1994).

15. Other differences involved the key role assigned in the Clinton plan to regional health purchasing alliances, which went well beyond that envisaged by the JHG for Health Insurance Purchasing Cooperatives both in their membership and their powers, as well as the system of price controls contemplated by Clinton if cost-control targets were not achieved.

16. The AMA's support for the Republican plan hinged upon the Republicans'

pledge to freeze planned reductions in the "conversion factors" used in determining physician remuneration under Medicare.

## Chapter 6  ·

1. This "unification" was, however, illusory in at least one respect: general practice continued to be, de facto, an "autonomous enclave" (Klein 1995: 88). The Family Practitioner Committees that held general practitioners' contracts shared boundaries with the AHAs but were in effect independent bodies dealing directly with the center.

2. For private insurance, these costs include sales, underwriting enrollment and policy service, claim adjudication, utilization review, actuarial functions, legal support services, investment functions, and corporate overhead and risk charges, as well as net additions to loss reserves and net underwriting gains or losses. For public administration, they include planning, regulation, monitoring, and evaluation—as well as implementation and managerial costs—of specific governmental programs of health care insurance and provision. For Britain, this includes expenditures of RHAs, DHAs, and FHAs as well as the central NHS administration, but not of hospitals, GPs, or other providers (Poullier 1992).

3. Ministerial statements emphasized the importance of maintaining a "steady state" as the reforms were being introduced—that is, maintaining similar patterns of clinical activity while developing the new purchaser–provider relationship. This "steady-state" requirement was interpreted somewhat differently by various RHAs in giving instructions to purchasers; but the general effect could be observed (as discussed in the text).

4. The major contracts surveyed by the NHS Review covered about 80% of total DHA expenditure.

5. Taking all contracts into account, survey data suggest that the proportion represented by simple block contracts declined from 43% in 1992–1993 to 20% in 1994–1995, while the proportion represented by block contracts with ceilings and floors rose from 19% to 48% (Appleby 1994: 26).

6. These figures, however, included contracts for mental health and community care. The proportion of specialty contracts in the acute services sector may have been somewhat higher.

7. Allowing for differences in the phrasing of questionnaires, the findings of these surveys were roughly comparable to those of similar surveys of American and Canadian physicians (Rappolt 1996: 184; Tunis et al. 1994; Woodward et al. 1995).

8. The fundholder's liability for expenditure on any given patient was limited to £5,000.

9. The Annual Representatives Meeting of the BMA in July 1993 passed a motion that "given the present reality, this meeting no longer asserts its opposition to fundholding" by a vote of 189–140 with 11 abstentions, after a heated debate. The BMA pointedly did not then (nor subsequently) go beyond a withdrawl of opposition to endorse the scheme (see "BMA Changes Its Attitude," *Fundholding* July 7, 1993: 5).

10. The summary of research on fundholding that follows draws heavily upon this excellent review article.

11. With the abolition of RHAs and the merger of DHAs and FHSAs in 1996, the point of accountability for fundholders became the HA.  ·

12. The question of whether these budgets were to be notional or real is potentially an important one, and it is one on which the major political parties differed. Labour, which consistently opposed the concept of fundholding as implying a two-tier system, favored notional budgets for all GPs, under the ultimate authority of the HA. The Conservatives and the Liberal Democrats favored real budgets for fundholders.

13. A third type of contract, the "cost-and-volume" contract, was essentially a hybrid of block and cost-per-case contracts. It specified a threshold level of activity to be funded on a block basis, with activity beyond that level to be funded on a cost-per-case basis. In 1994–1995, cost-per-case contracts accounted for just less than 8% of the value of contracts entered into by purchasing authorities, and cost-and-volume contracts accounted for just less than 25% (Appleby 1994: 26).

14. In 1994–1995 cost-per-case contracts accounted for 44% of the number (not the *value*) of GPFH contracts with acute care providers, according to an Audit Commission survey, and cost-and-volume contracts accounted for another 31% (Audit Commission 1996b: 34). This contrasts with proportions (again by number, not value) of 28% and 17% held by HAs with all provider types (Appleby 1994: 26).

15. In 1984, the "cost improvement program" (CIP) was inaugurated. With the advent of the internal market, the CIP was superseded by a program of targeted improvement in the "efficiency index." Under each of these programs, providers were expected to improve the ratio of a weighted sum of activity to real spending. Targets for efficiency improvements, established centrally, were in the range of 2% per year (Levitt et al. 1995: 41–44; Ham 1992: 61–62, 211–12). In 1994–1995, fewer than one-half of all providers estimated that they would achieve the efficiency target of 2.25% (Appleby 1994: 12), and the measure itself was the subject of intense criticism.

16. For example, one target was a reduction in the death rate from lung cancer in men under 75 by at least 30% and in women under 75 by at least 15% by 2010; another was to reduce conception in under-16s by at least 50% by the year 2000.

17. Copayments for dental services continued to increase over the course of the 1980s and 1990s. By 1996 patients who did not fall into exempt categories paid 80% of the cost of treatment up to a maximum of £300 for each course of treatment (Shepherd et al. 1996: 922).

18. This figure does not include abortions. More than one-third of all abortions performed on U.K. residents were privately financed and supplied in 1993 (Laing and Buisson 1995: A94).

19. About 800,000 people subscribed to private dental care plans in 1994, as compared with 25.4 million registered under NHS capitation. The number of dentists registered with the three largest plans increased from zero to 7,500 from the mid-1980s to the mid-1990s. (About 19,400 dentists participated in the general dental service of the NHS in 1994.) (Shepherd et al. 1996: 922).

20. These calculations do not include surgeons', anesthestists', and physicians' fees, which were similar in both pay-bed and independent hospital venues.

21. A complex monopoly was defined to exist where at least one-quarter of a certain type of service was supplied by members of the same group who "so conduct their respective affairs as in any way to prevent, restrict or distort competition in connection with the supply of these services" (Laing and Buisson 1995: A119).

22. Of the approximately 20,500 specialists with NHS consultant appointments in 1992 about 14,500 also engaged in private practice. An estimated 2,500 specialists who had retired from NHS positions also engaged in private practice. Only about 200 specialists engaging in private practice did not have NHS appointments. The proportion of the working week of NHS consultants devoted to private practice ranged from about 10% to about 33%, depending on the nature of their NHS appointment (Monopolies and Mergers Commission 1994: 13–14, 48).

23. While indulging in some rhetoric about "rejecting" the internal market and setting out a long litany of criticisms of its operation, Labour proposed changes that would in fact maintain it. The essential feature of the market—the purchaser–provider split—

would continue. Trust assets, however, were to be held owned and held nationally by the NHS (but not, as was the case prior to the internal market reforms, by the HAs), in order to make them less vulnerable to privatization. GP fundholding would be replaced by a system in which all GPs would participate in "GP commissioning" under the aegis of HAs— a development which, as noted earlier, would represent a particular path of evolution from the existing "purchaser plurality." Long-term "agreements" would replace annual contracts between purchasers and providers—a development that was also well underway by 1995. Performance indicators would be elaborated. And, not surprisingly, the emphasis in making appointments to the boards of health authorities and hospitals would ensure that the membership was "openly selected and broadly based to reflect the communities they serve," in contrast to the Conservative emphasis on business acumen.

24. As Propper (1995) has noted, the relationship between purchaser and provider managements and hospital doctors can be thought of as a set of overlapping pairs of principal-agent relationships: the provider management acts under contract as the purchaser's agent, and the hospital medical staff acts as the agent of provider management. One might also introduce into this mix the role of public health physicians, acting as the agents of purchaser management in dealing with hospital clinicians.

## Chapter 7

1. The German system functioned according to its own version of such a logic as well. But the German case was further complicated by the system of social insurance, in which the sickness funds as quasigovernmental organizations played an intermediate role between federal and state ministries and departments on the one hand and the medical profession on the other.

2. In eight provinces, private insurance coverage for services insured under the government plan was banned. But even in the absence of a formal ban, other features of the system made private coverage for publicly insured services uneconomical. After 1984, physicians could not "extra bill" for an amount beyond the government benefit: hence there was no need for "Medi-gap" insurance such as existed for Medicare recipients in the United States. Physicians could opt out of the public system entirely, but provincial regulations made this an unattractive option. In several provinces patients of opted-out physicians were denied any reimbursement from the public plan; in others, the rates that opted-out physicians could charge were regulated at the levels established under the government plan.

3. In Saskatchewan, professional "self-government" was also symbolized by allowing physician-sponsored medical care insurance plans to continue as "carriers" of government insurance. Other provinces varied in the extent to which the physician-sponsored plans chose to play what some saw as a "post office" role (Taylor 1979: 375–76). In any event, the "carrier" role was phased out after the first few years of medicare's operation.

4. Ontario physicians represented about 40% of all Canadian physicians, and both net professional incomes and medical fees were close to the Canadian average (Barer and Evans 1986: 78, 94).

5. I have discussed these provincial-level accommodations throughout the 1970s and 1980s in an earlier work (Tuohy 1992: 123–29). The present discussion draws heavily on that discussion.

6. The average annual increase in the Consumer Price Index in the 1970s was 8.0%, while hospital inflation was 10.9% and medical fees increased at an average annual rate of 5.3%. In the 1980s the corresponding figures were 5.9% for the CPI, 6.8% for hospital prices and 6.1% for medical fees (OECD 1995: 42).

7. Real per capita spending increased by 26.6% in the hospital sector and by 48.9% in the physician services sector between 1975 and 1990 (Health Canada 1997: table 5).

8. For a discussion of a somewhat more modest experiment in British Columbia using "Weighted Patient Days," see Haazen (1992).

9. As a share of total *public* expenditures on health, hospital spending declined from 54.3% in 1975 to 46.3% in 1990, and further to an estimated 42.9% in 1996. Over the same periods, the physician services share remained constant at about 20% (Health Canada 1997: table 6).

10. The summary of expenditure cap policies in the following paragraphs owes much to the comprehensive report prepared by Hurley et al. (1997).

11. These thresholds were established at relatively generous levels. In Ontario, for example, thresholds imposed during a stalemate in negotiations in 1996 were calculated at 40% above the median billings in each of thirty-two groups. This yielded thresholds roughly comparable to those that were previously and subsequently negotiated in Ontario and in other provinces. Across those provinces with individual billing thresholds in the mid-1990s, proration began at thresholds ranging from C$250,000–3000,000 for GPs and from C$325,000–400,000 for specialists (Hurley et al. 1997: table 2).

12. A similar policy was adopted on a short-term basis in Alberta, but never implemented.

13. The British Columbia provincial government had argued that any such limitations were necessary for the management of the health care system, and as such were consistent with the provision of the Charter that rights could be subject to such "reasonable limits, prescribed by law, as can be demonstrably justified in a free and democratic society"—an argument that it had not invoked in the mid-1980s case previously noted. The court, however, rejected this argument.

14. By 1993, further clinical trials had demonstrated a clear but marginal advantage to the use of tPA, but the provincial ministry continued to insist that it be funded, if at all, within global hospital budgets and not through extraglobal funding.

15. Candidates for deinsurance also included some services by nonphysicians that had been added to various provincial plans over time beyond the requirement to insure "medically necessary" services.

16. Another dramatic clash between the political interests of a government and the professional (not economic) interests of physicians occurred in Alberta in the mid-1990s, when the Conservative government announced that it would cover only those abortions deemed "medically necessary" according to guidelines to be developed by the Alberta College of Physicians and Surgeons. Both the college and the Alberta Medical Association refused to cooperate in this exercise, however, and the initiative was dropped.

17. The only significant exception involved services provided under workers' compensation insurance.

18. Even when the finance ministry was not formally present at the table, as in Quebec, it was clearly consulted by the government side (Lomas et al. 1992: 88).

19. That is, payment for a given service could be reduced or denied if the number of services provided to a given patient, or by a given physician, or within a given facility exceeded a prescribed maximum during a particular time period. The legislation also granted the government broad regulatory powers to control expenditures, limit the number of practitioners, and affect the geographic distribution of practitioners and facilities.

20. Notwithstanding the government's withdrawal of recognition from the OMA, it soon recognized that there was no feasible alternative agent to achieving a degree of peace with the profession.

21. As noted in chapter 5, international evidence suggested that Canadian physicians were more satisfied with their health system than were American physicians; the Canadians were less likely to complain of restrictions on clinical freedom but more likely to complain about limited facilities and equipment (Blendon et al. 1993: 1015).

22. See note 21.

23. In the mid-1990s there was a net migration from Canada to the United States of about 400–500 physicians a year, less than 1% of Canadian practicing physicians. But the disproportionate representation of certain subspecialties in the CMA survey sample suggests that the impact of out-migration on the Canadian physician stock may have been greater than the relatively small numbers would suggest (McKendry et al. 1996: 171).

24. The average annual rates of hospital medical, dental, and pharmaceutical inflation from 1980 to 1990 were 6.8%, 6.1%, 9.6%, and 6.6%, respectively (OECD 1995: 42; 1993, vol. 1: 151).

25. The extent to which the existence of governmental health insurance does provide firms with a competitive advantage is a matter of some dispute. Some economists maintain that health benefits simply form part of the compensation package for employees, and that as benefit costs decrease, wages will rise and vice versa (Fuchs 1993: 158–59). Others, however, point to the lower levels of health care price inflation and the lower administrative costs (for employers as well as public administrators) under governmental systems to demonstrate their cost advantages to business (Purchase 1996: 13). In the increasingly integrated North American economy, Canadian firms are more and more sensitive to such differentials.

26. These approaches were seen as efficiency enhancing, although the administrative costs of implementing them received little or no attention. Clearly, however, one reason that the administrative costs of Canada's public system were as low as they were, in international perspective, lies in the limited role that the monitoring of medical practice and the management of vertical and horizontal organizations played in the system.

27. There were a few exceptions in the hospital sector. Although hospital global budgets were largely historically based, some provincial governments contracted with hospitals to provide specified volumes of a few given procedures, such as coronary artery bypass surgery. Regional health authorities in Alberta also appeared to be attracted to the contracting mechanism.

## Chapter 8

1. For one review of such studies, see Tuohy (1994a).

2. Long-term and home care are financed separately from acute care under Medicare and Medicaid (Leutz et al. 1994). Overlaps between the two programs, moreover, have encouraged states to engage in various forms of cost-shifting with regard to their dually enrolled populations, and in some cases to press for federal waivers to allow funding from the two programs to be pooled to facilitate better integration (Kenney et al. 1998).

# References

Adams, Louise. 1995. "NHS Trusts." In *NHS Handbook 1995/96*. Birmingham: National Association of Health Authorities and Trusts.

Advisory Committee on Health Services. 1995. "A Model for the Reorganization of Primary Care and the Introduction of Population-based Funding." Report prepared for the Federal/Provincial/Territorial Conference of Deputy Ministers of Health (September). Ottawa: Health Canada Federal/Provincial Liaison.

Agnew, G. Harvey. 1974. *Canadian Hospitals, 1920 to 1970*. Toronto: University of Toronto Press.

Aldrich, Jonathan. 1982. "The Earnings Replacement Rate of Old-Age Benefits in 12 Countries, 1969–80." *Social Security Bulletin* 45, 11: 3–11.

Allsop, Judith. 1995. *Health Policy and the NHS: Towards 2000*. 2nd ed. London: Longman.

Alvi, Shahid. 1995. *Health Costs and Private Sector Competitiveness*. Ottawa: Conference Board of Canada.

American Hospital Association. 1995. *Hospital Statistics, 1994–95 Edition*. Chicago: American Hospital Association.

Amess, Moyra, Kieran Walshe, Charles Shaw, and James Cole. 1995. *The Audit Activities of the Medical Royal Colleges and Their Faculties in England*. London: CASPE Research.

Appleby, John. 1994. *Developing Contracting: A National Survey of Health Authorities, Boards, and NHS Trusts*. Birmingham, England: National Association of Health Authorities and Trusts.

Appleby, John, Paula Smith, Wendy Ranade, Val Little, and Ray Robinson. 1994. "Monitoring Managed Competition." In Ray Robinson and Julian Le Grand, eds., *Evaluating the NHS Reforms*. London: King's Fund Institute, 24–53.

Arthur, W. Brian. 1994. *Increasing Returns and Path Dependency in the Economy*. Ann Arbor: University of Michigan Press.

Atkinson, Rob and Stephen Cope. 1994. "Changing Styles of Governance since 1979." In Stephen P. Savage and Rob Atkinson, eds., *Public Policy in Britain*. New York: St. Martin's, 31–52.

Atkinson, Rob, and Stephen P. Savage. 1994. "The Conservatives and Public Policy." In Stephen P. Savage and Rob Atkinson, eds., *Public Policy in Britain*. New York: St. Martin's, 3–14.

Audit Commission. 1995. *For Your Information: A Study of Information Management and Systems in the Acute Hospital*. London: HMSO.

———. 1996a. *What the Doctor Ordered: A Study of GP Fundholders in England and Wales*. London: HMSO.

———. 1996b. *Fundholding Facts*. London: HMSO.

———. 1997. *Comparing Notes: A Study of Information Management in Community Trusts*. London: HMSO.

Baker, Laurence C., and Joel C. Cantor. 1993. "Physician Satisfaction under Managed Care." *Health Affairs* (Supplement): 258–70.

Baltzan, Marc A. 1983. "Why C.M.A. Opposes Canada Health Act." *Ontario Medical Review* (July): 345–47.

Banting, Keith. 1987. *The Welfare State and Canadian Federalism*. 2nd ed. Montreal: McGill-Queen's.

———. 1992. "Economic Integration and Social Policy: Canada and the United States." In Terrance M. Hunsley, ed., *Social Policy in the Global Economy*. Kingston, Ontario: Queen's University School of Policy Studies, 21–44.

Barer, Morris, and Robert G. Evans. 1986. "Riding North on a South-bound Horse: Expenditures, Prices, Utilization, and Incomes in the Canadian Health Care System." In Robert G. Evans and Greg L. Stoddart, eds., *Medicare at Maturity*. Calgary: University of Calgary Press, 53–164.

Barer, Morris L., Jonathan Lomas, and Claudia Sanmartin. 1996. "Re-Minding Our Ps and Qs: Medical Cost Controls in Canada." *Health Affairs* 15, 2 (Summer): 216–34.

Bartlett, Will. 1991. *Quasi-Markets and Contracts: A Markets and Hierarchies Perspective on NHS Reform*. Bristol: University of Bristol School for Advanced Urban Studies.

Baumgartner, Frank R., and Bryan D. Jones. 1993. *Agendas and Instability in American Politics*. Chicago: University of Chicago Press.

Beer, Samuel H. 1982. *Britain Against Itself*. New York: Norton.

———. 1998. "The Roots of New Labour: Liberalism Rediscovered." *The Economist* (February 7): 23–25.

Bell, Judith E. 1996. "Saving Their Assets: How to Stop Plunder at Blue Cross and Other Nonprofits." *The American Prospect* 25 (May/June): 60–66.

Benady, Susannah. 1993. "Succeed by Talking Doctor to Doctor." *Fundholding* (April 21): 20–23.

Bergthold, Linda. 1990. "The Frayed Alliance: Business and Health Care in Massachusetts." *Journal of Health Politics, Policy, and Law* 15, 4: 915–18

Berry, Charles H. 1965. *Voluntary Medical Insurance and Prepayment*. Background study for the Royal Commission on Health Services. Ottawa: Queen's Printer.

Besley, Timothy, John Hall, and Ian Preston. 1996. *Private Health Insurance and the State of the NHS*. London: Institute for Fiscal Studies.

Bhatia, V., S. West, and M. Giacomini. 1996. "Equity in Case-based Funding: A Case Study of Meanings and Messages in Hospital Funding Policy." Working Paper

No. 96–13, Centre for Health Economics and Policy Analysis. Hamilton, Ontario: McMaster University.

Björkman, James Warner. 1985. "Who Governs the Health Sector?" *Comparative Politics* 17 (July): 399–420.

Black, Sir Douglas. 1980. *Report of the Working Group on Inequalities in Health.* London: Secretary of State for Social Services.

Blackstone, Tessa, and William Plowden. 1988. *Inside the Think Tank.* London: Heinemann.

Blendon, Robert J. 1989. "Three Systems: A Comparative Survey." *Health Management Quarterly* XI, 1: 2–10.

Blendon, Robert J., and Karen Donelan. 1989. "British Public Opinion on National Health Service Reform." *Health Affairs* 8, 4 (Winter): 52–62.

Blendon, Robert J., Robert Leitman, Ian Morrison, and Karen Donelan. 1990. "Satisfaction with Health Systems in Ten Nations." *Health Affairs* 9, 2 (Summer): 185–92.

Blendon, Robert J., Karen Donelan, Robert Leitman, Arnold Epstein, Joel C. Cantor, Alan B. Cohen, Ian Morrison, Thomas Moloney, Christian Koeck, and Samuel Levitt. 1993. "Physicians' Perspectives on Caring for Patients in the United States, Canada, and West Germany." *New England Journal of Medicine* 328, 14: 1011–16.

Blendon, Robert J., Andrew Kohut, John M. Benson, Karen Donelan, and Carol Bowman. 1994. "Health System Reform: Physicians' Views on the Critical Choices," *Journal of the American Medical Association* 272, 19 (November 16): 1546–50.

Blendon, Robert J., John Benson, Karen Donelan, Robert Leitman, Humphrey Taylor, Christian Koeck, and Daniel Gitterman. 1995. "Who Has the Best Health Care System? A Second Look." *Health Affairs* 14, 4: 220–30.

Blewett, Lynn A. 1994. "State Report: Reforms in Minnesota: Forging the Path." *Health Affairs* 13, 4 (Fall): 200–9.

Boulding, Kenneth. 1968. *Beyond Economics.* Ann Arbor: University of Michigan Press.

Boycko, Maxim, Andrei Shleifer, and Robert W. Vishny. 1996. "A Theory of Privatization." *The Economic Journal* 106 (March): 309–19.

Brethour, Patrick. 1998. "Hospital Cures Computer Ailment." *The Globe and Mail.* Toronto (July 29): B27.

British Medical Association. 1995. *Core Values for the Medical Profession in the 21st Century: Survey Report.* London: British Medical Association.

Brodie, Mollyann, and Robert J. Blendon. 1995. "The Public's Contribution to Congressional Gridlock on Health Care Reform." *Journal of Health Politics, Policy, and Law* 20, 2 (Summer): 403–10.

Brown, Lawrence D. 1991. "Capture and Culture: Organizational Identity in New York Blue Cross." *Journal of Health Politics, Policy, and Law* 16, 4: 651–70.

Brown, Malcolm. 1996. "New Zealand Health Care Financing 'Reforms' Perceived in Ideological Context." *Health Care Analysis* 4: 293–308.

Burda, David. 1994. "How Much are Physicians Making?" *Modern Healthcare* (July 11): 43–49.

———. 1995. "How Much Depends on Who Asks." *Modern Healthcare* (July 10): 42.

Butler, Eamonn. 1994. "A Market Future for NHS Purchasing." In Eamonn Butler, ed., *Unhealthy Competition: The Public/Private Mix for Health.* London: Adam Smith Research Trust.

Butler, John. 1992. *Patients, Policies, and Politics.* Buckingham: Open University Press.

Buttery, Yvette, Kieran Walshe, James Coles, and Jennifer Bennett. 1994. *The Development of Audit: Findings of a National Survey of Healthcare Provider Units in England.* London: CASPE Research.

Buxton, Martin, Tim Packwood, and Justin Keen. 1991. *Final Report of the Brunel University Evaluation of Resource Management: Summary.* Uxbridge: Brunel University Health Economics Research Group.

Canadian Medical Association. 1998a. *Restoring Access to Quality Health Care: Brief Submitted to the House of Commons Standing Committee on Finance.* Ottawa: Canadian Medical Association.

———. 1998b. *Resolutions Adopted By CMA at 1998 General Council.* Ottawa: Canadian Medical Association.

Cantor, Joel C., Stephen H. Long, and M. Susan Marquis. 1995. "Private Employment-based Insurance in Ten States." *Health Affairs* 14, 2 (Summer): 199–211.

Cawson, Alan. 1982. *Corporatism and Welfare: Social Policy and State Intervention in Britain.* London: Heinemann.

Challis, Linda, Patricia Day, Rudolf Klein, and Ellie Scrivens. 1994. "Managing Quasi-Markets: Institutions of Regulation." In Will Bartlett et al., eds., *Quasi-Markets in the Welfare State.* Bristol: University of Bristol School for Advanced Urban Studies, 10–32.

Chernichovsky, Dov. 1995. "Health System Reforms in Industrialized Democracies: An Emerging Paradigm." *The Milbank Quarterly* 73, 3: 339–72.

Chisman, Forrest, Lawrence D. Brown, and Pamela J. Larson, eds. 1994. *National Health Forum: What Should the State Role Be?* Washington, D.C.: National Academy of Social Insurance.

Chrétien, Jean. 1994. "Opening Remarks to the National Forum on Health." Ottawa, Ontario (October 24).

Christianson, Jon, et al. 1995. "Managed Care in the Twin Cities." *Health Affairs* 14, 2 (Summer): 114–30.

Conference of Provincial/Territorial Ministers of Health. 1997. *A Renewed Vision for Canada's Health System.* Mimeograph.

Coombs, Rod, and David Cooper. 1992. "Accounting for Patients? Information Technology and the Implementation of the NHS White Paper." In Ray Loveridge and Ken Starkey, eds., *Continuity and Crisis in the NHS.* Buckingham: Open University Press, 118–25.

Cope, Stephen, and Rob Atkinson. 1994. "Changing Styles of Governance since 1979." In Stephen P. Savage and Rob Atkinson, eds., *Public Policy in Britain.* New York: St. Martin's, 31–52.

Coulter, Angela. 1995. "Evaluating General Practice Fundholding in the United Kingdom." *European Journal of Public Health* 5, 4: 233–39.

Coulter, Angela, and J. Bradlow. 1993. "The Effect of NHS Reforms on General Practitioners' Referral Patterns." *British Medical Journal* 306: 433–37.

Courchene, Thomas J. 1995. *Redistributing Money and Power: A Guide to the Canada Health and Social Transfer.* Toronto: C.D. Howe Institute.

———. 1996. *ACCESS: A Convention on the Canadian Economic and Social Systems.* A working paper prepared for the Ministry of Intergovernmental Affairs, Government of Ontario. Toronto: Ministry of Intergovernmental Affairs.

Coutts, Jane. 1995. "Support for Health-Care Principles Weaker among Well-off." *The Globe and Mail.* Toronto (October 26): A21.

———. 1996. "Doctors Tiptoe Toward Reforms." *The Globe and Mail.* Toronto (August 21): A1, A6.

Crittenden, Robert A. 1995. "State Report: Rolling Back Reform in the Pacific Northwest." *Health Affairs* 14, 2 (Summer): 302–5.

Curtis, Richard E., and Kevin Haugh. 1994. "Health Care Reform and Insurance Regulation." In Forrest Chisman, Lawrence D. Brown, and Pamela J. Larson, eds., *National Health Forum: What Should the State Role Be?* Washington, D.C.: National Academy of Social Insurance, 53–70.

David, Paul. 1985. "Clio and the Economics of QWERTY." *American Economic Review* 75: 332–37.

Davis, Karen, Karen Scott Collins, Cathy Schoen, and Cynthia Morris. 1995a. "Choice Matters: Enrollees' Views of Their Health Plans." *Health Affairs* 14, 2 (Summer): 99–112.

Davis, Karen, Diane Rowland, Drew Altman, Karen Scott Collins, and Cynthia Morris. 1995b. "Health Insurance: The Size and Shape of the Problem." *Inquiry* 32 (Summer): 196–203.

Day, Patricia, and Rudolf Klein. 1991. "Britain's Health Care Experiment." *Health Affairs* (Fall): 39–59.

———. 1992. "Constitutional and Distributional Conflict in British Medical Politics: The Case of General Practice, 1911–1991." *Political Studies* 40 (September): 462–78.

Department of Finance. 1995. *Budget Plan.* Ottawa: Department of Finance.

Department of Health. 1997. *The New NHS.* London: HMSO.

Department of National Health and Welfare. 1955. *Hospitals in Canada.* Ottawa: Department of National Health and Welfare.

———. 1958. *Voluntary Hospital and Medical Insurance in Canada, 1956.* Ottawa: Department of National Health and Welfare.

Desrosiers, Georges. 1986. "The Quebec Health Care System." *Journal of Health Politics, Policy, and Law* 11 (Summer): 211–17.

Dick, Andrew. 1994a. "Will Employer Mandates Really Work?" *Health Affairs* 13, 2 (Spring I): 343–49.

———. 1994b. "Hawaii: The Author Responds." *Health Affairs* 13, 4 (Fall): 232–35.

Döhler, Marian. 1989. "Physicians' Professional Autonomy in the Welfare State: Endangered or Preserved?" In Giorgio Freddi and James Warner Björkman, eds., *Controlling Medical Professionals: The Comparative Politics of Health Governance.* London: Sage, 178–244.

———. 1991. "Policy Networks, Opportunity Structures, and Neo-Conservative Reform Strategies in Health Policy." In Bernd Marin and Renate Mayntz, eds., *Policy Networks: Empirical Evidence and Theoretical Considerations.* Boulder, Colo.: Westview, 235–96.

———. 1994. "The State as Architect of Political Order: Policy Dynamics in German Health Care." Paper prepared for the Workshop on the State and the Health Care System, European Consortium for Political Research, Madrid, Spain, April 17–22.

Dunleavy, Patrick. 1990. "Government at the Centre." In Patrick Dunleavy, Andrew Gamble, and Gillian Peele, eds., *Development in British Politics.* New York: St. Martin's, 96–125.

Dunn, Mike, and Sandy Smith. 1994. "Economic Policy under the Conservatives." In Stephen P. Savage and Rob Atkinson, eds., *Public Policy in Britain.* New York: St. Martin's, 77–95.

Duplantie, Jean-Pierre. 1996. "Quebec's Responses to Regional Processes of Health Care Reform." Paper delivered at the conference on Reorganizing Canadian Health Care: Global Pressures/New Institutional Realities, Toronto, York University, April 1–2.

Dyck, Rand. 1988. "The Position of Ontario in the Canadian Federation." In R. D.

Olling and M. W. Westmacott, eds., *Perspectives on Canadian Federalism*. Scarborough, Ontario: Prentice-Hall, 326–45.

Elola, Javier. 1996. "Health Care System Reforms in Western European Countries: The Relevance of Health Care Organization." *International Journal of Health Services* 26, 2: 239–51.

Employer Committee on Health Care–Ontario. 1995. *A Perspective on Health Care.* Toronto: Employer Committee on Health Care–Ontario.

Enthoven, Alain C. 1978. "Consumer Choice Health Plan" (parts 1 and 2). *New England Journal of Medicine* 298, 12: 650–58, 13: 709–20.

———. 1985. *Reflections on the National Health Service.* London: Nuffield Provincial Hospitals Trust.

———. 1993. "The History and Principles of Managed Competition." *Health Affairs* (Supplement): 24–48.

———. 1994. "Why Not the Clinton Health Plan?" *Inquiry* 31 (Summer): 129–35.

Erichsen, Vibeke. 1995. "State Traditions and Medical Professionalization in Scandinavia." In Terry Johnson, Gerry Larkin, and Mike Saks, eds., *Health Professions and the State in Europe*. London: Routledge, 187–99.

Esping-Andersen, Gosta. 1990. *The Three Worlds of Welfare Capitalism*. Princeton, N.J.: Princeton University Press.

Evans, Robert G., Jonathan Lomas, Morris L. Barer, Roberta J. Labelle, Catherine Fooks, Gregory L. Stoddart, Geoffrey M. Anderson, David Feeney, Amiram Gafni, George W. Torrance, and William G. Tholl. 1989. "Controlling Health Expenditures—The Canadian Reality." *New England Journal of Medicine* 320, 9 (March 2): 571–7.

Fairfield, Gollian, and Rhys Williams. 1996. "Clinical Guidelines in the Independent Sector." *British Medical Journal* 312: 1554–55.

Feder, J., J. Hadley, and R. Mullner. 1984. "Falling through the Cracks: Poverty, Insurance Coverage, and Hospital Care for the Poor, 1980 and 1982." *Milbank Memorial Fund Quarterly* 62 (Fall): 544–66.

Feeny, David. 1994. "Technology Asessment and Health Policy in Canada." In Ake Blomqvist and David M. Brown, eds., *Limits to Care: Reforming Canada's Health System in an Age of Restraint*. Toronto: C.D. Howe Institute, 295–326.

Ferlie, Ewan. 1994. "The Evolution of Quasi-Markets in the NHS: Early Evidence." In Will Bartlett et al. eds., *Quasi-Markets in the Welfare State*. Bristol: University of Bristol School for Advanced Urban Studies, 209–24.

Ferrara, Maurizio. 1995. "The Rise and Fall of Democratic Universalism: Health Care Reform in Italy, 1978–1994." *Journal of Health Politics, Policy, and Law* 20, 2 (Summer): 275–302.

Figueras, Josep, Jennifer A. Roberts, and Colin F. Sanderson. 1993. "Contracting, Planning, Competition, and Efficiency." In M. Malek, P. Vacani, J. Rasquinha, and P. Davey, eds., *Managerial Issues in the Reformed NHS*. London: John Wiley, 223–36.

Flood, C. M. 1996. "Prospects for New Zealand's Internal Market." Paper prepared for the meeting of the International Health Economics Association, Vancouver, British Columbia, May, 19–20.

Fox, Daniel M. 1986. *Health Policies, Health Politics: The British and American Experience 1911–65*. Princeton, N.J.: Princeton University Press.

Fox, Daniel M., and Howard M. Leichter. 1993. "The Ups and Downs of Oregon's Rationing Plan." *Health Affairs* 12, 2 (Summer): 66–70.

Freddi, Giorgio, and James Warner Björkman, eds. 1989. *Controlling Medical Professionals: The Comparative Politics of Health Governance*. London: Sage.

Fubini, Sylvia. 1996. "Not-for-profit vs. For-profit: Reading the Tea Leaves." *Healthcare Trends Report* 10, 4 (April): 1–2, 16.

Fuchs, Victor. 1983. "The Battle for the Control of Health Care." *Health Affairs* 1, 3: 5–13.

———. 1993. *The Future of Health Policy*. Cambridge, Mass.: Harvard University Press.

Gagnon, Alain C., and Joseph Garcea. 1988. "Quebec and the Pursuit of Special Status." In R. D. Olling and M. W. Westmacott, eds., *Perspectives on Canadian Federalism*. Scarborough, Ontario: Prentice-Hall.

Gallup Canada. 1991. *The Gallup Report*. Toronto, August 1.

Gamble, Andrew. 1990. "The Thatcher Decade in Perspective." In Patrick Dunleavy, Andrew Gamble, and Gillian Peele, eds., *Developments in British Politics*. New York: St. Martin's, 333–58.

Gamliel, Sandy, Robert M. Politzer, Marc L. Rivo, and Fitzhugh Mullan. 1995. "Will Physicians Meet the Managed Care Challenge?" *Health Affairs* 14, 2 (Summer): 130–42.

Gardner, Annette, and Deane Neubauer. 1995. "State Report: Hawaii's Health QUEST." *Health Affairs* 14, 1 (Spring): 300–3.

Garland, Michael J. 1991. "Setting Health Care Priorities in Oregon." *Health Matrix* 1, 2 (Summer): 139–56.

Garpenby, Peter. 1995. "Health Care Reform in Sweden in the 1990s: Local Pluralism vs. National Coordination." *Journal of Health Politics, Policy, and Law* 20, 3 (Fall): 695–718.

General Accounting Office. 1991. *Canadian Health Insurance: Lessons for the United States*. Report to the Chairman, Committee on Government Operations, House of Representatives. Washington, D.C.: United States GAO, June.

Gilbert, Neil, and Kwong Leung Tang. 1995. "The United States." In Norman Johnson, ed., *Private Markets in Health and Welfare: An International Perspective*. Oxford: Berg, 203–23.

Gillam, Steve. 1998. "Clinical Governance." In Rudolf Klein, ed., *Implementing the White Paper: Pitfalls and Opportunities*. London: The King's Fund, 66–73.

Ginsburg, Paul B. 1996. "RWJF Community Snapshops Study: Introduction and Overview." *Health Affairs* 15, 2 (Summer): 7–20.

Glazner, Judith, William R. Braithwaite, Steven Hull, and Dennis C. Lezotte. 1995. "Questionable Value of Medical Screening in the Small-Group Market." *Health Affairs* 14, 2 (Summer): 224–34.

Glennerster, Howard, and Julian Le Grand. 1995. "The Development of Quasi-Markets in Welfare Provision in the United Kingdom." *International Journal of Health Services* 25, 2: 203–18.

Glennerster, Howard, Manos Matsaganis, Pat Owens, and Stephanie Hancock. 1994. "GP Fundholding: Wild Card or Winning Hand?" In Ray Robinson and Julian Le Grand, eds., *Evaluating the NHS Reforms*. London: King's Fund Institute, 74–197.

Gold, Marsha R., Robert Hurley, Timothy Lake, Todd Ensor, and Robert Berenson. 1995. "A National Survey of the Arrangements Managed-care Plans Make with Physicians." *New England Journal of Medicine* 333, 25 (December 21): 1678–83.

Gold, Marsha, Michael Sparer, and Karyen Chu. 1996. "Medicaid Managed Care: Lessons from Five States." *Health Affairs* 15, 3 (Fall): 153–66.

Gottlieb, Martin. 1995. "The Managed Care Cure-All Shows Its Flaws and Potential." *New York Times* (October): 1; 10.

Granovetter, Mark. 1992. "Economic Institutions as Social Constructions: A Framework for Analysis." *Acta Sociologica* 35: 3–11.

Gray, Gwendolyn. 1996. "Reform and Reaction in Australian Health Policy." *Journal of Health Politics, Policy, and Law* 21, 3 (Fall): 587–615.

Greene, Jay. 1995. "Tax-exempts Feeling the Heat." *Modern Healthcare* (November 20): 46–52.

Greene, Jay, and Sandy Lutz. 1995. "A Down Year at Not-for-profits; For-profits Soar." *Modern Healthcare* (May): 22, 43–50.

Greenspon, Edward, and Hugh Winsor. 1997. "Spending Increase Favoured, Poll Finds." *The Globe and Mail*. Toronto (January 23): A1, A8.

Groenewegen, Peter P. 1994. "The Shadow of the Future: Institutional Changes in Health Care." *Health Affairs* 13, 5 (Winter): 137–48.

Haazen, Dominic S. 1992. "Redefining the Globe: Recent Changes in the Financing of British Columbia Hospitals." In Raisa B. Deber and Gail G. Thompson, eds., *Restructuring Canada's Health Services System: How Do We Get There from Here?* Toronto: University of Toronto Press, 73–84.

Hacker, Jacob. 1997. *The Road to Nowhere*. Princeton, N.J.: Princeton University Press.

Hall, Peter. 1986. *Governing the Economy: The Politics of State Intervention in Britain and France*. New York: Oxford.

Ham, Christopher. 1992. *Health Policy in Britain: The Politics and Organization of the National Health Service*. 3rd ed. London: Macmillan.

———. 1997. "Reforming the New Zealand Health Reforms." *British Medical Journal* 314 (June 28): 1844–45.

Harrison, Stephen. 1995. "Clinical Autonomy and Planned Markets: The British Case." In Richard B. Saltman and Casten von Otter, eds., *Implementing Planned Markets in Health Care: Balancing Social and Economic Responsibility*. Buckingham: Open University Press, 156–76.

Harrison, Stephen, and Christopher Pollitt. 1994. *Controlling Health Professionals: The Future of Work and Organization in the NHS*. Buckingham: Open University Press.

Harrison, Stephen, and Rockwell I. Schulz. 1989. "Clinical Autonomy in the United Kingdom and the United States: Contrasts and Convergence." In Giorgio Freddi and James Warner Björkman, eds., *Controlling Medical Professionals: The Comparative Politics of Health Governance*. London: Sage, 198–243.

Hartz, Louis. 1955. *The Liberal Tradition in America*. Toronto: Longman.

Hatch, S., and I. Mocroft, 1983. *Components of Welfare*. London: Bedford Square.

Health Canada. 1996. *National Health Expenditures in Canada 1975-1994*. Policy and Consultation Branch. Ottawa: Health Canada.

———. 1997. *National Health Expenditures in Canada 1975–1996*. Health System and Policy Division. Ottawa: Health Canada.

Health Care Financing Administration (HCFA). 1995a. *Health Care Financing Review: 1995 Statistical Supplement*. Washington, D.C.: Health Care Financing Administration.

———. 1995b. "Minnesota Health Care Demonstrations Approved." Press Release, April 27.

———. 1995c. "Kentucky Medicaid Demonstration Amendment Approved." Press Release, October 11.

Health Services Utilization and Research Commission. 1995. *A Closer Look*. Saskatoon, Saskatchewan: Health Services Utilization and Research Commission (Summer).

Heclo, Hugh. 1981. "Toward a New Welfare State?" In Peter Flora and Arnold J. Heidenheimer, eds., *The Development of Welfare States in Europe and America*. New Brunswick, N.J.: Transaction Books Flora, 383–406.

———. 1995. "The Clinton Health Plan: Historical Perspective." *Health Affairs* 14, 1 (Spring): 86–95.

Henke, Klaus-Dirk, Margaret A. Murray, and Claudia Ade. 1994. "Global Budgeting in Germany: Lessons for the United States." *Health Affairs* 13, 4 (Fall): 7–21.

Hinrichs, Karl. 1995. "The Impact of German Health Insurance Reforms on Redistribution and the Culture of Solidarity." *Journal of Health Politics, Policy, and Law* 20, 3 (Fall): 653–88.

Hoffenberg, Sir Raymond. 1987. *Clinical Freedom*. London: Nuffield Provincial Hospitals Trust.

Hogg, Peter. 1985. *Constitutional Law of Canada*. Toronto: Carswell.

Holahan, John, Colin Winterbottom, and Shruti Rajan. 1995a. "A Shifting Picture of Health Insurance Coverage." *Health Affairs* 14, 4 (Winter): 253–74.

Holahan, John, Teresa Coughlin, Leighton Ku, Debra J. Lipson, and Shruti Rajan. 1995b. "Insuring the Poor through Medicaid 1115 Waivers." *Health Affairs* 14, 1 (Spring): 199–216.

Hollingsworth, J. Rogers, Jerald Hage, and Robert A. Hanneman. 1988. *State Intervention in Medical Care: Consequences for Britain, France, Sweden, and the United States, 1890–1970*. Ithaca, N.Y.: Cornell University Press.

Horowitz, Gad. 1966. "Conservatism, Liberalism, and Socialism in Canada." *Canadian Journal of Economics and Political Science* 42 (May): 143–71.

Hurley, Jeremiah, and Robert Card. 1996. "Global Physician Budgets as Common-Property Resources: Some Implications for Physicians and Medical Associations." *Canadian Medical Association Journal* 154, 8 (April 15): 1161–68.

Hurley, Jeremiah, Laurie Goldsmith, Jonathan Lomas, Humaira Khan, and Victoria Vincent. 1996. "A Tale of Two Provinces: A Case Study of Physicians Expenditure Caps as Financial Incentives." Working Paper No. 96–12, Centre for Health Economics and Policy Analysis. Hamilton, Ontario: McMaster University.

Hurley, Jeremiah, Robert Card, and Laurie Goldsmith. 1997. "Physician Expenditure Cap Policies in Canada: Development, Design, and Implications for Analysing Their Effects." Final report submitted to the National Health Research and Development Program. Hamilton, Ontario: McMaster University Centre for Health Economics and Policy Analysis, mimeograph.

Hurley, Jeremiah, Jonathan Lomas, and Laurie J. Goldsmith. n.d. "Physician Responses to Global Physician Expenditure Budgets in Canada: A Common Property Perspective." Hamilton, Ontario: McMaster University Centre for Health Economics and Policy Analysis, mimeograph.

Iglehart, John [K.]. 1990. "Canada's Health Care System Faces Its Problems." *New England Journal of Medicine* 322, 8 (Feb. 22): 562–68.

———. 1991. "Health Policy Report: Germany's Health Care System." *New England Journal of Medicine* 324, 7: 503–8; 324, 24: 1750–56.

———. 1994. "Changing Course in Turbulent Times: An Interview with David Lawrence." *Health Affairs* 13, 5 (Winter): 65–77.

———. 1997. "Health Issues, the President, and the 105th Congress." *New England Journal of Medicine* 336, 9: 671–75.

Immergut, Ellen M. 1991. "Institutions, Veto Points and Policy Results: A Comparative Analysis of Health Care." *Journal of Public Policy* 10: 391–416.

Independent Healthcare Association. 1989. *IHA Acute Hospital Survey 1989*. London: Independent Healthcare Association.

———. 1995. *IHA Acute Hospital Survey 1995*. London: Independent Healthcare Association.

Institute of Medicine. 1986. *For-profit Enterprise in Health Care*. Washington, D.C.: National Academy Press.

Jackson, Peter M. 1992. "Economic Policy." In David Marsh and R. A. W. Rhodes, eds., *Implementing Thatcherite Policies: Audit of an Era*. Buckingham: Open University Press, 11–31.

Jacobs, Alan. 1998. "Seeing Difference: Market Health Reform in Europe." *Journal of Health Politics, Policy, and Law* 23, 1: 1–34.

Jacobs, Lawrence R. 1993. *The Health of Nations: Public Opinion and the Making of American and British Health Policy*. Ithaca: Cornell University Press.

Jacobs, Lawrence R., and Robert Y. Shapiro. 1995. "Don't Blame the Public for Failed Health Care Reform." *Journal of Health Politics, Policy, and Law* 20, 2 (Summer): 411–23.

Jacobs, Lawrence R., Theodore Marmor, and Jonathan Oberlander. 1998. "The Oregeon Health Plan and the Political Paradox of Rationing." *Health Affairs* forthcoming.

Jaklevic, Mary Chris. 1995. "PHOs Fall Short of Expectations." *Modern Healthcare* (October 9): 77–82.

James, John. 1995. "Reforming the British National Health Service: Implementation Problems in London." *Journal of Health Politics, Policy, and Law* 20, 1 (Spring): 191–210.

Johnson, Haynes, and David S. Broder. 1996. *The System: The American Way of Politics at the Breaking Point*. Boston: Little Brown.

Johnson, Norman. 1995. Conclusion to Norman Johnson, ed., *Private Markets in Health and Welfare: An International Perspective*. Oxford: Berg, 225–44.

Johnson, Terry, Gerry Larkin, and Mike Saks, eds. 1995. *Health Professions and the State in Europe*. New York: Routledge.

Johnston, Richard, and André Blais. 1988. "A Resounding Maybe." *The Globe and Mail*. Toronto (December 19): A7.

Jones, Dee, Carolyn Lester, and Robert West. 1994. "Monitoring Changes in Health Services for Older People." In Ray Robinson and Julian Le Grand, eds., *Evaluating the NHS Reforms*. London: King's Fund Institute, 130–54.

Judge, Ken, and Michael Solomon. 1993. "Public Opinion and the National Health Service: Patterns and Perspectives in Consumer Satisfaction." *Journal of Social Policy* 22, 3: 299–327.

Judis, John B. 1995. "Abandoned Surgery: Business and the Failure of Health Reform." *The American Prospect* 21 (Spring): 65–73.

Kammerling, Robert M., and Andrew Kinnear. 1996. "The Extent of Two-tier Service for Fundholders." *British Medical Journal* 312: 1399–1401.

Katz, Steven J., Cathy Charles, Jonathan Lomas, and H. Gilbert Welch. 1997. "Physician Relations in Canada: Shooting Inward as the Circle Closes." *Journal of Health Politics, Policy, and Law* 22, 6: 1413–32.

Katzenstein, Peter J. 1987. *Policy and Politics in West Germany: The Growth of a Semi-Sovereign State*. Philadelphia: Temple University Press.

Kemper, Tony, and Gordon Macpherson. 1994. *The NHS—a Kaleidoscope of Care—Conflicts of Service and Business Values*. London: Nuffield Provincial Hospitals Trust.

Kenney, Genevieve, Shruti Rajan, and Stephanie Soscia. 1998. "State Spending for Medicare and Medicaid Home Care Programs." *Health Affairs* 17, 1: 201–12.

Kerrison, Susan, Tim Packwood, and Martin Buxton. 1994. "Monitoring Medical Audit." In Ray Robinson and Julian Le Grand, eds., *Evaluating the NHS Reforms*. London: King's Fund Institute, 155–77.

Kertesz, Louise. 1995. "Kaiser Retools to Fight for Lost Ground." *Modern Healthcare* (July 17): 34–40.

Kingdon, John. 1984. *Agendas, Alternatives, and Public Policies*. Boston: Little, Brown.

Kirkman-Liff, Bradford L. 1990. "Physician Payment and Cost-Containment Strategies in West Germany: Suggestions for Medicare Reform." *Journal of Health Politics, Policy, and Law* 15, 1 (Spring): 69–99.

Klein, Rudolf. 1991. "Risks and Benefits of Comparative Studies: Notes from Another Shore." *The Milbank Quarterly* 16, 2: 275–91.

———. 1993. "The NHS Reforms So Far." *Annals of the Royal College of Physicians of England* 75: 74–78.

———. 1995. *The New Politics of the National Heath Service*. 3rd ed. London: Longman.

———. 1997. "Learning from Others: Shall the Last Be the First?" *Journal of Health Politics, Policy, and Law* 22, 5: 1267–78.

———. 1998. "Why Britain Is Reorganizing Its National Health Service—Yet Again." *Health Affairs* 17, 4 (July/August): 111–25.

Klein, Rudolf, and Michael O'Higgins. 1988. "Defusing the Crisis of the Welfare State." In Theodore R. Marmor and Jerry L. Mashaw, eds., *Social Security: Beyond the Rhetoric of Crisis*. Princeton, N.J.: Princeton University Press, 203–26.

Klein, Rudolf, Patricia Day, and Sharon Redmayne. 1996. *Managing Scarcity: Priority Setting and Rationing in the National Health Service*. Buckingham: Open University Press.

Krasner, Stephen D. 1988. "Sovereignty: An Institutional Perspective." *Comparative Political Studies* 21: 66–94.

Krieble, Todd. 1997. "Contracting and Management in the New Zealand Health Sector." Paper given at the conference From Program to Contract Management: New Trends in Public Administration. Faculty of Law, University of Toronto, February 20.

Labour Party. 1996. "Renewing the National Health Service: Labour's Agenda for a Healthier Britain." Reprinted in *International Journal of Health Services* 26, 2: 269–308.

Laing and Buisson. 1995. *Laing's Review of Private Healthcare 1995*. London: Laing and Buisson.

Le Grand, Julian. 1997. "Knights, Knaves, or Pawns? Human Behaviour and Social Policy." *Journal of Social Policy* 26, 2: 149–69.

Lee, Philip R., and Lynn Etheredge. 1989. "Clinical Freedom: Two Lessons for the U.K. from U.S. Experience with Privatization of Health Care." *The Lancet* (February 4): 263–65.

Leichter, Howard M., ed. 1992. *Health Policy Reform in America: Innovations from the States*. London: M. E. Sharpe.

———., ed. 1997. *Health Policy Reform in America: Innovations from the States*. 2nd ed. London: M. E. Sharpe.

Leman, Christopher. 1977. "Patterns of Policy Development: Social Security in the United States and Canada." *Public Policy* 25: 261–91.

Leutz, Walter N., Merwyn R. Greenlick, and John A. Capitman. 1994. "Integrating Acute and Long-term Care." *Health Affairs* 13, 4: 58–74.

Levitt, Ruth, Andrew Wall, and John Appleby. 1995. *The Reorganized National Health Service*. 5th ed. London: Chapman and Hall.

Lewin, Lawrence, R. A. Derzon, and R. Marguiles. 1981. "Investor-owned and Non-profits Differ in Economic Performance." *Hospitals* (July 1): 52–58.

Lewis, Steven. 1996. "Issues in the Evolution of Decision-making at Regional Levels." Paper delivered at the symposium on Globalization, State Choices, and Citizens' Participation in Canadian Health Care. Sponsored by the Robarts Centre for Canadian Studies and the Centre for Health Studies, York University, Toronto, April 1–2.

Leyerle, Betty. 1994. *The Private Regulation of American Health Care*. Armonk, N.Y.: M. E. Sharpe.

Light, Donald. 1995. "Countervailing Powers: A Framework for Professions in Transition." In Terry Johnson, Gerry Larkin, and Mike Saks, eds., *Health Professions and the State in Europe*. London: Routledge, 25–41.

Lindblom, Charles E[dward]. 1966. *The Intelligence of Democracy*. New York: Free Press.

———. 1977. *Politics and Markets*. New York: Basic Books.

Linton, Adam, and David C. Naylor. 1990. "Organized Medicine and the Assessment of Technology: Lessons from Ontario." *New England Journal of Medicine* 323: 1463–67.

Lipset, Seymour Martin. 1990. *Continental Divide: The Values and Institutions of the United States and Canada*. New York: Routledge.

Lipson, Debra J., and Jeanne M. De Sa. 1996. "Snapshots of Change in Fifteen Communities: Purchasers." *Health Affairs* 15, 2 (Summer): 62–76.

Lomas, Jonathan. 1996. "Devolving Authority for Health In Canada's Provinces: IV. Emerging Issues and Future Prospects." Working Paper 96-5. Hamilton, Ontario: McMaster University Centre for Health Economics and Policy Analysis.

Lomas, Jonathan, Catherine Fooks, Tom Rice, and Roberta J. Labelle. 1989. "Paying Physicians in Canada: Minding Our P's and Q's." *Health Affairs* 8, 1 (Spring): 80–102.

Lomas, Jonathan, Cathy Charles, and Janet Greb. 1992. "The Price of Peace: The Structure and Process of Physician Fee Negotiations in Canada." Working Paper No. 92-17, Hamilton, Ontario: McMaster University Centre for Health Economics and Policy Analysis.

Lomas, Jonathan, Julia Abelson, and Brian Hutchison. 1995. "Registering Patients and Paying Capitation in Family Practice: Lessons from Canada." *British Medical Journal* 311 (November 18): 1317–18.

Lomas, Jonathan, Gerry Veenstra, and John Woods. 1996a. "Devolving Authority for Health in Canada's Provinces: II. Backgrounds, Resources, and Activities of Board Members." Working Paper 96-3. Hamilton, Ontario: McMaster University Centre for Health Economics and Policy Analysis.

———. 1996b. "Devolving Authority for Health in Canada's Provinces: III. Motivations, Approaches, and Attitudes of Board Members." Working Paper 96-4. Hamilton, Ontario: McMaster University Centre for Health Economics and Policy Analysis.

Lutz, Sandy. 1995a. "1995: A Record Year for Hospital Deals." *Modern Healthcare* (December 18–25): 43.

———. 1995b. "Joint Provider Budget Protest Fractured." *Modern Healthcare* (November 27): 14.

MacBride-King, Judith L. 1995. *Managing Corporate Health Care Costs: Issues and Options*. Ottawa: Conference Board of Canada.

Maioni, Antonia. 1995. "Nothing Succeeds Like the Right Kind of Failure: Postwar National Health Insurance Initiatives in Canada and the United States." *Journal of Health Politics, Policy, and Law* 20, 1 (Spring): 5–30.

Majeed, Fazeem, and Simon Voss. 1995. "Performance Indicators for General Practice." *British Medical Journal* 311: 209–10.

Major, Michael J. 1995. "For Profit or Not for Profit." *Managed Healthcare* (May): 24–28.

*Managed Healthcare*. 1995. "A Push in the Pacific." *Managed Healthcare* (March): 34–35.

Mansfield, Caroline D. 1995. "Attitudes and Behaviours towards Clinical Guidelines: The Clinicians' Perspective." *Quality in Health Care* 4: 250–55.

Marmor, Theodore R. 1973. *The Politics of Medicare*. New York: Aldine-Atheron.

———. 1998. "Forecasting American Health Care: How We Got Here and Where We

Might Be Going." In Mark Peterson, ed., *Healthy Markets? The New Competition in Medical Care*. Durham, N.C.: Duke University Press.

Marmor, Theodore, with Mark Goldberg. 1994. "American Health Reform: Separating Sense from Nonsense." In Theodore R. Marmor, *Understanding Health Care Reform*. New Haven: Yale University Press, 1–18.

Marmor, Theodore R., with James A. Morone. 1983. "The Health Programs of the Kennedy–Johnson Years: An Overview." In Theodore R. Marmor, *Political Analysis and American Medical Care*. Cambridge: Cambridge University Press, 131–44.

Marmor, Theodore R., Richard Boyer, and Julie Greenberg. 1983. "Medicare and Pro-competitive Reform." In Theodore R. Marmor, *Political Analysis and American Medical Care*. Cambridge: Cambridge University Press, 239–61.

Marmor, Theodore R., with Mark Schlesinger and Richard W. Smithey. 1994. "Nonprofit Organizations and Health Care." In Theodore R. Marmor, *Understanding Health Care Reform*. New Haven: Yale University Press, 48–87.

Marsh, David. 1991. "Privatization under Mrs. Thatcher." *Public Administration* 69: 459–80.

———. 1992. *The New Politics of British Trade Unionism: Union Power and the Thatcher Legacy*. London: Macmillan.

Martin, Cathie Jo. 1997. "Markets, Medicare, and Making Do: Business Strategies after National Health Care Reform." *Journal of Health Politics, Policy, and Law* 22, 2 (Summer): 557–93.

———. 1993. "Together Again: Business, Government, and the Quest for Cost Control." *Journal of Health Politics, Policy, and Law* 18, 2: 359–93.

———. 1995. "Stuck in Neutral: Big Business and the Politics of National Health Reform." *Journal of Health Politics, Policy, and Law* 20, 2: 431–36.

Mays, Nicholas, and Jennifer Dixon. 1996. *Purchaser Plurality in the U.K.* London: King's Fund.

McCracken, Mike. 1996. "Federal Transfer Scenarios: What are the Choices?" Paper delivered at the Symposium on Globalization, State Choices, and Citizens' Participation in Canadian Health Care. Sponsored by the Robarts Centre for Canadian Studies and the Centre for Health Studies, York University, Toronto, April 1–2.

McKendry, Robert J. R., George A. Wells, Paula Dale, Owen Adams, Lynda Buske, Jill Strachan, and Lourdes Flor. 1996. "Factors Influencing the Emigration of Physicians from Canada to the United States." *Canadian Medical Association Journal* 154, 2 (January 15): 171–81.

McRae, Kenneth. 1964. "The Structure of Canadian History." In Louis Hartz, ed., *The Founding of New Societies*. Toronto, Longman.

McVicar, Malcolm, and Lynton Robins. 1994. "Education Policy: Market Forces or Market Failure?" In Stephen P. Savage and Rob Atkinson, eds., *Public Policy in Britain*. New York: St. Martin's, 203–20.

Merry, Peter, ed. 1997. *The 1997/98 NHS Handbook*. 12th ed. Tunbridge Wells: JMH Publishing.

Monopolies and Mergers Commission. 1994. *Private Medical Services*. London: HMSO.

Moran, Michael. 1994. "Reshaping the Health-Care State." *Government and Opposition* 29, 1: 48–63.

Morone, James A. 1990. *The Democratic Wish: Popular Participation and the Limits of American Government*. New York: Basic Books.

———. 1995. "Nativism, Hollow Corporations, and Managed Competition: Why the Clinton Health Care Reform Failed." *Journal of Health Politics, Policy, and Law* 20, 2 (Fall): 391–98.

Morone, James A., and Janice M. Goggin. 1995. "Health Policies in Europe: Welfare States in a Market Era." *Journal of Health Politics, Policy, and Law* 20, 3 (Fall): 557–70.

Morrisey, Michael A. 1994. *Cost Shifting in Health Care: Separating Evidence from Rhetoric.* Washington, D.C.: AEI Press.

Morrissey, John. 1994. "Providers Get Their Due." *Modern Healthcare* (November 7): 60–66.

———. 1995. "Info Systems Refocus Priorities." *Modern Healthcare* (February 13): 65–72.

Mueller, Keith J. 1993. *Health Care Policy in the United States.* Lincoln, NB: University of Nebraska Press.

National Academy of Social Insurance. 1993. "Legislative Developments," *Update* 31 (September): 1.

National Forum on Health. 1994. *Fact Sheet.* Ottawa: National Forum on Health.

———. 1997. *Canada Health Action: Building on the Legacy.* 2 vols. Ottawa: Minister of Public Works and Government Services.

National Health Service. 1993a. *Review of Contracting—Guidance for the 1994–95 Contracting Cycle.* EL(93)103. Leeds: NHS Executive.

———. 1993b. *Improving Clinical Effectiveness.* EL(93)115. Leeds: NHS Executive (December 21).

———. 1994a. *1995–96 Contracting Review: Handbook.* Leeds: NHS Executive.

———. 1994b. *Clinical Involvement in Contracting: Report of the Task Group.* Leeds: NHS Executive.

———. 1994c. *Comparative Cost Data: The Use of Costed HRGs to Inform the Contracting Process.* EL(94)51. Leeds: NHS Executive.

———. 1996. *Priorities and Planning Guidance for the NHS: 1996/97.* Leeds: NHS Executive.

Naylor, C. David. 1986. *Private Practice, Public Payment: Canadian Medicine and the Politics of Health Insurance 1911–1966.* Montreal: McGill-Queen's University Press.

Neubauer, Deane. 1992. "Hawaii: The Health State." In Howard M. Leichter, ed., *Health Policy Reform in America: Innovations from the States.* London: M. E. Sharpe, 147–72.

———. 1993. "Hawaii: A Pioneer in Health System Reform." *Health Affairs* 12, 2 (Summer): 31–39.

Newman, Penny. 1995. "Interview with Alain Enthoven: Is There Convergence between Britain and the United States in the Organization of Health Services?" *British Medical Journal* 310 (June 24): 1652–55.

Niskanen, William A. 1971. *Bureaucracy and Representative Government.* Chicago: Aldine.

Olson, Mancur. 1982. *The Rise and Decline of Nations.* New Haven: Yale University Press.

Orchard, Carol. 1995. *Using HRGs in Hospital Management.* Internal document. Winchester: NHS Executive National Casemix Office.

Orfield, Gary. 1988. "Race and the Liberal Agenda: The Loss of the Integrationist Dream, 1965–1974." In Margaret Weir, Ann Shola Orloff, and Theda Skocpol, eds., *The Politics of Social Policy in the United States.* Princeton, N.J.: Princeton University Press, 313–55.

Organization for Economic Cooperation and Development (OECD). 1992. *The Reform of Health Care: A Comparative Analysis of Seven OECD Countries.* Paris: OECD.

———. 1993. *OECD Health Systems: Facts and Trends 1960–1991.* Paris: OECD.

———. 1994. *New Orientations for Social Policy.* Paris: OECD.

———. 1995. *Internal Markets in the Making: Health Systems in Canada, Iceland, and the United Kingdom.* Paris: OECD.

Orloff, Ann Shola. 1988. "The Political Origins of America's Belated Welfare State." In Margaret Weir, Ann Shola Orloff, and Theda Skocpol, eds., *The Politics of Social Policy in the United States.* Princeton, N.J.: Princeton University Press, 37–80.

Oxman, Andrew D., Mary Ann Thompson, David A. Davis, and R. Brian Haynes. 1995. "No Magic Bullets: A Systematic Review of 102 Trials of Interventions to Improve Professional Practice." *Canadian Medical Association Journal* 153, 10 (November 15): 1423–31.

Packwood, T., J. Keen, and M. Buxton. 1991. *Hospitals in Transition: The Resource Management Initiative.* Milton Keynes: Open University Press.

———. 1992. "Process and Structure: Resource Management and the Development of Sub-Unit Organizational Structure," *Health Services Management Research* 5, 1: 66–76.

Pallarito, Karen. 1995. "New Health Systems Hungry for Capital." *Modern Healthcare* (April 10): 44.

Pattison, Robert V., and Hallie M. Katz. 1983. "Investor-owned and Not-for-profit Hospitals: A Comparison Based on California Data." *New England Journal of Medicine* 309, 6: 347–53.

Pear, Robert. 1998. "High Rates Hobble Law to Guarantee Health Insurance." *New York Times* (March 17): A1, A14.

Peterson, Mark A. 1993. "Political Influence in the 1990s: From Iron Triangles to Policy Networks." *Journal of Health Politics, Policy, and Law* 18, 2 (Summer): 395–438.

———. 1995. "How Health Policy Information Is Used in Congress." In Thomas E. Mann and Norman J. Ornstein, eds., *Intensive Care: How Congress Shapes Health Policy.* Washington, D.C.: AEI/Brookings, 79–126.

———. 1997. "Health Care Into the Next Century." *Journal of Health Politics, Policy, and Law* 22, 2 (April): 291–313.

———. 1998. "Introduction—The Next Century in Health Care." In Mark Peterson, ed., *Healthy Markets? The New Competition in Medical Care.* Durham, N.C.: Duke University Press.

Pfaff, Martin. 1996. "Health Policy Formulation and the Role of Information in Managing Change, in Consumer Choice and in Resource Allocation: A German Perspective." Paper prepared for the Four Country Conference on Health Reform, Health Policy—Towards 2000, Montebello, Quebec, May 16–18.

Pierson, Paul. 1994. *Dismantling the Welfare State? Reagan, Thatcher, and the Politics of Retrenchment.* New York: Cambridge University Press.

———. 1997. "Path Dependence, Increasing Returns, and the Study of Politics." Cambridge, Mass.: Harvard University Center for European Studies, mimeograph.

Pierson, Paul, and R. Kent Weaver. 1993. "Political Institutions and Loss Imposition: The Case of Pensions." In R. Kent Weaver and Bert A. Rockman, eds., *Do Institutions Matter?* Washington: The Brookings Institution, 110–50.

Pollitt, Christopher. 1993. *Managerialism and the Public Services: Cuts or Cultural Change in the 1990s?* 2nd ed. Oxford: Blackwell.

Pope, Gregory C., and John E. Schneider. 1992. "Trends in Physician Income." *Health Affairs* 11, 1 (Spring): 181–93.

Poullier, Jean-Pierre. 1992. "Administrative Costs in Selected Industrialized Countries." *Health Care Financing Review* 13, 4 (Summer): 167–72.

Pressman, Jeffrey, and Aaron Wildavsky. 1973. *Implementation.* Berkeley: University of California Press.

Primary Care Reform Advisory Group. 1996. *Primary Care Reform: A Strategy for Stability.* Toronto, Ontario: Ontario Medical Association.

Prince, Michael J. 1991. "From Meech Lake to Golden Pond: The Elderly, Pension Reform, and Federalism in the 1990s." In Frances Abele, ed., *How Ottawa Spends: The Politics of Fragmentation, 1991–92*. Ottawa: Carleton University Press.

Propper, Carol. 1995. "Agency and Incentives in the NHS Internal Market." *Social Science and Medicine* 40, 12: 1683–90.

Punnett, R. M. 1994. *British Government and Politics*. 6th ed. Aldershot: Dartmouth.

Purchase, Bryne. 1996. "Health Care and Competitiveness." Background paper commissioned for the National Health Care Policy Summit. Sponsored by the Canadian Medical Association, Liberty Health, MDS Health Group Limited, and SHL Systemhouse, Montebello, Quebec, March 18–19.

Purdum, Todd S. 1996. "Facets of Clinton." *The New York Times Magazine* (May 19): 35–41, 62, 77–78.

Putnam, Robert. 1993. *Making Democracy Work*. Princeton, N.J.: Princeton University Press.

Quadagno, Jill. 1988. *The Transformation of Old Age Security*. Chicago: University of Chicago Press.

Radical Statistics Health Group. 1995. "NHS 'Indicators of Success': What Do They Tell Us?" *British Medical Journal* 310: 1045–50.

Ramsay, Craig R., ed. 1995. *U.S. Health Policy Groups: Institutional Profiles*. Westport, Conn.: Greenwood.

Rappolt, Susan G. 1996. "In the Name of Science: The Effects of the Clinical Guidelines Movement on the Autonomy of the Medical Profession in Ontario." Ph.D. diss., University of Toronto.

————. 1997. "Clinical Guidelines and the Fate of Medical Autonomy in Ontario." *Social Science and Medicine* 44, 7: 977–87.

Redmayne, Sharon. 1996. *Small Steps, Big Goals: Purchasing Policies in the NHS*. University of Bath: Centre for the Analysis of Social Policy.

Rehnberg, Clas. 1995. "The Swedish Experience with Internal Markets." In Monique Jérôme-Forget, Joseph White, and Joshua M. Wiener, eds., *Health Care Reform through Internal Markets: Experience and Proposals*. Montreal: Institute for Research on Public Policy, 49–74.

Rein, Martin, and Lee Rainwater. 1987. "From Welfare State to Welfare Society." In Gösta Esping-Andersen, Martin Rein, and Lee Rainwater, eds., *Stagnation and Renewal in Social Policy*. Armonk, N.Y.: M. E. Sharpe, 143–59.

Relman, Arnold S. 1980. "The Medical-Industrial Complex." *New England Journal of Medicine* 303: 963–70.

Rich, Robert E., and William D. White, eds. 1996. *Health Policy, Federalism, and the American States*. Washington, D.C.: Urban Institute.

Robinson, James C. 1993. "Payment Mechanisms, Nonprice Incentives and Organizational Innovation in Health Care." *Inquiry* 30 (Fall): 328–33.

Robinson, James C., and Lawrence P. Casalino. 1996. "Vertical Integration and Organizational Networks in Health Care." *Health Affairs* 15, 1 (Spring): 7–22.

Robinson, Ray, and Philippa Hayter. 1995. "Why Do GPs Choose Not to Apply for Fundholding?" University of Southampton, Institute for Health Policy Studies, mimeograph.

Robinson, Ray, and Julian Le Grand. 1995. "Contracting and the Purchaser–Provider Split." In Richard B. Saltman and Casten von Otter, eds., *Implementing Planned Markets in Health Care: Balancing Social and Economic Responsibility*. Buckingham: Open University Press, 25–44.

Rodríguez, Josep. 1995. "The Politics of the Spanish Medical Profession: Democratization and the Construction of the National Health System." In Terry Johnson, Gerry Larkin, and Mike Saks, eds., *Health Professions and the State in Europe*. London: Routledge, 141–61.

Rogal, Deborah L., and W. David Helms. 1993. "Tracking States' Efforts to Reform Their Health Systems." *Health Affairs* 12, 2 (Summer): 27–30.

Roos, Noralou, Charlyn D. Black, Norman Frohlich, Carolyn DeCoster, Marsha M. Cohen, Douglas J. Tataryn, Cameron A. Mustard, Fred Toll, Keumhee C. Carriere, Charles A. Burchill, Leonard MacWilliam, and Bogdan Bogdanovich. 1995. "A Population-Based Health Information System." *Medical Care* 33, 12 (December Supplement): DS 13–20.

Rothman, David J. 1993. "A Century of Failure: Health Care Reform in America." *Journal of Health Politics, Policy, and Law* 18, 2 (Summer): 271–86.

———. 1997. *Beginnings Count: The Technological Imperative in American Medicine*. New York: Oxford University Press.

Rovner, Julie. 1995. "Congress and Health Care Reform, 1993–94." In Thomas E. Mann and Norman J. Ornstein, eds., *Intensive Care: How Congress Shapes Health Policy*. Washington, D.C.: AEI/Brookings, 179–226.

Rowland, Diane, and Kristina Hanson. 1996. "Medicaid: Moving to Managed Care." *Health Affairs* 15, 3 (Fall): 150–52.

Royal Commission on Health Services. 1964. *Final Report*. Ottawa, Ontario: Queen's Printer.

Rueschemeyer, Dietrich. 1986. "Comparing Legal Professions Cross-nationally: From a Professions-centered to a State-centered Approach." *American Bar Foundation Research Journal* (Summer): 415–46.

Ruggie, Mary. 1996. *Realignments in the Welfare State: Health Policy in the United States, Canada, and Britain*. New York: Columbia University Press.

Rumsey, Moira, Kieran Walshe, Jennifer Bennett, and James Coles. 1994. *The Role of the Commissioner in Audit: Findings of a National Survey of Commissioning Authorities in England*. London: CASPE Research.

Salmon, J. Warren, ed. 1994. *The Corporate Transformation of Health Care: Perspectives and Implications*. Amityville, N.Y.: Baywood.

Salmon, J. Warren, William D. White, and Joe Feinglass. 1994. "The Futures of Physicians: Agency and Autonomy Reconsidered." In J. Warren Salmon, ed., *The Corporate Transformation of Health Care: Perspectives and Implications*. Amityville, N.Y.: Baywood, 125–38.

Schepers, Rita. 1995. "The Belgian Medical Profession since the 1980s: Dominance and Decline?" In Terry Johnson, Gerry Larkin, and Mike Saks, eds., *Health Professions and the State in Europe*. London: Routledge, 162–77.

Schick, Allen. 1971. "Toward the Cybernetic State." In Dwight Waldo, ed. *Public Administration in a Time of Turbulence*. New York: Chandler.

———. 1995. "How a Bill Did Not Become Law." In Thomas E. Mann and Norman J. Ornstein, eds., *Intensive Care: How Congress Shapes Health Policy*. Washington, D.C.: AEI/Brookings, 227–72.

Schieber, George, and Jean-Pierre Poullier. 1987. "Recent Trends in International Health Spending." *Health Affairs* 6, 3 (Fall): 105–12.

Schieber, George, Jean-Pierre Poullier, and Leslie M. Greenwald. 1994. "Health System Performance in OECD Countries, 1980–1992." *Health Affairs* 13, 4 (Fall): 100–12.

Schlesinger, Mark, Bradford Gray, and Elizabeth Bradley. 1996. "Charity and Community: The Role of Nonprofit Ownership in a Managed Care System." *Journal of Health Politics, Policy, and Law* 21, 4 (Winter): 697–752.

Schoen, Cathy, and Karen Scott Collins. 1996. "Turbulent Times: Physicians' Practice Experiences in an Era of Managed Care." Working paper. New York: Commonwealth Fund.

Schurman, Donald. 1997. "Primary Care Reform in Canada: Promise or Reality." Paper prepared for the Four Country Conference on Primary Care and Health Care Reform, Boppard, Germany, June 5–8.

Schut, Frederik T. 1995. "Health Care Reform in the Netherlands: Balancing Corporatism, Etatism, and Market Mechanisms." *Journal of Health Politics, Policy, and Law* 20, 3 (Fall): 615–52.

Scott, Lisa. 1995. "AmHS, Premier to Merge." *Modern Healthcare* (August 7): 2–3.

Secretaries of State for Health, Wales, Northern Ireland, and Scotland. 1989. *Working for Patients*. London: HMSO.

Secretary of State for Social Services. 1989. *Working for Patients: Medical Audit*. Working paper 6. London: HMSO.

Shapiro, Evelyn. 1994. " Community and Long-Term Health Care in Canada." In Ake Blomqvist and David M. Brown, eds., *Limits to Care: Reforming Canada's Health System in an Age of Restraint*. Toronto: C. D. Howe Institute, 327–62.

Shepherd, Jonathan P., David W. Thomas, and Paul Shepherd. 1996. "Privatising the NHS: Dentistry Paves the Way." *British Medical Journal* 312 (April 13): 922–23.

Sheppard, Robert. 1995. "The Premiers' Best Face." *The Globe and Mail*. Toronto (August 28): A11.

Shock, Maurice. 1994. "Medicine at the Centre of the Nation's Affairs." *British Medical Journal* 309: 1730–33.

Shortell, Stephen M., Robin R. Gillies, and David A. Anderson. 1994. "The New World of Managed Care: Creating Organized Delivery Systems." *Health Affairs* 13, 5 (Winter): 46–64.

Shortell, Stephen M., Robin R. Gillies, David A. Anderson, Karen Morgan Erickson, and John B. Mitchell. 1996. *Remaking Health Care in America: Building Organized Delivery Systems*. San Francisco: Jossey-Bass.

Sicotte, Claude, Charles Tilquin, and Marie Valois. 1992. "The Quebec Experience." In Marion Ogilvie and Eleanor Sawyer, eds., *Managing Information in Canadian Health Care Facilities*. Ottawa, Ontario: Canadian Hospital Association Press, 229–49.

Simon, Carol J., and Patricia H. Born. 1996. "Physician Earnings in a Changing Managed Care Environment." *Health Affairs* 15, 3 (Fall): 124–33.

Simon, Herbert. 1956. *Administrative Behaviour*. 2nd ed. New York: Macmillan.

Siriwardena, A. N. 1995. "Clinical Guidelines in Primary Care: A Survey of General Practitioners' Attitudes and Behaviour." *British Journal of General Practice* (December): 643–47.

Skocpol, Theda. 1993. "Is the Time Finally Ripe? Health Insurance Reform in the 1990s." *Journal of Health Politics, Policy, and Law* 18, 3 (Fall): 531–50.

———. 1995. "The Rise and Resounding Demise of the Clinton Plan." *Health Affairs* 14, 1 (Spring): 66–85.

———. 1996. *Boomerang: Clinton's Health Security Effort and the Turn Against Government in U.S. Politics*. New York: W. W. Norton.

Sloan, Frank A., and Robert A. Vraciu. 1983. "Investor-owned and Not-for-profit Hospitals: Addressing Some Issues." *Health Affairs* 2, 1 (Spring): 25–37.

Smee, Clive. 1995. "Self-governing Trusts and GP Fundholders: The British Experience." In Richard B. Saltman and Casten von Otter, eds., *Implementing Planned Markets in Health Care*. Buckingham: Open University Press, 177–208.

Smeeding, Timothy, Barbara Torrey, and Martin Rein. 1988. "Patterns of Income and Poverty: The Economic Status of Children and the Elderly in Eight Countries." In Isabel Palmer, Timothy Smeeding, and Barbara Torrey, eds., *The Vulnerable*. Washington, D.C.: The Urban Institute, 89–119.

Smith, Helen E., G. I. Russell, A. J. Frew, and P.T Dawes. 1992. "Medical Audit: The Differing Perspectives of Managers and Clinicians." *Journal of the Royal College of Physicians of London* 26, 2 (April): 177–80.

Soderstrom, Lee. 1994. "Health Care Reform in Canada: Restructuring the Supply Side." In Ake Blomqvist and David M. Brown, eds., *Limits to Care: Reforming Canada's Health System in an Age of Restraint*. Toronto: C. D. Howe Institute, 217–65.

Somers, Herman Miles, and Anne Ramsay Somers. 1961. *Doctors, Patients, and Health Insurance: The Organization and Financing of Medical Care*. Washington, D.C.: The Brookings Institution.

Sparer, Michael S. 1998. "Devolution of Power: An Interim Report Card." *Health Affairs* 17, 3 (May/June): 1–16.

Srinivasan, Srija, Larry Levitt, and Jane Lundy. 1998. "Wall Street's Love Affair with Health Care." *Health Affairs* 17, 4 (July/August): 126–31.

Starr, Paul. 1982. *The Social Transformation of American Medicine*. New York: Basic Books.

———. 1991. *The Logic of Health-Care Reform*. Knoxville, Tenn.: Grand Rounds Press.

Steinmo, Sven. 1989. "Political Institutions and Tax Policy in the United States, Sweden, and Britain." *World Politics* 41: 500–35.

Steinmo, Sven, and Jon Watts. 1995. "It's the Institutions, Stupid! Why Comprehensive National Health Insurance Always Fails in America." *Journal of Health Politics, Policy, and Law* 20, 2 (Summer): 329–72.

Stevenson, H. Michael, Eugene Vayda, and A. Paul Williams. 1987. "Medical Politics after the Canada Health Act: Preliminary Results of the 1986 Physicians' Survey." Paper delivered at the annual meeting of the Canadian Political Science Association, McMaster University, Hamilton, Ontario.

Stoddart, G. L., and J. R. Seldon. 1983. "Publicly Financed Competition in Canadian Health Care Delivery: A Viable Alternative to Increased Regulation?" In J. A. Boan, ed., *Proceedings of the Second Annual Conference on Health Economics*. University of Regina, Regina, Saskatchewan, September 9–11, 121–160.

Stoker, Gerry. 1990. "Government Beyond Whitehall." In Patrick Dunleavy, Andrew Gamble, and Gillian Peele, eds., *Development in British Politics*. New York: St. Martin's, 126–49.

Stone, Deborah. 1977. "Professionalim and Accountability: Controlling Health Services in the United States and West Germany." *Journal of Health Politics, Policy, and Law* 2, 1 (Spring): 32–47.

Strong, Philip, and Jane Robinson. 1990. *The National Health Service: Under New Management*. Buckingham: Open University Press.

Sullivan, Michael. 1992. *The Politics of Social Policy*. London: Harvester Wheatsheaf.

Sullivan, Michael, Kathryn Harvey, and David Fletcher. 1995. "Physician Survey on Health Care Reform." *Ontario Medical Review* (January): 22–29.

Suttie, Boyd. 1988. "The Future of Utilization Analysis." Paper presented at the First Annual Health Policy Conference of the Centre for Health Economics and Policy Analysis, McMaster University, Hamilton, Ontario, May 26–27.

Taylor, Malcolm G. 1979. *Health Insurance and Canadian Public Policy: The Seven Decisions that Created the Canadian Health Insurance System*. Montreal: McGill-Queen's University Press.

Taylor-Goodby, Peter. 1996. "The Future of Health Care in Six European Countries." *International Journal of Health Services* 26, 2: 203–20.

Thorpe, Kenneth. 1997. "The Health Care System in Transition: Care, Costs, and Coverage." *Journal of Health Politics, Policy, and Law* 22, 2 (April): 339–62.

Tilley, Leslie. 1994. "Contracting is Expanding—But is the Infrastructure There to Support It?" *HMFA Newsletter.* London: Healthcare Financial Management Association, 8–10.

Timmins, Nicholas. 1995. *The Five Giants: A Biography of the Welfare State.* London: Harper Collins.

Toynbee, Polly. 1984. "The Patient and the NHS." *The Lancet* (June 23): 1399–1401.

Troy, Timothy N. 1995. "Managed Care's Merger Mania." *Managed Healthcare* (November): 30–32.

Tunis, S. R. R. S. Hayward, M. C. Wilson, H. R. Rubin, E. B. Bass, and W. Johnson. 1994. "Internists' Attitudes About Clinical Practice Guidelines." *Annals of Internal Medicine* 120: 956–63.

Tuohy, Carolyn. 1976. "Medical Politics after Medicare: The Ontario Case." *Canadian Public Policy* 11, 2 (Spring): 192–210.

————. 1982. "Does a Claims Monitoring System Influence High Volume Medical Practitioners? Attitudinal Data from Ontario." *Inquiry* (Spring): 18–31.

————. 1986. "Conflict and Accommodation in the Canadian Health Care System: Comparisons and Contrasts with the United States." In R. G. Evans and G. L. Stoddard, eds., *Medicare at Maturity.* Calgary: University of Calgary Press, 393–434.

————. 1988. "Medicine and the State in Canada: The Extra-billing Issue in Perspective." *Canadian Journal of Political Science* 21 (June): 268–96.

————. 1992. *Policy and Politics in Canada: Institutionalized Ambivalence.* Philadelphia: Temple University Press.

————. 1993. "Social Policy: Two Worlds." In Michael M. Atkinson, ed. *Governing Canada: Institutions and Public Policy.* Toronto: Harcourt Brace Jovanovich, 275–306.

————. 1994a. "Interests and Institutions: Making the Match." In Bryne Purchase, ed., *Policy Making and Competitiveness.* Kingston, Ontario: Queen's University School of Policy Studies.

————. 1994b. "Principles and Power in the Health Care Arena: Reflections on the Canadian Experience." *Health Matrix* 4, 2 (Summer): 205–42.

————. 1996. "Variation in Health Care Policy in the American States: The Dog That Didn't Bark." In Robert E. Rich and William D. White, eds., *Health Policy, Federalism, and the American States.* Washington, D.C.: The Urban Institute, 203–29.

Tuohy, Carolyn, and Alan D. Wolfson. 1977. "The Political Economy of Professionalism: A Perspective." In Michael J. Trebilcock, ed., *Four Aspects of Professionalism.* Consumer Research Council, Department of Consumer and Corporate Affairs, Government of Canada, 41–86.

van de Ven, Wynand P. M. M., René C. J. A. van Vliet, Erik M. van Barneveld, and Leida M. Lamers. 1994. "Risk-adjusted Capitation: Recent Experience in the Netherlands." *Health Affairs* 13, 5 (Winter): 120–36.

van der Wilt, Gert Jan. 1995. "Towards a Two Tier System: How to Put Theory into Practice." *Journal of Medicine and Philosophy* 20, 6 (December): 617–30.

Volpp, Kevin G., and Bruce Siegel. 1993. "New Jersey: Long-Term Experience with All-Payer State Rate Setting." *Health Affairs* 12, 2 (Summer): 59–65.

Walker, William. 1996. "Ontarians Think Services Poorer, Poll Reveals." *The Toronto Star* (April 27): A9.

Walshe, Kieran, and James Coles. 1993. *Evaluating Audit: A Review of Initiatives.* London: CASPE Research.

Warden, John. 1991. "Patients First." *British Medical Journal* 303: 1153.

———. 1997a. "NHS Gets £1.2bn Cash Boost." *British Medical Journal* 315 (July 12): 76.

———. 1997b. "Review of NHS Spending Begins." *British Medical Journal* 314 (June 21): 1781.

Wareham, N. J. 1994. "External Monitoring of Quality of Health Care in the United States." *Quality in Health Care* 3: 97–101.

Weale, Albert. 1990. "Social Policy." In Patrick Dunleavy, Andrew Gamble, and Gillian Peale, eds., *Developments in British Politics.* New York: St. Martin's.

Weiner, Jonathan P., and Gregory de Lissovoy. 1993. "Razing a Tower of Babel: A Taxonomy for Managed Care and Health Insurance Plans." *Journal of Health Politics, Policy, and Law* 18, 1 (Spring): 75–103.

Weinrib, Lorraine E. 1996. "The Exercise of Public Power Under the *Savings and Restructuring Act, 1995* (Bill 26)." *CanadaWatch* 4, 3 (January/February): 61-62.

Weissenstein, Eric. 1994. "A Second Opinion on PROs." *Modern Healthcare* (May 9): 45–50.

———. 1995a. "Big Health PACs Bet Heavily against Reform." *Modern Healthcare* (August 21): 102.

———. 1995b. "Managed Care Eats at Hospital Cost Shifts." *Modern Healthcare* (April 24): 3.

White, Joseph. 1995. "The Horses and the Jumps: Comments on the Health Care Reform Steeplechase." *Journal of Health Politics, Policy, and Law* 20, 2 (Summer): 373–84.

White, William D., J. Warren Salmon, and Joe Feinglass. 1994. "The Changing Doctor–Patient Relationship and Performance Monitoring: An Agency Perspective." In J. Warren Salmon, ed., *The Corporate Transformation of Health Care: Perspectives and Implications.* Amityville, N.Y.: Baywood, 195–224.

Whitehead, Margaret. 1994. "Is It Fair? Evaluating the Equity Implications of the NHS Reforms." In Ray Robinson and Julian Le Grand, eds., *Evaluating the NHS Reforms.* London: King's Fund Institute, 208–42.

Whitty, Geoff. 1990. "The Politics of the 1988 Education Reform Act." In Patrick Dunleavy, Andrew Gamble, and Gillian Peele, eds., *Developments in British Politics.* New York: St. Martin's, 305–30.

Williamson, Oliver E. 1975. *Markets and Hierarchies: Analysis and Anti-trust Implications.* New York: Free Press.

Wilsford, David. 1994. "Path Dependency, or Why History Makes it Difficult but Not Impossible to Reform Health Care Systems in a Big Way." *Journal of Public Policy* 14, 3: 251–83.

———. 1995. "States Facing Interests: Struggles over Health Policy in Advanced Industrial Democracies." *Journal of Health Politics, Policy, and Law* 20, 3 (Fall): 571–14.

Wilson, P. R., D. Chappell, and R. Lincoln. 1986. "Policing Physician Abuse in British Columbia." *Canadian Public Policy* 12 (March): 236–44.

Wofford, Harris. 1995. Seminar delivered at the Department of Political Science, University of Toronto, March 16.

Wolfson, A. D., and Carolyn J. Tuohy. 1980. *Opting Out of Medicare: Private Medical Markets in Ontario.* Toronto: University of Toronto Press.

Woodward, C. A., B. Ferrier, A. P. Williams, and M. Cohen. 1995. "Attitudes of a Cohort of Family Physicians Towards Practice Guidelines." *Canadian Family Physicians* 41: 2104–2111.

Yungblut, Robert M. 1992. "Managing Information and the Hospital Medical Records Institute." In Marion Ogilvie and Eleanor Sawyer, eds., *Managing Information in Canadian Health Care Facilities.* Ottawa, Ontario: Canadian Hospital Association Press, 195–213.

Zysman, John. 1983. *Governments, Markets, and Growth.* Ithaca: Cornell University Press.

# Index

305

## DATE RETURN